ALTERNATIVE MEDICINE AND AMERICAN RELIGIOUS LIFE

Alternative Medicine and American Religious Life

ROBERT C. FULLER

New York   Oxford
OXFORD UNIVERSITY PRESS
1989

Oxford University Press

Oxford New York Toronto
Delhi Bombay Calcutta Madras Karachi
Petaling Jaya Singapore Hong Kong Tokyo
Nairobi Dar es Salaam Cape Town
Melbourne Auckland

and associated companies in
Berlin Ibadan

Published by Oxford University Press, Inc.,
200 Madison Avenue, New York, NY 10016

Oxford is a registered trademark of Oxford University Press

Library of Congress Cataloging-in-Publication Data
Fuller, Robert C., 1952–
    Alternative medicine and American religious life/
Robert C. Fuller.
        p. cm.
    ISBN 0-19-505775-9
    1. Alternative medicine—United States. 2. United States—
Religion—1965–   I. Title.
    R733.F85 1989
    615.5′0973—dc19   88-30120 CIP

9 8 7 6 5 4 3 2 1

Printed in the United States of America
on acid-free paper

To Matt

Acknowledgments

Writing is never the solitary enterprise that many mistake it to be. For every hour of solitude before the word processor there is an enlivening discussion or gesture of support from a colleague, friend, or loved one. It is for this reason that scholars want to acknowledge the many persons who participated in the completion of their project. The research for this book prompted me to contact a long-admired medical and cultural historian, Ron Numbers of the University of Wisconsin. Ron offered numerous suggestions and was of invaluable help in supplying several of the photographs that appear in this book. I was also fortunate to receive timely assistance from Norman Gevitz of the University of Illinois at Chicago and from Dr. Joseph Donahue, D. C., a chiropractic physician and historian of chiropractic medicine. I might note that although Dr. Donahue took exception to some of my interpretations, his careful explanations were of great help.

Bradley University is an ideal place for a scholar-teacher to work in. Undergraduate teaching is taken very seriously here and, importantly, so is scholarly research. This is the fourth book that I have written while on Bradley's faculty and I gratefully acknowledge the continued support of its professional librarians, text processing department, and Office for Research and Sponsored Programs.

I appreciate the assistance I received in assembling the photographs that appear in this book. The Palmer College of Chiropractic

Library in Davenport, Iowa and the A. T. Still Memorial Library at the Kirksville College of Osteopathic Medicine in Missouri were especially congenial in responding to my requests. Michael Sellon graciously provided his drawings of Therapeutic Touch, which originally appeared in the book *The Therapeutic Touch* by Janet Macrae and published by Alfred Knopf. Both Janet and Toinette Lippe, a Knopf editor, cheerfully and quickly made these drawings accessible to me. Ms. Linda Laing, a crystal healer in Indianapolis, enabled me to include a vivid scene of the fusion of spirituality and empathy found in New Age medicine. All along the way Jim Brey, a photographer on Bradley's professional staff, offered his continued assistance in reproducing photographs.

Finally, I would like to dedicate this book to my son, Matt, who has patiently waited his turn as other books have been dedicated to his mother, older brother, and grandparents. Blessed with a calm and independent spirit, he has taught me much about finding some serenity amidst the hectic moments of life.

Contents

ALTERNATIVE MEDICINE AND AMERICAN RELIGIOUS LIFE

1

Introduction

AMERICANS HAVE BEEN both bewildered and amused at the number of offbeat "metaphysical movements" that the media have publicized in recent years. One of the best known has been a cluster of beliefs and practices commonly referred to as the New Age movement. *Time* magazine, for example, devoted a cover story to this loosely knit amalgam of unconventional spirituality. Major bookstore chains have devoted large display sections to "Religion/New Age" books and report burgeoning sales. Most of these books, which would formerly have appeared under the now-abandoned "Occult" heading, discuss such varied subjects as meditation, spirit "channeling," the mind's hidden parapsychological powers, and self-help techniques designed to help persons achieve some combination of spiritual growth and economic success. But perhaps what has most aroused public interest is the New Age movement's belief in nonmedical forms of healing. Herbal remedies, acupuncture, crystal healing, and psychic mending of the "astral body" are all being touted by the movement's adherents.

Consider, for example, actress Shirley MacLaine's belief that "natural, holistic approaches worked better for me than medicines or drugs. . . . Orthodox Western medicine relied far too heavily on drugs."[1] Abandoning medical pharmacology, Miss MacLaine has instead availed herself of the healing powers to be found in acupuncture, spirit messages, and crystal rocks. She now bathes with "four

3

quartz crystals sitting on each corner of the tub," and claims, "I have been learning to work with the power of crystals and that discipline has become part of my daily life."[2] This discipline has transformed Miss MacLaine's life to the point where she feels the presence of "spirit guides," has vivid memories of her past incarnations, and studies techniques for releasing the body's own healing energies.

Another Hollywood actress, Jill Ireland, credits meditation techniques combined with the healing power of crystals for her successful recuperation from cancer. She writes:

> I recalled the moment when I learned I had cancer. At the instant I had heard those fateful words, something in me had kicked over. It was as if a switch had been thrown. I felt myself gather all my forces and begin to fight. The energy was there waiting to be tapped. It knew what to fight. The enemy was within my body. The question was how.
>
> I also grasped the healing properties of quartz crystals for focusing and energizing my mind and body. A crystal is the only thing in the world that has a perfect molecular order; it is, in fact, perfect order. Sue Colin [her holistic health practitioner] used them for healing. She would hold a crystal in her hand, drawing the healing energy into her. Sometimes when I was with her, I would meditate using the energy of the crystal [and] held them during my cancer meditation.[3]

Like MacLaine and Ireland, several hundred thousand Americans have turned to some form of alternative healing in hopes of integrating body, mind, and spirit. And their pursuit of the "secret" of physical health has inevitably taken them beyond the mysteries of the body to those of the psyche and soul. In short, Americans' involvement with unorthodox medical practices often leads them to a variety of unorthodox religious beliefs.

This book is an attempt to put contemporary Americans' interest in metaphysical healing systems into a historical and interpretive context. It shows, for example, that the connection between unconventional medical ideas and unconventional religious ideas is not at all new in American culture. And although the practitioners of metaphysical healing operate according to ideas vastly different from those underlying either the medical establishment or the biblically based ministry, they nonetheless possess a tradition of their own. The story of this tradition is, as we shall see, a fascinating chapter in the history of American medical and religious life.

Religion and Medicine: Cultural Relationships

To most modern Americans, religion and medicine would appear to have little in common. Religion speaks to our beliefs in a reality that transcends the physical. Medicine entails systematic efforts to repair organic damage caused by natural disease and injury. Whenever the media report an attempt to relate the two, most people react with skepticism and amusement and sometimes with indignation. The vast majority of the educated American public has little sympathy for Jehovah's Witnesses who refuse to let their children receive blood transfusions, Christian Scientists who decline immunizations, or charismatic healers who prefer blind faith to scientific medicine. The advent of modern science has tended to relegate religion and medicine to separate spheres, and most people feel quite comfortable with the assumption that religious beliefs are irrelevant to matters of healing and health.

What must be kept in mind, however, is that our culture's tendency to separate healing from religion is just as historically conditioned as were previous eras' efforts to unite them. Healing is a profoundly cultural activity. Labeling a disease and prescribing treatment express a healer's commitment to a particular set of assumptions about the structure and properties of physical existence. For this reason, the notion of orthodoxy pertains to medical systems as surely as it does to religious or political traditions. Ever since Descartes and the Enlightenment, medical orthodoxy has been defined by a commitment to the causal role of organic, or "material," factors in the etiology of disease. Western medical science is thus historically as well as conceptually opposed to the pre-Enlightenment world view within which the church supplied culturally compelling explanations of nonmaterial or spiritual causes of disease (e.g., sin or spirit possession) as well as corresponding schemas for therapeutic intervention (e.g., confession or exorcism). The continuous successes of medical science have had the cumulative effect of providing evidence for the superiority of its underlying conceptions and world view. As a consequence, religious explanations of health and disease have been relegated to the realm of superstition. Pehaps in no other arena has the capitulation of Western religion to the forces of secularization been more complete, and religious and medical orthodoxies have for the most part been content with a clear-cut division of labor whereby the cure of souls and bodies is entrusted to their respective professions.

The fact that certain medical systems continue late in the twentieth century to espouse theories that defy scientific orthodoxy is thus of particular interest to the cultural historian. For example, popular fascination with holistic healing methods, laying on of hands, and Oriental systems for self-purification seems to indicate that a fairly large number of Americans subscribe to beliefs that belong neither to science nor to the more genteel theologies of our mainstream churches. By contradicting what might be called the "monistic materialism" underlying medical science, practitioners of unorthodox medicine become defenders of a point of view that by "official" cultural definition should be considered irrational and superstitious. Yet, strictly speaking, any medical system is rational insofar as its methods of treatment are logically entailed by its fundamental premises or assumptions about the nature of disease. We might, for example, recognize at least four different types of explanations that could "rationally" be used to describe the cause of disease and, therefore, healing: physiological, environmental, attitudinal/psychological, and spiritual or supernatural (i.e., caused by the activity of entities or forces that are considered to be both extrasomatic and extrapsychological). Those propounding "supernatural-cause" explanations of healing are thus not necessarily less rational than those engaged in medical science. They are, however, advancing a metaphysical claim concerning the existence of causal forces not recognized by contemporary scientific theory. It is also clear that, whether they conceptualize this "higher" spiritual agency in categories of transcendence or of immanence, they are providing their clientele with both empirical (i.e., experiential) and pragmatic grounds for adopting a religiously charged interpretation of reality.

Thus, it is not simply that unorthodox medicine draws its constituency from the ranks of those who are either educationally disenfranchised from scientific knowledge or so desperately ill that they no longer expect hope from the methods of conventional medicine. The persistence and popularity of unorthodox medical systems is at least equally attributable to their articulation of a religiously significant way of viewing the world. Indeed, from a cross-cultural perspective it is clear that one of the most important functions of healing rituals is their capacity to induce an existential encounter with a sacred reality. In primitive societies, healing rituals involve participants in the reenactment of cosmological dramas; the shaman is both a healer and a mystagogue, or mediator between the divine and human realms. And in the case of Christianity, healing was thought to be a sign of Jesus's divine nature and was thereafter institutionalized as a function of Christian proclamation and ministry.[4] Yet, with the gradual divorce of physical healing from the church's routine activities, this means of introducing individuals to a higher spiritual reality necessarily shifted to the fringes of cultural orthodoxy.

Of course, not every system of healing that falls outside of the American Medical Association's sanctioned activities propounds a supernatural cause of healing. Nutritional and exercise therapies, for example, seek to strengthen and regulate basic metabolic processes through diet and sundry fitness regimens. Many massage and breathing systems likewise make no claims concerning the presence or activity of extrasomatic energies when explaining their programs for producing deep muscle relaxation and an overall sense of well-being.[5] It might be noted, however, that unorthodox systems of the nonsupernaturalist variety tend to emphasize preventive rather than curative practices. They are also not as likely to ask their clientele to make fundamental revisions in their conceptions of the causal forces at work in the universe. It is for this reason that this book is primarily concerned with those systems of unorthodox medicine that offer supernatural-cause explanations of healing. A distinguishing character of these systems is that they utilize vocabularies and techniques designed to induct individuals into a world view predicated upon the "fact" that under certain conditions extramundane forces enter into, and exert sanative influences upon, the human realm. They are, therefore, substantively religious in that they seek to induce consciousness of a sudden, felt intrusion of a "More" that is experienced as "other" than the material world and thereafter replaces all other forms of reality as normative or ultimately meaningful.[6]

The fact that many contemporary healing systems seek to inculcate supernaturalist beliefs in an essentially ad hoc and nonecclesiastical way does not detract from their ability to have a recognizable impact on American religious life. On the contrary, they are important reminders that many of our nation's religious beliefs are of the unchurched, or "folk," variety. For example, such decidedly supernaturalist systems of belief as astrology, spiritualism, and parapsychology are perduring sources of Americans' world views even though they have no formal relationship to normative cultural institutions.[7] Moreover, even though these groups have distinct historical lineages and utilize different terminology, they are nonetheless understood by their American adherents to be advocating quite similar conceptions of reality.[8] Historian Sydney Ahlstrom has described the kind of spirituality that Americans acquire from these self-proclaimed New Age movements as "harmonial piety" insofar as their doctrines articulate a view of the world "in which spiritual composure, physical health, and even economic well-being are understood to flow from a person's rapport with the cosmos."[9] Among the metaphysical doctrines supporting the harmonial interpretation of life are belief in the existence of unseen levels or realms of reality; the "correspondence" of the physical realm with higher metaphysical realms, enabling lawful patterns of interaction among them; the possibility that under certain conditions there might occur a flow of energies from higher dimensions into lower ones; and an emanationist cosmology that pictures the universe as an expression of an evolving divine force continuously seeking to move life onward and upward.

Americans' interest in medical systems based on a harmonial interpretation of the relationship between the physical and metaphysical spheres of life is hardly new. More than eighty years ago William James noted that a metaphysical healing system gives "to some of us serenity, moral poise, and happiness, and prevents certain forms of disease as well as science does, or even better in a certain class of persons."[10] What made these groups so significant in James's opinion was that they overthrew the pretension of positivistic science as the sole method for defining reality. These groups advocated a kind of science that embraced higher spiritual realities and thus portended a New Age in which humanity's scientific and religious needs were reconciled in a single intellectual system. By using healing methods that purported to show that under certain conditions "higher energies filter in" and that "work is actually done upon our finite personality," practitioners of unorthodox medicine were furnishing empirical evidence in support of a religious outlook very similar to James's own radical empiricism.[11] He further observed that these groups were generating a wave of religious enthusiasm among those seeking a felt sense of an unseen order of reality, and he predicted that metaphysical healers would play as great a role in the evolution of popular religion in the twentieth century as Luther and Calvin had in their day.[12]

James's comparison of metaphysical healing systems with the Protestant Reformation was a bit exaggerated. He did nonetheless identify a certain strand of unchurched, or popular, religious thought that appears to have a particular affinity with American culture. This book attempts to examine this enduring strain of American religiosity and to set it in historical, cultural, and sociological contexts. Chapter 2 will treat the development of unorthodox medicine in the nineteenth century. Prior to the 1830s "regular," or orthodox, medicine had not become sufficiently institutionalized to make the notion of self conscious commitment to a countervailing system a meaningful historical or cultural concept. By the mid-nineteenth century, however, America was awash in "irregular," sectarian, healing systems, among them homoeopathy, Thomsonianism, hydropathy, and sundry dietary regimens inspired by the unflagging efforts of Sylvester Graham. All of these movements resonated with the progressivist and perfectionist tendencies of early nineteenth-century American Protestantism, yet none logically entailed a "spiritual" or "metaphysical" causal explanation of healing. This is not, however, to imply that Americans failed to educe such religiously edifying notions from them. They did so largely by uniting, at the level of popular culture, ideas born of two new metaphysical systems competing for adherents in nineteenth-century America: Swedenborgianism and mesmerism.

The third chapter will examine the influence of the Swedish mystic Emanuel Swedenborg and the Viennese physician Anton Mesmer on developments in unorthodox medicine in this country. Swedenborgianism and mesmerism offered late nineteenth-century Americans new terms for describing their relationship to the higher forces and energies upon which human well-being is thought to be ultimately dependent. The diffusion of Swedenborgian and mesmerist terminology into the American metaphysical vocabulary brought exciting new dimensions to the references to the healing powers of nature found in homoeopathy, Thomsonianism, hydropathy, and Grahamism. The Swedenborgian and mesmerist systems articulated a locus of interconnection between the physical and spiritual realms—the human psyche—providing Americans with a profound sense of their own inner capacity for receiving an ecstatic influx of divine spirit into their systems. As a result, these movements gave birth to such quintessentially American religious philosophies as New Thought and Christian Science.

The fourth chapter will examine the emergence of two new unorthodox healing systems in the late nineteenth century: chiropractic and osteopathic medicine. As we will see, they are both indebted to the mesmeric model of human well-being and thus have at their core an explicitly metaphysical notion of healing. And although each has over the years gradually muted references to metaphysical concepts of disease, the origins of chiropractic and osteopathic medicine nonetheless constitute remarkable case studies in the intermingling of religion and medicine in American culture.

The fifth chapter will treat the twentieth century's concern with "holistic healing" techniques. The concept of a holistic approach to medicine does not in and of itself necessarily entail acknowledging the kind of metaphysical view of reality central to so many unorthodox healing systems in America. However, underlying such diverse healing practices as Ayurvedic medicine, Yoga, Shiatsu, rolfing, psychic healing, Therapeutic Touch, Alcoholics Anonymous, and New Age crystal healing is a conceptual system that recognizes that "every human being is a unique, wholistic, interdependent relationship of body, mind, emotions, and spirit."[13] And by introducing "spirit" as a causal agent alongside somatic and psychic factors in the determination of health and disease, these groups have emerged and functioned as prime carriers of the kind of popular religion to which William James so presciently pointed some ninety years ago.

The sixth and final chapter will attempt to make sense of Americans' continuing advocacy of medical theories and techniques that clearly run against the grain of scientific orthodoxy. This, the most analytical section of the book, will attempt to set these groups in their larger social and cultural contexts. Employing both current theory in the field of psychosomatic medicine and psychological perspectives drawn from what is known as object relations theory, I will argue that these groups are particularly effective in bringing the resources of religion to bear upon the healing process. Far from promulgating religious notions inherently detrimental to their adherents' capacity for effective functioning in life, many of these groups appear to be fostering as mature and vivid a form of spirituality as might be expected in an age so dominated by secular rationality.

A few qualifications are in order. First, I would like to caution the reader that this is by no means intended to be an exhaustive treatment of "fringe" medicine in America. Its concern is with tracing the various ways in which medical systems have served as carriers of an unchurched strain of American religious thought. Groups have been selected or excluded not on the basis of their intrinsic significance to the history of medicine but rather on their ability to illuminate the patterns whereby sectarian healing movements come to articulate religious visions of reality. Second, let me repeat a word of caution from above. I am not arguing that every unorthodox medical group evokes a religiously salient world view. Nor am I maintaining that the groups discussed in this book were relegated to an unorthodox status solely because of the religious dimension of their theories. My project is more modest and seeks only to demonstrate the vast extent to which unorthodox medical systems have provided their adherents with beliefs and practices that together constitute an enduring tradition of unchurched American religious life. And third, nowhere does this book address what is commonly referred to as "faith healing." The concern here is not with religious groups that include healing in their ministries but with medical systems that dispense heavy doses of unconventional religion. Thus, although the presence of healing practices in our churched religious traditions is a fascinating topic, this book restricts its focus to the presence of religious symbolism in the therapeutic activities of groups with no formal religious affiliation. In fact, a major thesis of this book is that some unorthodox medical systems enable modern individuals to experience the sacred in ways that are more rejuvenating than can be found in many of our established churches. For this reason, they deserve special attention as a mode of religion which not only survives but actually thrives in our secular society.

2

Sectarian Healing and Protestant Perfectionism in the Nineteenth Century

INSTITUTIONS AND PROFESSIONS are expressions of sociological structures. A developing nation consequently has few institutions and professions that possess widespread authority and prestige. In the United States, only the church and ministry had well-defined cultural functions throughout the colonial and early national periods, and it was not until the late eighteenth or early nineteenth century that anything resembling an orthodox medical profession emerged.

The medical practices of the indigenous Indian population varied by tribal organization and contributed very little to the ongoing development of medicine in this country—except, perhaps, as a somewhat naive symbol by which later generations of Americans would occasionally voice a nostalgic yearning for a return to harmony with nature.[1] Nor was the seventeenth- and eighteenth-century colonial period able to produce much in the way of a cohesive medical profession. Nearly all educated men of the colonial era acquired some medical knowledge in the course of their normal reading. The ministry, as the most learned of colonial professions, was also the most knowledgeable in medicine and readily dispensed advice for the body as well as the soul. Thus, for example, Cotton Mather is remembered not only for his lofty theological acumen but also for the fact that he recommended the application of a poultice made of dung and urine. Apothecaries, bone setters, midwives, barber-surgeons, and African tribal healers among the slave population also provided a range of healing services.[2] None, however, wielded sufficient influence to form anything that might be considered "orthodoxy."

After the Revolution, as Americans set themselves to the task of building a republic, a medical profession slowly emerged that for the most part mirrored the intellectual and cultural outlook of the pace-setting educated citizenry of the Northeast. The ideals of the Enlightenment held sway among those who devoted themselves to medical theory. Following the model of Isaac Newton, Enlightenment philosophers believed that the workings of the universe could be reduced to a single set of governing principles. The goal of science was to use empirical methods to find a single fundamental force or principle responsible for what otherwise appear to be complex phenomena. Ironically, it was this same Enlightenment notion—in a popularized form—that would give later "sectarian" systems of medical science such as Thomsonianism, mesmerism, and Grahamism their plausibility. Among the learned members of early nineteenth-century New England, however, this Enlightenment quest for a rational medical science gave rise to a more or less empirical effort to discern regular patterns in the body's interactions with the physical environment.

American medical orthodoxy, then, emerged as committed to the view that health is a function of the interaction between a person's constitutional endowment and the physical environment. This point of view was supported by a corollary theoretical assumption and carried with it a fairly distinct orientation to therapeutic activities.[3] First, it built upon the assumption that every part of the body is inextricably related to every other part—that is, health and disease were understood as having more to do with one's overall state of well-being than with particular causes. It must be remembered that it was not until 1876 that Pasteur and Koch finally discovered the role of microorganisms in producing disease. Nineteenth-century medicine thus did not—indeed, could not—concern itself with diagnosing the specific causes of disease. Second, and following from this, there were very few disease-specific therapies. Because the body was viewed in terms of its overall interaction with the environment, health was synonymous with equilibrium in these transactions. Disease was defined as a loss of equilibrium in the interactions between the organism and its environment. Medicine consequently amounted to a set of procedures for regulating the systems of "intake" and "outflow" through which a person assimilated and discharged substances from the environment.

The physician, operating without the benefit of modern diagnostic techniques, had to rely primarily on his own visual observation of the patient's assimilations and excretions. By charting changes in the quantity and coloration of blood, urine, menstruation, or feces, a physician could hope to monitor the overall system of intake and outflow. The therapeutic arsenal at his disposal consisted of drugs and various invasive techniques that could influence a patient's ability to assimilate or excrete fluids. Bleedings, sweating, blistering, and the use of drugs aimed at inducing either vomiting or diarrhea were the most common therapeutic techniques. Thus, for example, calomel was the most widely used drug in the first half of the nineteenth century. Containing the chloride of mercury, calomel breaks down in the intestines into its poisonous, and even lethal, components. In so doing it irritates the bowels and serves as a violent laxative, producing effects consistent with the assumptions that antebellum Americans held concerning the etiology of diseases. It was therefore embraced as part of a fully rational system of medicine, along with the incessant bleedings, blisterings, and purgatives that comprised the period's dominant therapeutic activities.

The emerging corps of physicians who operated on the basis of this "rational" approach to medical science came to be referred to as practitioners of "regular" medicine. What regular physicians stood for above all else was a vehement scorn for the healing powers of nature. Regular medicine was allopathic—that is, it worked by seeking to counteract or even combat the forces of nature. As the preeminent physician Benjamin Rush put it, regular medical practice was predicated upon "believing in direct and drastic interferences" with the patient's system.[4] The regular physicians' weaponry of alcohol, opium, mercury, arsenic, and strychnine—let alone the continual bloodletting—eventually earned them the apt designation as practitioners of "heroic" medicine. Doctors literally assaulted their patients in an effort to stimulate and reinvigorate their constitutions. Those hardy patients who did not die in the course of these largely futile endeavors were at the very least weakened by the ordeal.

Fortunately, heroic medicine began to lose favor somewhat by the late 1830s. The influence of Parisian medical schools and their increased emphasis upon anatomical research, the art of diagnosis, and the use of the stethoscope began to diminish the dogmatic application of heroic assaults upon the patient. More controlled clinical trials and advances in physiological knowledge helped regular physicians to become more adept in their diagnoses and treatments. Medical historian John Warner reminds us that "nineteenth-century medical therapeutics *did work;* though perhaps not when judged by criteria of efficacy satisfying to a twentieth-century pharmacologist. Physicians were not ordinarily simpleminded, passive, or duplicitous, nor were they unobservant of the results of their therapies."[5] The point is not so much that medicine became increasingly scientific during the nineteenth century as that what counted as scientific changed and evolved. Medical therapeutics followed and benefited from changing conceptions of what constituted scientific study.

The damage wrought by heroic therapeutics was also circumscribed by recognition of the self-limiting character of many diseases and the accompanying willingness to allow nature to take its course. In addition, changes in therapeutic practice stemmed not only from scientific progress stimulated by "high" culture, but also from the competition that "low" culture provided in the crowded medical marketplace. John Duffy comments: "As much as anything, it was the public's decision to turn from the regular profession to the herbalists, homeopaths, hydropaths, and other medical sects eschewing heroic practices which literally forced orthodox physicians to reconsider their position."[6]

It is important to note that regular physicians, unlike those following systems whose underlying assumptions fell outside the purview of the dominant medical model, possessed sufficient socioeconomic clout to be at the forefront of early efforts to organize the kinds of societies, schools, and regulatory legislation that would protect their vested professional interests. Regular physicians began to establish both local and state societies as early as the eighteenth century.[7] The purpose of these societies was to standardize medical practice both by promoting the sharing of professional knowledge and by actively attempting to legislate competitors out of the marketplace. Most of the early regulatory legislation proved ineffective and was, in fact, later repealed under the pressure of the Jacksonian era's confidence in the common person's right to pursue his or her self-interest unfettered by restraints imposed by the privileged classes. Nonetheless, regular physicians continued to institutionalize their own rational and scientific approach to medicine. The American Medical Association (AMA), while largely ineffective until the twentieth century, was founded in 1847 to uphold the ideal that physicians "should study, also, in their deportment, so to unite tenderness with firmness, and condescension with authority, as to inspire the minds of the patients with gratitude, respect, and confidence."[8] The AMA code also detailed the obligations of patients to their physicians. The counseled its members to instruct patients to confide in them freely, without, however, bothering them "with a tedious detail of events or matters not appertaining to his disease" nor with "the details of his business nor the history of his family concerns." The patient was further warned that his "obedience . . . to the prescriptions of his physician should be prompt and implicit" and "after his recovery, [he should] entertain a just and enduring sense of the value of the services rendered him by his physician; for these are of such a character that no mere pecuniary acknowledgment can repay or cancel them."[9] It would thus appear that, from its outset, the AMA sought not only to promote scientific progress but to ensure for its members a preeminent cultural status.

What medical societies and early legislative efforts failed to achieve in the way of promoting medical uniformity was gradually accomplished by the proliferation of medical schools. In the first few decades of the nineteenth century, only 4 medical schools existed in the United States; by the end of the century 157 existed, all but 31 of which were dominated by regular physicians.[10] Of course, medical school education during these years differed greatly from what we know today. Most schools required attendance at only two four-month lecture sessions. There were generally no clinical training sessions, no laboratories, and for that matter no admissions requirements. Even as late as 1870, only a very small percentage of medical students had earned a bachelor's degree. But, significantly, the very existence of medical schools served to standardize medical practice in this country. The publication of new textbooks designed to complement the basic lecture sequence promulgated a common core of medical knowledge. And as the established medical schools finally began to perceive the need for clinical training and entered into cooperative agreements with hospitals to establish internships and residencies, they gained ever more control over who would be allowed entrance into the profession. Thus, without question, the regular physicians and their "material-cause" outlook on health and disease attained in the 1800s the position of medical orthodoxy.

Thomsonianism and the Rise of Sectarian Medicine

Even as state and local medical societies were growing, licensing laws being enacted, and medical schools being standardized, the first real challenge to the orthodoxy of regular medicine appeared in the form of Thomsonianism. Samuel Thomson (1769–1843) came from a poor farming family in rural New Hampshire. In early adulthood he saw his mother die from what he took to be excessive doses of mercury and opium prescribed by a physician. A few years later his wife fell ill from complications following childbirth and barely survived the mercurial drugs and relentless bleedings forced upon her by a regular doctor. At least Thomson called upon two local "root and herb" doctors, and credited their botanical compounds with effecting her recovery. Thomson's experiences led him to the study of the medicinal value of herbs, and in 1805 he struck out on his own as an itinerant botanical healer.

The healing philosophy that Thomson gradually evolved was in many respects little more than a variant of regular medical theory. In line with the period's penchant for deducing a single fundamental principle to account for the whole of medicine, he surmised that there was only one cause of disease, cold, and one cure, heat.

> Heat, I found was life; and Cold, death. . . . Our life depends on heat [and when the body loses heat] the man is sick in every part of the whole frame.
>
> This situation of the body shows the need of medicine, and the kind needed; . . . raise the heat again, and nourish the whole man. All the art required to do this is, to know what medicine will do it, and how to administer it, as a person knows how to clear a stove and the pipe when clogged with soot, that the first may burn free, and the whole room be warmed as before.[11]

To perform this "clearing out" function Thomson used botanics (e.g., sumac, spruce, bayberry) that served as emetics, purgatives, or diuretics. Combining steam baths with other botanics such as cayenne pepper, he was able to restore "heat" to the system and gain control over the general intake and outflow of vital body fluids. One great differences between Thomsonianism and regular medicine was that it did not utilize harsh bleedings or mercurial drugs. Nor did it require economic dependence on physicians who cloaked themselves in an aura of cultural superiority.

Thomson began issuing circulars and pamphlets explaining his system and, in 1822, published a book entitled *New Guide to Health; or Botanic Family Physician*. He commissioned agents to help him sell his book for $20 per copy. The purchase price entitled the buyer to practice this "entirely new" system of botanic medicine within his or her own family. Thomson claims to have sold about 100,000 copies of this book. Its readers organized into local Friendly Botanic Societies to help promote its healing philosophy, and new disciples founded journals such as the *Boston Thomsonian Manual* and *The Boston Thomsonian Medical and Physiological Journal*. The Thomsonian system could be easily and inexpensively incorporated into family medical practice. For this reason, as medical historian William Rothstein notes, "of the various alternatives to regular therapy, only botanical medicine was widely used and understood by the public."[12] Before long the movement spread throughout the Northeast and Midwest.

It is surely not surprising that, with the deplorable condition of regular medicine, the nineteenth century spawned a number of alternative, or sectarian, healing systems such as Thomsonianism. What is remarkable is the extent to which these movements were implicated in the period's moral and religious life; and, as we shall see, a good many of the period's unorthodox medical systems were fraught with notions of metaphysical causality that ran counter to the general tide of secularization then gaining momentum not only in the burgeoning fields of science but in institutionalized religion as well.

The Thomsonian system appealed to Americans in the first few decades of the nineteenth century because of its ability to convey a number of salient cultural themes. First, and most obviously, it gave succinct popular expression to the fierce democratizing spirit of Jacksonian America. Samuel Thomson was a living symbol of the period's belief in the resourcefulness and natural wisdom of the common man. He repeatedly spoke out for seizing medicine back from the rich and powerful and returning it to the private citizen. The *Boston Thomsonian Manual* pronounced that the movement intended nothing less than "To make every man his physician."[13] Another Thomsonian advocate wrote that this would put an end to the system of regular medicine, whose practices operated exclusively to "make the rich,—richer, the poor,—poorer."[14] Understanding well the larger cultural forces symbolized by his medical reformation, Thomson wrote that "The priest, the doctor, and the lawyer" were all guilty of "deceiving the people."[15] The Thomsonian system thus gave the average person a tool of political power. It enabled men and, to an even greater extent, women to express their yearning for freedom from elitism, institutionalism, and remote sources of authority and power.[16] The *New Guide to Health* returned medicine to the domestic unit. All of this played well in an era in which the common person yearned for common remedies to common ailments.

Medical systems are multivalent phenomena. As Charles Rosenberg has observed, "Therapeutics is after all a good deal more than a series of pharmacological or surgical experiments. It involves emotions and personal relationships, and incorporates all of those cultural factors which determine belief, identity, and status."[17] Insofar as sectarian medical systems are successful in attracting a popular following, they are necessarily making new and creative use of "those cultural factors" determining our beliefs and identities. Particularly dramatic instances of sectarian medical formation are thus prime instances or expressions of what cultural historian William McLoughlin calls "awakenings."[18] According to McLoughlin, awakenings are periodic phases of social life in which a people reshapes its identity, transforms its patterns of thought and action, and redefines the means for sustaining a healthy relationship with the wider powers upon which its well-being is dependent. Awakenings typically give rise to a number of sectarian religious, political, and social movements that seek to give inherited belief systems a new and more functional expression. Such was the case, McLoughlin tells us, in the 1830s (when Thomsonianism, homoeopathy, Grahamism, and hydropathy all began to surface in American life), the 1880s (which witnessed the emergence of New Thought, Christian Science, and the beginnings of chiropractic and osteopathic medicine), and the 1960s (which gave rise to holistic health awareness, an avid appropriation of Oriental systems of self-purification, and a rebirth of New Age thinking).

Of central importance is the fact that the major periods of cultural renewal or awakening in American history have all entailed the reinvigoration of a fairly small core of conceptions that have shaped our country's experience. Among the most salient of these core beliefs are

> the covenant with God; the higher (biblical or natural) law, against which private and social behavior is to be judged; the laws of science, presumed to be from the Creator, and evolutionary or progressive in their purpose; the free and morally responsible individual; and the benevolence of nature under the exploitative or controlling hand of men.[19]

Each major awakening reinterprets these shaping symbols in ways befitting contemporary patterns of social, economic, and political change. In the 1820s and 1830s, the demand to push forward the frontiers of a spanking new nation made the older, Calvinist version of these ideas untenable for a good many Americans. The revivalist preachers of the era had done much to sway popular opinion away from the Calvinist preoccupation with humanity's helplessness and depravity. Instead, the theological climate promoted emphasis upon our particular sins (e.g., intemperance, Sabbath breaking, unchastity); by overcoming these sins we might—by our own will and effort—restore our rightful relationship to God and the providential forces that God has implanted for us in nature. At the core of all of this was a renewed faith in human perfectibility.

Medical sectarians like the Thomsonians were thus supplying the physiological counterpart to the period's theological perfectionism. Paralleling the revivalist preachers, they too told their audiences that worldly happiness is intended by both divine and natural law. It followed that all we had to do to avail ourselves of God's progressive plan was to assume willful responsibility for our own physiological salvation. The medical sectarians insisted that disease is by no means a deserved reprimand from a wrathful God, but was instead a natural phenomenon and thus subject to laws that human reason could discover and systematically apply. Small wonder, then, that much of the interest in medical sectarianism was linked with the revival-born enthusiasm for finding new and more efficient ways of doing God's work on earth.[20] In fact, Thomsonianism spread along precisely the same geographical lines that revivalist preachers had traveled (i.e., roughly from Vermont and New Hampshire into western New York State and into the Ohio Valley) spreading the new theological mood of optimism and perfectionism.[21]

Those infected by the prevailing theological mood—especially the clergy—were understandably prone to ask more of medical theory than the regular physicians were able to supply. They sought what might be described as a physiological Arminianism, that is, a patented panacea whereby individuals could take control of their own physical and spiritual salvation. Thomsonianism presented individuals with the opportunity to renounce self-defeating practices and instead align themselves systematically with the lawful patterns that God had established for the continuing improvement of His world. The national mood thus conjoined themes that were logically separable. Confidence in progress, trust in nature, and distrust of elitist authority were united in the period's outlook in a way that enabled the peculiar tenets of Thomsonianism to attract a far more loyal following than its therapeutic record alone warranted. Consider, for example, the testimony of a New York State senator in 1844 as he hailed the virtues of Thomson's system:

> The study of the healing art may be pursued to as great advantage by the inquiring and enlightened mind, by reading the great book of nature, which a wise and bountiful providence has spread before him; and obtain from it as great a knowledge of healing . . . as can be obtained from the study of musty books in the halls of institutions of materia medica.[22]

The Thomsonian system aimed at nothing less than "reform in medicine, dietetics and morals, or, in short, a reform in physiology and morality."[23] It eschewed the "poisoning, bleeding, blistering, or physicing" of the regular physicians and instead countenanced "the use of those remedies only, that act in harmony with Nature's laws."[24] In so doing, it not only endorsed a set of medical practices, but articulated the very "cultural factors" that oriented the general public to issues of identity, status, and belief. Medical sectarians bespoke newer, more progressive interpretations of the covenant linking individuals to those transcendent forces upon which they believed their lives to be dependent. In the final analysis, a major reason Thomsonianism was able to win the allegiance of nineteenth-century popular audiences was that it promised them wholeness in ways that resonated clearly with the theological symbols by which they took their bearings on life.

Homoeopathy

A second form of "irregular" medicine, homoeopathy, began to emerge more or less concurrently with the public's gradual loss of enthusiasm for the Thomsonian system. A major difference between the two was that while Thomsonianism was advocated by persons clearly outside the orthodox, or regular, medical system, practitioners of the homoeopathic system often came from the ranks of the regular physicians themselves. Moreover, while the clients or patients of Thomsonianism tended to be rural and poor, homoeopathy thrived among the urban upper classes. This latter fact led to direct economic competition with the regular system; and thus from its very inception in American culture, homoeopathy existed in self-conscious opposition to the orthodox medical profession.

The homoeopathic system of medicine was the creation of the German physician Samuel Christian Hahnemann (1755–1843). Hahnemann grew increasingly critical of the indiscriminate prescription of drugs by his contemporaries. He was particularly disturbed by the tendency of allopathic physicians to combat disease with heavy doses of several drugs taken in combination. Believing that much more needed to be learned about the therapeutic effects of each individual drug, he began taking doses of the purest samples of various drugs in an effort to observe the particular physiological changes they brought about. When he swallowed a dose of cinchona, a bark commonly used to combat fever, he broke out in a fever himself. Hahnemann deduced from this that a drug that causes an illness in a healthy person will cure that same illness in a sick person. This principle, which he termed *similia similbus curantur,* or "like is cured by like," became the cornerstone of his homoeopathic doctrine.

Hahnemann set forth a thorough exposition of his healing system

in an 1810 volume entitled *Organon of the Rational Art of Healing.*
Hahnemann's healing art was based upon the premise that a disease
is synonymous with its symptoms. As he put it, "A disease in its
whole range is represented only by the complex of morbid symptoms. . . . in disease there is nothing to lay hold of except these phenomena."[25] He reasoned that physicians should carefully study the
symptoms that different drugs produce in healthy persons and, following his "like is cured by like" principle, prescribe drugs that
produce effects most similar to a patient's symptoms—because, to
again quote Hahnemann, "the healing power of medicines depends
on the resemblance of their symptoms to the symptoms of disease."[26]

Hahnemann went on to enunciate a second fundamental principle of homoeopathic medicine, which came to be known as the
doctrine of infinitesimals. It was his conviction that the greatest
therapeutic benefit was to be obtained by administering diluted
doses of a drug. He claimed, for example, that even $1/500,000$ or $1/1,000,000$
of a gram was in actuality more potent than a larger dose. Interestingly, regular physicians were somewhat at a loss to argue against
homoeopathy on the grounds of its "like is cured by like" principle.
After all, they too sought to attack symptoms through the use of
selected drugs and really had no theoretical basis upon which to
attack homoeopathy's major premise. The notion of diluted doses,
however, struck regular physicians as nonsense and gave them opportunity to denounce homoeopathy as therapeutically ineffectual.
Though, ironically, the homoeopathic physicians' use of small doses
undoubtedly negated any therapeutic value their drugs might have
had, at least these small doses had the virtue of not assaulting the
patient's own recuperative powers as did the regular physicians' use
of bleeding and poisonous drugs. It is thus not surprising that so
many ailing persons turned to homoeopathy as a viable alternative
to orthodox medicine. It should also be noted that homoeopathy's
popular appeal was a major factor in the formation and success of
the American Medical Association, as economic motives joined
with scientific ones to rally regular physicians in opposition to their
irregular competitors.

Homoeopathy spread quite rapidly in the United States.[27] It was
first introduced by Hans Gram, who opened an office in New
York after studying the homoeopathic system in Europe. By 1835
a homoeopathic college had been formed, and in 1844 the Ameri-

can Institute of Homoeopathy was organized and constituted the first national medical association in the country (predating the AMA by three years). Throughout the 1800s, ten to twelve percent of the total number of the country's medical schools and medical school graduates were adherents of homoeopathy.[28] The spread and relative popularity of the homoeopathic system provide an instructive lesson in the functions of alternative medicine in American culture. A first, and not insignificant, reason for homoeopathy's popular appeal was its use of less invasive forms of therapy. The infinitesimal doses used by homoeopathic physicians proved far more beneficial in cases where the bleedings and purgings of regular physicians so weakened patients that they failed to overcome illnesses that if left alone, would have run their natural courses and receded. Thus, for example, in cholera epidemics homoeopathic advocates could point to demonstrably better results among their patients.

A second reason for homeopathy's popularity is reflected in medical historian Joseph Kett's observation that it flourished in the same areas in which Thomsonianism had been successful earlier.[29] Kett persuasively argues that homoeopathy offered a new outlet for those whose enthusiasm had been previously aroused by the Friendly Botanic Societies. Homoeopathy's tirades against regular physicians went even further than Thomsonianism in appealing to the period's faith in the beneficence and progressive tendencies of the laws of nature. As one of the movement's spokespersons put it, "We Homoeopathic physicians abjure Allopathia for this—she ignores nature and her powers, in her practice violates her, and in her place sets up the supremacy of her own art."[30] In stark contrast, homoeopathic physicians sought to strengthen nature's own tendencies toward healing and perfection and, in so doing, articulated a philosophy that satisfied the public's desire to learn how they might best align themselves with providential laws and purposes.

Having noted that homoeopathy had certain similarities with Thomsonianism, it is all the more important to focus upon their significant differences. Thomsonians made little or no real effort to part from a material-cause view of healing. They simply substituted their herbs for the regular physicians' noxious drugs. Homoeopaths, however, moved increasingly in the direction of advocating a spiritual or metaphysical view of healing and for this reason were among the first to align alternative medicine with powerful currents in the period's unchurched religious thought. Hahnemann had from the start imbued homoeopathy with a thinly veiled vitalism. In the *Organon* he observed that "the action upon the living human body of the remedial counter-force which constitutes a medicine is so profound . . . that this action must be called spirit-like."[31] Hahnemann's writings, which finally became available in English translations in the 1840s, encouraged progressive thinkers to envision a subtle form of interaction between the material and spiritual dimensions of life. Homoeopathic medicine had unveiled the secret whereby humanity might bring physical events under the action of a "higher law." As Hahnemann wrote, his system of therapeutics possessed the power to affect the vital spirit responsible for organic life: "Homeopathic dynamizations are processes by which the medicinal properties of drugs, which are in a latent state in the crude substance, are excited and enabled to act spiritually [i.e., dynamically] upon the vital forces."[32]

These cryptic references to the "spirit-like" activity of certain medical substances caught the imagination of many intellectuals seeking innovative answers to the perennial question of the relationship of the world of matter to the world of spirit. Hence, although the names of Thomsonian supporters are barely known to us today, homoeopathy won the endorsement of some of the leading philosophers and religious thinkers of the day. Homoeopathy gave its advocates a medium in which to exercise their metaphysical imaginations. Most of the directions in which they pushed were soon to be reinforced by Swedenborgianism and mesmerism, as we shall see. A contemporary, writing about Hans Gram's followers and the new ideas they were coming to embrace, noted:

> In each of these directions Gram led the way to a wider and deeper knowledge of the relations between soul and body, the human and divine, the transitory and the permanent, than can be entertained by purely materialistic researches.[33]

The homoeopaths were flirting with an overtly metaphysical view of the causal forces influencing human health and well-being. By contrast, Thomsonians stuck to the commonsense view that matter is matter and spirit is spirit, thereby aligning themselves with the orthodox world view held not only by Western science but by the churches as well. Homoeopaths seemed to insinuate a more mystical view in which matter, if not exactly an expression of spirit, was at least receptive to spiritual infusions. For this reason, their healing system was avidly investigated by many followers of Transcendentalism and others who had become disillusioned with the static conceptual categories of Enlightenment rationality. Whatever the therapeutic benefit of homoeopathic practice, it certainly struck a number of educated Americans as a sanative philosophy.

Hydropathy

References to the curative power of water can be found in almost every culture throughout world history. In India, the waters of the Ganges are thought to purify both body and soul. In Western culture, Greek and Roman physicians praised the healing properties of water administered either internally or externally. And in the United States, faith in the restorative powers of mineral springs had long existed among the native Indians; by the 1660s, numerous mineral water sites were commonly used by the early European settlers of the New World.[34] It was not, however, until the mid-1840s that the healing practices of Vincent Priessnitz made their way across the Atlantic from his native Austria and that a fully articulated system of hydropathy, or water-cure, evolved in the United States. For Priessnitz, hydropathy consisted primarily of the external application of cold water to ailing parts of the body. Showers, baths, and wet-packs were all used to apply water's intrinsic therapeutic powers to bodily infirmities. The first American proponents of Priessnitz's system saw in it a viable alternative to allopathic medicine's excessive use of drugs and sought to make it the nucleus of an encompassing medical philosophy that would include also the essential insights of Thomsonianism, homoeopathy, and Grahamism.

The first major spokesman for hydropathy in the United States was Joel Shew. Shew, along with his associate Russell Trall, opened a water-cure institute in Lebanon Springs, New York, in 1845. Two years later Shew began publishing *The Water-Cure Manual* to promote his conviction that "too much, indeed, cannot be said in praise of cold water. . . . [for nowhere else] has Providence provided any thing as a beverage so grateful."[35] Shew advised his clientele to combine the therapeutic benefits to be had from the internal and external applications of water with the curative powers of fresh air, exercise, diet, sleep, and proper clothing. The comprehensive water-cure regimen was, in Shew's opinion, a veritable panacea. It could cure fever, hiccups, cholera, stomach bleeding, constipation, poisoning, as well as improve the digestion. Other water-curists added to this list malaria, whooping cough, diseases of the ear, gout, bladder infections, obesity, and excessive sexual desire.

The theoretical rationale of hydropathy centered upon the power of water to restore humans to a condition of purity. Whether taken internally or applied externally by wrapping the patient in what was known as a "wet sheet," water had an almost sacramental power to remove impurities. The hydropathists' wet sheets brought the skin into direct contract with pure water and thus made possible a sanative flow of vital fluids in and out of the body. Impurities from the patient's body could be eliminated through the skin while pure water could be ingested from the sheet or bath and restore purity to the physical system. The "philosophy of water-cure," then, was based not so much on combatting illness as on enhancing the natural vitality intrinsic to living organisms.[36] Water-curists were ideologically opposed to regular medicine. Dr. Henry Nichols, a leading hydropathist of the time, wrote an article for the *Water-Cure Journal* in which he compared the underlying rationale of all the various "pathies." While finding homoeopathy and Thomsonianism sound, if somewhat less profound than hydropathy, he launched a vituperative tirade against allopathic medicine and its principle of counterirritation. He charged that the drugs, emetics, and bleedings of allopathic medicine act as "paralyzers" and "stupefacients." Hydropathy, on the other hand, is based upon the "application of the principles and agency of nature to the preservation of health and the cure of disease."[37]

Hydropathy made harmony with nature the cornerstone of a comprehensive vision of human nature. One editorial pronounced:

The natural state of man, as of all plants and animals, is one of uninterrupted health. The only natural death is the gradual and painless decay of old age. Such a life and death are in happy harmony with nature; pain, and disease, and premature mortality are the results of violated laws.[38]

In the final analysis, disease is the lawful consequence of humanity's failure to abide by the providential structures that God has stamped onto the natural order of things. As another hydropathist put it:

> We regard Man, in his primitive and natural condition as the most perfect work of God, and consider his present degenerated physical state as only the natural and inevitable result of thousands of years of debauchery and excess, of constant and wilful perversions of his better nature, and the simple penalty of outraged physical law, which is as just and more severe than any other.[39]

Hydropathy was thus suggesting that all impediments to health and human progress could be removed by a better understanding of physical law. Its investigations, therefore, were both physiological and moral. The principles of life it uncovered were proclaimed to be the true foundation of any reform of the human condition since they sought to "purify the body as well as educate the mind ... reforming the whole man."[40] The *Water-Cure Journal* carried the apt subtitle "Herald of Reforms Devoted to Physiology, Hydropathy and the Laws of Life," and in one issue informed its readers that "the Water-Cure revolution is a great revolution. It touches more interests than any revolution since the days of Jesus Christ."[41]

Hydropathy eventually became entangled with so many "interests" that it gradually lost its distinctive character and became loosely incorporated into a number of diet and exercise philosophies. Russell Trall, along with editing *The Hydropathic Encyclopedia* and establishing a Hygieo-Therapeutic College in New York, also helped found the American Vegetarian Society. In this latter connection Trall aligned the principles of hydropathy with the crusading themes of the likes of William Alcott, Lucy Stone, Amelia Bloomer, Susan B. Anthony, and Horace Greeley. Trall also formed a partnership with the New York publishers Orson Fowler, Lorenzo Fowler, and Samuel R. Wells. The Fowlers and Wells were metaphysical dilettantes and make for an interesting story in their own right. Not only did they personally dabble in water-cure, phrenology, vegetarianism, mesmerism, Grahamism, and spiritualism, but they also published the most significant books on these topics. Of further interest is the fact that they brought all these diverse beliefs to the attention of the American reading public on the same advertisement pages. In doing this, Wells and the Fowlers were undoubtedly justified. For whether logically compatible or not, metaphysical theories of all kinds were linked by the popular intellectual climate. A good many Americans were dissatisfied with orthodox theology and were seeking progressive-minded insights into the higher laws of nature. Eclecticism and broad-minded synthesis appealed to those seeking a philosophy fit for a new age in which religion and science might be combined in some kind of transcendent intellectual synthesis. The Fowlers and Wells saw to it that unorthodox medical systems contributed to promoting this metaphysical mélange.

The water-cure movement thus attracted a number of mid-century Americans seeking a more encompassing vision of the forces upon which our health or well-being depends. Susan Cayleff has shown that several interconnected factors contributed to hydropathy's ideological appeal: it offered noninvasive hygienic principles in place of drug-based therapeutics; it provided distinct opportunities for a "conversion" to a new world view in a revival-like setting; and it fostered self-determination through changes in personal habits, as well as promoted a reformist and even emancipationist social outlook toward the class- and gender-based status quo.[42] Particularly interesting is the last of these, hydropathy's overt concern with overturning the hierarchical class and gender structures associated with allopathic medicine and substituting a more egalitarian model of social organization. The hydropathic movement rejected university training or professional membership as necessary criteria for restoring a patient's health. By emphasizing home self-doctoring and by offering sliding fees and other cost-reducing innovations, hydropathists broke down barriers between healers and clients and thereby fostered a sense of cooperation in the healing process. Hydropathy's reformist impulse was especially pronounced in its articulate attention to women's physiology. Water-cure writers such as Mary Gove Nichols and Russell Trall advocated a demystification of women's physiology and stressed the "naturalness" of the female reproductive system. Insisting, in fact, that "the sexual orgasm on the part of the female is just as normal as on the part of the male," Trall underscored hydropathy's commitment to a new and self-consciously progressive ideological matrix.[43]

One final hydropathist deserves to be singled out: James Caleb

Jackson, who established a water-cure in Dansville, New York. Seeking to outdo the other water-cure establishments throughout the country, Jackson constructed a palatial resort in which he combined hydropathic facilities, organized exercise programs, educational lectures, theater, and health food meals. One interesting sidelight is that Jackson began to produce health foods as a commercial venture, and among his first packaged products was a dry cereal he called "Granula," for which he ultimately won a trademark lawsuit against John Harvey Kellogg. Of greater importance is the fact that Jackson's resort, "Our Home on the Hillside," served as the meeting place for the individuals who were to join hydropathic principles to those of the fourth of our countervailing healing systems, the health food regimen inspired by Sylvester Graham.

Grahamism and the Christian Health Movement

Sylvester Graham represents something of a case study in the confluence of religious intentions and health reform during the first half of the nineteenth century. As Stephen Nissenbaum has shown in his critical study of Grahamism, Graham's life affords a microcosm of "Victorian physiological theory and practice in the very act of coming into being—as a complete ideological system governing every aspect of private routine."[44] Graham's health-reform system was essentially preventive rather than curative in design and therefore lies somewhat outside the scope of this book. Yet his ideas were so avidly appropriated by those espousing Thomsonianism, homoeopathy, hydropathy, and mesmerism that they can scarcely be separated from the nineteenth century's legacy to countervailing medical traditions.

Sylvester Graham (1794–1851) began his career as an ordained Presbyterian minister and itinerant evangelical preacher. Typical of the Arminian-leaning theological spirit of his day, Graham believed that humans have an important role in effecting their own salvation and, therefore, that the ministry is obligated to become involved in any reform movement dedicated to the progressive improvement of the human condition. Graham's primary interest lay in the temperance movement. His impassioned lectures and writings brought the zeal of Protestant piety to bear upon individuals' ability to take control of their physical well-being. James Whorton notes in his *Crusaders for Fitness* that "temperance lecturers such as Graham were in reality evangelical preachers mixing rum with brimstone and demanding total abstinence from alcohol as a prerequisite for Christian perfection."[45] What was novel in Graham's approach was that he not only detailed the eternal consequences of unregenerate behavior such as the consumption of alcohol, but enumerated the worldly wages of sin as well. He denounced "every liquid stimulant stronger than water" on the ground that they were "disturbing to the body, wearing it out sooner, and . . . detrimental to the health."[46]

Graham's commitment to the complete regeneration of every individual made it impossible for him to limit his attention to the unrestrained consumption of alcohol. He soon broadened the sphere of his prophetic witness to include the dangers of masturbation and sexual excess. While not unmindful of how the passions might lead one to trespass against God's revealed moral laws, Graham pricked the conscience of his audiences by drawing their attention to the bodily defilement wrought by carnal desires. In his 1832 *Lectures to Young Men on Chastity* he described how overstimulation of the sexual organs causes diabetes, jaundice, acne, bad hearing, and the loss of teeth. His research on the connections between moral conduct and physical health, he claimed, proved "that the Bible doctrine of marriage and sexual continence and purity is founded on the physiological principles established in the constitutional nature of man."[47]

In time Graham came to concentrate on the area of hygienic reform in which his contributions were to be the most original and long lasting: diet. He studied the physiological research of the French medical theorists Xavier Bichet and François Broussais, as well as the work of Benjamin Rush, and concluded that health depends upon the activity of the stomach. The stomach, it seems, is the physiological agent responsible for delivering "vital power" to the organism in its quest to overcome the various causes of disease and death. The stomach must be supplied with pure, nutritive substances, but must under no condition be "overstimulated." This purported physiological fact led Graham to embrace vegetarianism. While Graham was not the first proponent of vegetarianism in the United States, he became its most distinctive nineteenth-century advocate owing to the strictly physiological arguments he presented in its behalf. Earlier vegetarians such as Rev. William Metcalfe had provided religious and moral reasons for abstaining from meat eating. Graham's advocacy of a strictly vegetarian diet, like all his health-reform suggestions, was derived "purely by my physiological investigations."[48] To be sure, Graham was incapable of understanding human physiology in ways that would be inconsistent with his era's religious morality. But in his lectures and writings he professed that his various hygienic proposals were based upon a scientific rationale.

At the heart of Graham's dietary crusade was his insistence that the stomach required a steady supply of "well-made bread" in order to provide the system sufficient organic vitality without overstimulation. Denouncing the bread baked from the heavily refined flour manufactured by the country's burgeoning bakery industry, Graham insisted on the use of unbolted wheat flour. This coarse bread, later produced in cracker form, carries his name to this day. Graham was not content with simply telling his readers and listeners what they should eat; he offered advice on how it was to be prepared and eaten as well. Bread, for example, owing to the "intimate relation between the quality of the bread and the moral character of a family," should ideally be baked by "a devoted wife and mother."[49] And, to avoid overstimulating the stomach, meals were to be taken at least six hours apart; one should never eat before going to bed; one should avoid spicy condiments; and one should abstain from tea and coffee as they stunt growth and poison the body. Added to all of this were lengthy instructions on proper sleep, exercise, dress, personal hygiene, and avoidance of medicine ("All medicine, as such, is itself an evil").

The significance of Graham's regimen was not altogether confined to its explicitly stated goals. His audiences read a great deal more into his systematic program for health reform than the modern reader is likely to appreciate. To nineteenth-century Protestants seeking "new measures" whereby the entire universe might be reformed so as to be befitting to God, Grahamism had all the trappings of a sure-fire path to the millennial dawn. The Grahamite American Health Convention assembled in Boston in 1838 resolved:

> That the blessed cause of human improvement, the spread of the Gospel, and the universal regeneration of the world, can never be successfully

carried forward without the aid of the great work which we are now assembled to advance.[50]

Graham's ideas were among the most widely circulated of all the nineteenth century's health philosophies. They were implemented at hundreds of hydropathic clinics and spread into homoeopathic health counsels as well. The widely traveled evangelist Charles G. Finney became a convert to the Grahamite cause and brought it squarely into the perfectionist program that pervaded the nation's religious outlook. Several of the period's communitarian experiments—Brook Farm, Fruitlands, the Shakers—based their dietary programs on Graham's principles. The most intriguing extension of Grahamism, however, is undoubtedly its extension into the second largest religious denomination ever to emerge in the United States, the Seventh Day Adventists. The prophetess and foundress of Seventh Day Adventism, Ellen Gould White, was an occasional visitor at James C. Jackson's "Our Home on the Hillside" hydropathic resort in Dansville, New York.[51] Several years after her exposure to Graham's dietary program at Dansville, Ellen White had a mystical vision in which God revealed to her that his hygienic laws were to be kept as faithfully as the Ten Commandments. Thereafter all of those who joined her in awaiting the Second Coming of Christ were admonished to keep the body temple pure through adherence to Grahamite principles.

Ellen White was, as Gerald Carson has wryly observed, perhaps the only individual who could state with the full force of prophetic authority that "The health food business is one of the Lord's own instrumentalities."[52] Her concern for the "health food business" was inspired both by divine and pecuniary interests. She had taken under her wing a young Seventh Day Adventist who had studied medicine at Trall's Hygieo-Therapeutic College (where Grahamism was firmly ensconced) before earning a medical degree from New York's Bellevue Hospital. This young protégé, John Harvey Kellogg, soon took over the Western Health Reform Institute in Battle Creek, Michigan, which Ellen White had founded as an Adventist counterpart to the Dansville hydropathic resort. The Adventist sanitarium (affectionately referred to as the "San" by its patrons) grew into a large and diverse health resort and, under Kellogg's direction, attracted such luminaries as J. C. Penney, Montgomery Ward, Alfred DuPont, John D. Rockefeller, and President Taft. As described in an advertising brochure, its operating philosophy was that

> no drugs whatever, will be administered, but only such means employed as NATURE can best use in her recuperative work, such as Water, Air, Light, Heat, Food, Sleep, Rest, Recreation, &c. Our tables will be furnished with a strictly healthful diet.[53]

In his efforts to provide this "strictly healthful diet" to a wider audience, John Harvey Kellogg and a former patient of the San, C. W. Post, began to develop dry, prepackaged breakfast cereals such as corn flakes, shredded wheat, and variations upon Jackson's Granula. The rest, as they say, is history.

Summary and Prospectus

Thomsonianism, homoeopathy, hydropathy, and Grahamism all thrived as countervailing medical voices in the nineteenth century for many reasons. For one thing, they were generally less expensive than their "regular" competition. Second, they did not assault the patient through heavy doses of poisonous drugs and bleeding, thereby allowing the patient's own recuperative powers the chance to effect cure. A third reason, as Stephen Nissenbaum has so ably pointed out, is that they also offered an essentially nostalgic vision that placed healing in the hands of a loved family member rather than yet another representative of the steadily growing industrial and professional classes. Thus, for example, Graham's appeal to eat homemade bread was a powerful symbolic appeal to the ethic of self-sufficiency in an age in which the industrial revolution was shifting the production of basic commodities from the home to the factory.

And yet, as we have seen, above and beyond all of these factors was the ability of these healing movements to appeal to the core conceptions of American culture and to do so in ways that resonated with the progressivist temperament of the time. All four movements had deep roots in the Second Great Awakening, which accentuated the role of humans in effecting the Kingdom of God on earth. In both the ideas they embraced and the persons who articulated them, these movements carried the ideological thrust of that religio-cultural awakening to its most practical applications. These movements, like so many other "pseudosciences" of the nineteenth century, resonated well with the nation's utilitarianism, its egalitarianism, its implicit faith in America's special destiny, and the widespread anticipation that Americans would some day witness the complete transformation of their physical and spiritual beings.[54] Thus, when they asked their clientele to trust the progressive powers of nature to restore them to purity, they needed little in the way of empirical proof. The ideas carried about them the aura of self-evident truths.

There were, of course, considerable differences among these healing systems (although most of these differences were ignored by the general public that interpreted them with its own agenda in mind). We have already noted that Thomsonianism was a philosophy prone to acceptance by the poor, ill-educated, and rural. Homoeopathy, on the other hand, appealed mostly to the upper classes, the well educated, and urban. In his study of Grahamism, Nissenbaum makes much of the sharp contrasts between Sylvester Graham and his contemporary Ralph Waldo Emerson.[55] While each emphasized that the source of true authority is to be found in the individual, they understood the "inner person" in completely different ways. Emerson was a mystic and Transcendentalist. He believed that beneath the conscious intellect was an inner faculty for becoming receptive to a higher power. The final source of all regenerative and progressive actions, then, was the spiritual emanations of the Over-Soul which filtered through the mind's inner recesses. To Emerson, true spirituality had nothing at all to do with the Bible or traditional Christian morality. It instead entailed an aesthetic appreciation of one's own inner connection with the fundamental laws of the universe. In sharp contrast, Graham was a Protestant moralist. For him, all progressive activity was in the final analysis due to strict conformity with divine will. Graham called for scrutiny, control, discipline, and regimen in living, for the purpose of guarding against our tendency to fall away from conformity with God's lawful patterns. Emerson thought that consistency—as with all narrowing activities of the rational mind—was precisely what prevented humanity from letting go and becoming receptive to the forces hidden in the psyche's depths. In this contrast we have the two principal temperaments of American Protestantism—the ascetic (Graham) and the aesthetic (Emerson). And, in turn, we have the key to the different paths that alternative medical philosophies might travel as they make their way through the collective American mind.

Upon closer analysis, little in the four nineteenth-century healing systems we have examined could be called overtly or distinctively religious. The means of healing—herbs, minute drug doses, water, and nutritive food—all fall into the category of "material" therapeutic causes. True, the substances they utilized were not recognized by regular physicians as having curative power, but none of these unorthodox healing systems challenged the conceptual basis of regular medicine by explicitly professing belief in the therapeutic power of nonmaterial agents. And thus, although all four shared the Second Great Awakening's mission to narrow the great gulf that Calvinism had posited between a stern, wrathful God and His weak, depraved creation, none did anything to eliminate this gulf altogether. Ironically, the more overt their connection with institutional Christianity, the less likely were these theories to espouse anything resembling a spiritual- or metaphysical-cause explanation of healing. Instead, they conformed with ascetic Protestantism and its emphasis upon willful obedience to divine law. Almost entirely absent was anything that a historian of religion might describe as bearing the imprint of ecstasy or mystical encounter with the holy. For this to come to the fore, the aesthetic style of religious thought and its belief in humanity's inner capacity to become receptive to an "influx" of divine spirit had to make its way into popular healing practices.

Catherine Albanese has written of the metaphysical turn taken by many medical theorists in the nineteenth century. These theorists, she observes, learned to perceive hidden spiritual depths in nature and steadily linked this numinous nature to theories of the mind.[56] The homoeopaths, as might be expected, were among the first to strike out in this direction. In an essay appearing in *The Homoeopathic Advocate and Guide to Health* in 1851, W. O. Woodbury ventured that

> The *mind* is the power which produces in the human body, not only the intellectual and moral but also the vital phenomena. As the *almighty*

mind produces all the wondrous and mysterious workings throughout the material universe, . . . all in accordance with its own inherent impressions of love, mercy, justice, goodness, wisdom and truth, so does the *human mind* produce in its own little universe, the body, all its varied phenomena, from the lowest action of vitality to the most powerful physical motions, and thence upward to the highest grade of intellectual and moral phenomena.[57]

This homoeopathic advocate had identified a fundamental correspondence between the macrocosm (universal mind) and the microcosm (human mind), but he had still not educed any physiological or psychological interconnection that might explain interaction between the two spheres. The world view that his theory expressed was simply too one-dimensional to permit notions of spiritual or metaphysical causality.

It was to this need that Americans would apply the ideological resources of yet two more European-born "isms." Swedenborgianism and mesmerism were all but destined to be pulled into the center of nineteenth century America's metaphysical musings. Both, as we shall see, lent scientific and intellectual authority to an aesthetic spirituality that looked to humanity's psychic depths for a point of interconnection with a higher spiritual power.

3

From Physic to Metaphysic:
The Spiritualizing of
Alternative Medicine

A MUCH ABUSED and fad-weary public awaited Charles Poyen at
the beginning of his American lecture tour in 1836. Inundated with
"doctors of the people" out to capitalize on their physical suffer-
ings, many Americans had learned to regard all medical theories
with a skepticism mitigated only by their desperate desire for a
more reliable program of cure. Poyen's audiences knew virtually
nothing about his subject and, by his account, seemed to prefer it
that way. Poyen consoled himself with the knowledge that all great
truths—even when espoused by the likes of Galileo, Columbus, or
Christ—are initially dismissed by the general populace. His confidence and evangelical zeal emanated from the conviction that he
was speaking on the basis of "well-authenticated facts concerning
an order of phenomena so important to science and so glorious to
human nature."[1] Knowing that his audience's indifference was
rooted in simple ignorance, Poyen persisted in his prophetic mission
to acquaint Americans with Franz Anton Mesmer's science of animal magnetism.

Mesmer (1734–1815) had attracted a good deal of attention
when he presented himself to European intellectual circles as the
bearer of an epoch-making discovery.[2] The Viennese physician
claimed to have detected the existence of a superfine substance or
fluid that had until then eluded scientific notice. Mesmer referred to
this invisible fluid as animal magnetism and postulated that it per-

meated the physical universe. He explained that animal magnetism constituted the etheric medium through which forces of every kind—light, heat, magnetism, electricity—passed as they traveled from one physical object to another. Every event transpiring in nature depended upon the fact that animal magnetism linked physical objects together and made possible the transmission of influences from one to another.

Mesmer believed that his discovery had removed the basic impediment to scientific progress and that every area of human knowledge would soon undergo rapid transformation and advancement. He was most concerned with its application to the treatment of disease. Animal magnetism was said to be evenly distributed throughout the healthy human body. If for any reason an individual's supply of animal magnetism was thrown out of equilibrium, one or more bodily organs would consequently be deprived of sufficient amounts of this vital force and eventually begin to falter. "There is," Mesmer reasoned, "only one illness and one healing."[3] Therefore, since any and all illnesses can ultimately be traced back to a disturbance in the body's supply of animal magnetism, medical science could be reduced to a simple set of procedures aimed at supercharging a patient's nervous system with this mysterious life-giving energy.

Before Mesmer's theory reached American shores, his pupils had introduced significant changes that would drastically alter the science of animal magnetism. The Marquis de Puysegur exerted the greatest influence upon subsequent interpretations of his teacher's remarkable healing talents. Puysegur faithfully imitated Mesmer's techniques, only to have his patients fall into unusual, sleeplike states of consciousness. They had, so to speak, become "mesmerized." These entranced individuals exhibited the most extraordinary behaviors. Puysegur's subjects responded to his questions with more intelligent and nuanced replies than could possibly be expected given their educational and socioeconomic background. Many subjects suddenly remembered long-forgotten experiences with astonishing accuracy. A select few appeared to drift into a much deeper state of consciousness, which Puysegur described as one of "extraordinary lucidity." These subjects spontaneously performed feats of telepathy, clairvoyance, and precognition. Puysegur had stumbled upon the existence of a stratum of mental life just below the threshold of ordinary consciousness and quite different than anything of which humanity had yet been aware. In discovering the means of inducing persons into this unconscious mental realm, he had initiated a revolution in the study of human nature.

Animal Magnetism Enters the American Mind

Charles Poyen had studied directly under Puysegur and thus confidently stood before his American audiences as a self-appointed Professor of Animal Magnetism. Like his mentor, Poyen believed that mesmerism's single most important discovery was that of the somnambulic, or mesmeric, state of consciousness. His public lectures consequently centered upon on actual demonstrations of the mesmeric state and all of its attendant phenomena. For these demonstrations Poyen depended in part upon the services of an assistant who was particularly adept at entering into the entranced state. He also made a practice of enlisting a few volunteers from the audience. He would explain to his subjects that his manual gestures heightened the activity of their body's own supply of animal magnetism to the point where their "external sensibilities" temporarily receded from consciousness, inducing a sleeplike condition. Poyen usually succeeded in putting about half of his volunteers into a trance that rendered them peculiarly unresponsive to their surroundings. Loud hand clapping and jars of ammonia passed under their noses failed to evoke even the slightest response. To all appearances, their minds had withdrawn from the physical world.

Staged exhibitions of mesmerism proved to be great theater. Crowds gathered to see their friends and relatives transformed before their eyes. The entertainment value of these demonstrations obviously outstripped their application to contemporary medical science. The frivolity that inevitably accompanied the demonstrations predictably alienated mesmerism from the established medical and scientific communities. Despite their unintended disservice to the science of animal magnetism, however, Poyen's lecture-demonstrations stimulated the public's imagination with novel "facts" about human nature—facts that, if not as "important to science" as Poyen had hoped, were soon thought to be more "glorious to human nature" than even he had dreamed.

Many of Poyen's volunteers came in hope of a medical cure. He obliged by making repeated "passes" with his hands in an effort to direct the flow of animal megnetism to the appropriate part of the body. A large proportion of those receiving this treatment awoke from their mesmeric sleep and, remembering nothing of what had transpired, claimed cure. Poyen's own account, in many cases supported by newspaper reports and letters to the editor, lists successful treatment of such disorders as rheumatism, nervousness, back troubles, and liver ailments.

Roughly ten percent of the subjects mesmerized by Poyen attained the "highest degree" of the magnetic condition. Their behavior went beyond the peculiar to the extraordinary. The onset of this stage in the mesmerizing process was marked by the formation of an especially intense rapport between the subject and the operator. A crucial ingredient of this rapport was the establishment of some nonverbal means of communication by which the subject telepathically received unspoken thoughts from the operator. Most subjects obligingly attributed this ability to a heightened receptivity to animal magnetism flowing into their system from without. Some actually reported feeling animal magnetism act upon their nervous systems; they felt prickly sensations running up and down their bodies. Others claimed up to "see" dazzling bright lights. Nor was it uncommon for subjects to perform feats of clairvoyance and extrasensory perception. They would locate lost objects, describe events transpiring in distant locales, or read the minds of persons in the audience. Upon returning to the waking state, they remembered little of their trance-bound experiences. It was as if they had temporarily existed in an altogether different realm. They knew only that they were now refreshed, energetic, and healed of their former ailments.

Word of Poyen's fantastic healing methods spread throughout New England. His 1837 treatise on the progress of animal magnetism in New England declares that "nineteenth months have elapsed since that period and already Animal Magnetism has sprung from a complete state of obscurity and neglect into general notice, and become the object of a lively interest throughout the country."[4] Newspapers began to take notice. The *Providence Journal* reported that more than one hundred cases of "Magnetic Somnambulism" had been reported in Rhode Island alone. Poyen's system was, according to one observer, fast becoming a "steady theme of interest in New England papers" and making "a deep impression upon some of the soundest and best balanced minds."[5] Poyen cited articles published in Rhode Island, Maine, and Connecticut supporting his contention that the science of animal magnetism had become a topic of conversation in all classes of society, especially—as he was quick to point out—among the learned and well-to-do.

It is not difficult to see why. Poyen was an able and evocative speaker. A former activist in the abolition movement and the author of a pamphlet detailing methods for promoting the spirit of Christianity, Poyen was merely shifting the focus of his evangelic zeal. He now played upon the growing public confidence in the ability of science to help initiate a utopian order. He prophesied that, when fully accepted by the "intelligent and fast progressing" American people, mesmerism was destined to make America "the most perfect nation on earth."[6] In this way Poyen not only launched mesmerism into the surging tide of American nationalism, but also associated it with the Jacksonian era's belief in the ultimate perfectibility of society through the progressive improvement of its individual citizens. By appealing to deeply rooted beliefs concerning the nation's manifest destiny, Poyen quite unwittingly hastened the identification of magnetic cures with other programs for personal rejuvenation then enjoying the enthusiastic support of various New England constituencies.

Poyen returned to his native France in 1839. His efforts had attracted a host of American followers eager to become spokesmen for the science of animal magnetism. According to one estimate, by 1843 more than two hundred "magnetic healers" were selling their services in the city of Boston alone.[7] Claims of successful cures accumulated. Among the conditions for which cure was claimed were rheumatism, loss of voice, stammering, nervousness, epilepsy, blindness, insomnia, St. Vitus's Dance, and the abuse of coffee, tea, and alcohol.[8] Growing public interest in this new medical science stimulated demand for books and pamphlets, and the American mesmerists willingly complied. Most of the dozens of works to appear over the next twenty years followed a common format: an introductory exhortation to open-mindedness; a short history of Mesmer's discovery; a catalogue of typical cures; documented reports of clairvoyance and telepathy; and last, but not least, a set of do-it-yourself instructions. One widely circulated pamphlet bore the appropriate title *The History and Philosophy of Animal Magnet-*

ism with Practical Instruction for the Exercise of this Power. Another included in its title the promise to explain "the system of manipulating adopted to produce ecstasy and somnambulism."[9]

A consensus about the scientific principles established by mesmeric phenomena soon emerged in the literature. Relying heavily on the writings of a British mesmerist named Chauncy Townshend, American investigators came to view the mesmerizing process as a technique for shifting mental activity along a continuum.[10] Each stage or point along the continuum was said to correspond to a successively deeper level of consciousness. The mesmerizing process dismantled the normal waking state of consciousness and induced individuals to shift their attention inward, away from events occurring in the physical world. As the sensations by the five physical senses gradually receded from consciousness, subjects entered the beginning stage or level of the mesmeric state. In this relatively light trance state subjects would appear totally insensible to any external sensation other than the voice of the mesmerist. This condition, which today we might call light hypnotic trance, facilitated the mesmerists' ability to use "passes" to stimulate the flow of animal magnetism within the body and to transmit willfully this spiritual fluid from his own body to that of the patient.

The most distinctive claim made by the mesmerists, however, was that the mind could be moved even farther along this continuum until, freed at last from its bondage to the five physical senses, it opened up to wholly new ranges of experience. As Townshend had put it, mesmerism brings about "the inaction of the external operations of the senses, coexistent with the life and activity of some inner source of feeling."[11] The mesmeric state had made possible a giant breakthrough in the scientific study of the human constitution. The mesmerists' experiments were hailed as having empirically proven that there exists "a sense in man which perceives the presences and qualities of things without the use of . . . the external organs of sense."[12] At this deeper level, the mind detects orders of sensation never monitored by the physical senses. The patient is now freed from dependence upon the mesmerists insofar as he or she is in a condition uniquely receptive to the unmediated inflow of animal magnetism. Healings occur spontaneously in this exalted state of consciousness. The activation of what Townshend called "the inner source of feeling" was also said to afford clairvoyance, prevoyance, telepathy, and intuitive knowledge of universal laws and structures.

These deeper realms of the mesmeric state had a decidedly mystical element. Subjects felt that they had transcended the mundane affairs of ordinary existence and entered into an intimate rapport with the cosmos. In the mesmeric state individuals temporarily felt endowed with omnipresent and omniscient powers. One investigator reported that mesmerized subjects "speak as if, to their consciousness, they had undergone an inward translation by which they had passed out of a material into a spiritual body. . . . The state into which a subject is brought by the mesmerizing process is a state in which the spirit predominates for the time being over the body."[13]

In mesmerism, the healing process was propaedeutic to spiritual discovery. The mesmerists' psychological continuum defined both an experiential path initiated by the healing process and a metaphysical hierarchy. That is, the "deeper" levels of consciousness achieved during the mesmerizing process put individuals into contact with qualitatively "higher" planes of reality. The mesmerists were thus articulating a healing philosophy that attributed the true cause of healing and personal growth to a distinctively metaphysical, as opposed to physiological or psychological, agent.

Linking Matter, Mind, and Spirit

The mesmerists were launching their medical theory into uncharted cultural waters. Their commitment to the causal agency of animal magnetism (often referred to as vital fluid, vital force, divine electricity, etc.) placed their theoretical endeavors equally far outside the spheres of Protestant orthodoxy and regular medicine. The problems inherent in uniting matter, mind, and spirit (i.e., animal magnetism) in a single cosmological system were at once its major liability and its major attraction. Thus, for example, a Midwestern physician and self-styled progressivist by the name of Joseph Buchanan embraced mesmerism as the key to a "neurological anthropology" that would encompass medical science, philosophy, and religion. To Buchanan, mesmerism was a hermeneutic principle unveiling humanity's psychosomatic unity. The doctrine of animal magnetism taught that "positive material existence and positive Spiritual existence—however far apart they stand, and however striking the contrast between their properties—are connected by these fine gradations . . . both are subject to the same great system of laws which each obeys in its own sphere."[14]

According to Buchanan, strictly physiological theories of human nature lead inevitably to materialism, pessimism, and atheism. He rejected contemporary medical science as an inadequate framework for describing the human constitution, "since it lacks the essential perspective of the modus operandi of life power."[15] Theological dogma, while recognizing humanity's higher, spiritual nature, was likewise unacceptable because it undermined the inductive spirit of any true anthropology. Mesmerism signaled an intellectual breakthrough of the highest magnitude. It forged the relative contributions of medical physiology and theology into a higher synthesis. At last Buchanan could confidently affirm that "the power of disembodied mind and intellectual manifestations . . . fall within the scope of the fundamental principles of the constitution of man, and spiritual mysteries, too, are beautifully elucidated by the complete correspondence, and mathematical harmony, between the spiritual and material laws of our being."[16]

Buchanan's interest in mesmerism's religious and metaphysical implications was widely shared. As early as February 1837 a letter addressed to the editor of the *Boston Recorder* had testified:

> George was converted from materialism to Christianity by the facts in Animal Magnetism developed under his [Poyen's] practice . . . it proves the power of mind over matter . . . informs our faith in the spirituality and immortality of our nature, and encourages us to renewed efforts to live up to its transcendent powers.[17]

A high school teacher wrote to the *Providence Journal* that "God and eternity are the only answer to these mysterious phenomena—these apparitions of the Infinity and the Unknown."[18] An early tract on the science of animal magnetism drew attention to the ways in which it casts "light on how we are constituted, how nearly we are related to, and how far we resemble our original . . . God who is a pure spiritual essence."[19] The same author went on to boast that mesmerism "shows that man has within him a spiritual nature, which can live without the body . . . in the eternal NOW of a future existence."[20]

Those who experienced the mesmerizing process described it as a decidedly numinous experience. Direct contact with the instreaming animal magnetic forces was thought to momentarily transform and elevate a person's being. A typical account relates that

> the whole moral and intellectual character becomes changed from the degraded condition of earth to the exalted intelligence of a spiritual state. The external senses are all suspended and the internal sense of spirit acts with its natural power as it will when entirely freed from the body after death. No person, we think, can listen to the revelations of a subject in a magnetic state, respecting the mysteries of our nature, and continue to doubt the existence of a never dying soul and the existence of a future or heavenly life.[21]

It is evident that Americans saw mesmerism as rejuvenating individuals in ways that went well beyond the healing of isolated complaints. They believed that the mesmerizing process helped them to reestablish inner harmony with the very source of physical and emotional well-being. In the mesmeric state, they learned that disease and even moral confusion were the unfortunate consequences of having fallen out of rapport with the invisible spiritual workings of the universe. Conversely, health and personal virtue were the innate rewards of living in accordance with the cosmic order. When patients returned from their ecstatic mental journey, they saw themselves as having been raised to a higher level of participation in the life force that "activates the whole frame of nature and produces all the phenomena that transpire throughout the realms of unbounded space."[22]

Mesmerism had no overt connections with institutional religion. It was nonetheless interpreted as a progressive variation of the religious revivals which had by then become the most effective institution in American religious life. Appearing in the mid-1830s, mesmerism— with other antebellum sectarian medical systems—was swept along in the wake of the religious enthusiasm unleashed by the outburst of revivalist activity that historians call the Second Great Awakening. Numerous revivalist preachers had disposed the popular religious climate toward an "alleviated Calvinism." In this view sin, rather than being thought to originate in humanity's inherent depravity, was instead understood as a function of ignorance, lack of self-discipline, or the result of faulty social institutions. Humankind's "lower nature" was therefore considered to be correctable through humanly initiated reforms. American religious thought during this period thus implicitly sanctioned experimental doctrines seeking the immediate and total renovation of humanity.

The period's most successful revivalist, Charles Grandison Finney, epitomized the changing outlook that made a healing philosophy such as mesmerism so religiously salient. Finney's *Lectures on Revivals,* published in 1835, outlined what he believed to be an empirically tested system of techniques designed to turn the conversion process into a lawful science. In Finney's estimation, a conversion "is not a miracle or dependent on a miracle in any sense . . . it consists entirely in the right exercise of the powers of nature."[23] By implication, religious experience can be humanly engineered. His was a scientific pneumatology predicated on the fact that "God had connected means with ends through all departments of his government—in nature and in grace."[24]

Finney was articulating a progressivist religiosity that matched the sense of expansion and discovery so predominant in the 1820s and 1830s. "New measures," he wrote, "are necessary from time to time to awaken attention and to bring the gospel to bear upon the public mind."[25] The "new measures" Finney had in mind were emotionally charged techniques whereby a charismatic individual might bring others to the point of ecstatic religious experience. According to Whitney Cross, the instrumental role of the revivalist in initiating the regenerative process established "the notion that special efforts under a person of particular talents would create a keener spirituality than the ordinary course of events could achieve."[26]

Historians have referred to the religious innovations set in motion by revivalists such as Finney the "burned-over" phenomenon. Between 1800 and 1850 religious fervor reached a stage of intensity that prompted many to compare the spread of experiential forms of religion with the ravaging flames of a forest fire. Termed "ultraism" by contemporaries, this peculiarly American religious creation has been described by Whitney Cross as a "combination of activities, personalities, and attitudes creating a condition of society which could foster experimental doctrines." Mormonism, Shakerism, Adventism, communitarianism, and millenarianism all emerged among those engaged in a protracted search for new ways of getting "the automatically operant Holy Spirit to descend and symbolize the start of the New Life."[27] Innovation was, as Cross documents, at the very heart of the period's religious quest:

> Popular demand, whetted by constant revivals, invited ever-more-novel departures. Finney's relatively sane popularizing tendency grew among his emulators into a mania. More than one itinerant may have claimed to be "recipient and channel of a sensible divine emanation, which he caused to pass from him by a perceptible influence, as electricity passes from one body to another."[28]

That mesmerism—more than any other nineteenth-century sectarian medical system—was able to stimulate Americans' metaphysical imaginations in "ever-more-novel" directions is not at all surprising. The mesmerists traveled from town to town on a New England circuit nearly identical to that of the revivalists. Some came to hear them out of sheer curiosity, but many came out of desperation. Those suffering from prolonged illness or from an inability to get a firmer hold on life were naturally vulnerable to the mesmerists' impassioned rhetoric concerning an invisible spiritual power with which they were in all likelihood out of touch. Like the revivalists, the mesmerists were preaching that individuals would continue to be plagued by sundry physical and emotional ills so long as they refused to open themselves up to a higher spiritual power. Mesmerism provided inwardly troubled individuals with an intense experience thought to restore them to harmony with unseen spiritual forces. The mesmeric state, no less than the emotion-laden conversion experience, gave powerful and convincing experiential grounds for the belief that humanity's lower nature can be utterly transformed and elevated when brought under the guiding influence of spirit.

Yet the mesmerists differed from the revivalists in at least one important respect. Far from reproaching individuals for challenging orthodox religious thinking, they encouraged them to do so. Mesmerism's doctrines tended to appeal to those whose religious sensibilities could not be constrained by scriptural piety and who yearned instead for a progressive, co-scientific religious outlook. As one advocate put it, mesmerism "not only disposes the mind to adopt religious principles, but also tends to free us from the errors of superstition by reducing to natural causes many phenomena."[29] Mesmerism's ability to help individuals fashion a way of viewing the world that was at once religiously and scientifically satisfying was greatly assisted by its unofficial alliance with yet another European-born metaphysical system—Swedenborgianism.

Swedenborgianism and American Harmonial Piety

The teachings of Emanuel Swedenborg (1688–1771) were not inherently germane to the unorthodox medical systems emerging in nineteenth-century American culture. It was their form and vision, not their substance, that gave them their poignancy. Their influence was much like that exerted by the writings of Teilhard de Chardin, which in the 1960s and 1970s helped pull together the religious and scientific interests of many involved in holistic and psychic healing. That is, they lent an ideological matrix to a wide array of activities and gave them a certain plausibility they might otherwise have lacked.

An eminent scientist in his day, Emanuel Swedenborg had made significant contributions in such varied fields as physics, astronomy, and anatomy before finally dedicating himself to the study of the secret mysteries contained in Christian scripture. By this time he had, however, moved beyond the inductive methods of laboratory science. Swedenborg claimed that, while in states of mystical reverie, he had been granted "perfect inspiration." He was not nearly as reticent as mystical seers are usually wont to be and wrote more than thirty volumes purporting to uncover the spiritual essence buried beneath the literal sense of Christian doctrine.

Swedenborg's writings carried with them a gnostic intrigue that appealed to those wishing to find a spirituality that went beyond routine church affairs. His revelations freed the essence of the Christian message from bondage to ancient scripture. Swedenborg was himself living proof that the truths of religion could be known directly through inward illumination. He explained that the universe is composed of several interpenetrating dimensions—physical, mental, spiritual, angelic, among others. Each of these dimensions is in some imperceptible way connected with every other. It follows, then, that complete harmony in any one dimension of life depends upon establishing rapport with other levels on the cosmic scale. All true progress proceeds according to influences received from above. The physical body achieves inner harmony by first becoming attuned with the mind, the mind through contact with the soul, the soul through connection with superior angelic beings, and so on up the spiritual hierarchy. Through diligent study and prolonged introspection, anyone might obtain the requisite gnosis to make contact with higher spiritual planes. The benefits to be obtained were numerous: spontaneous insight into cosmological secrets; conversations with angelic beings; intuitive understanding of the hidden spiritual meaning of scripture; and the instantaneous healing of both physical and emotional disorders.

Swedenborg's undaunted confidence in the soul's capacity for limitless development contrasted sharply with the Calvinists' insistence upon human depravity. His doctrines thus complemented and appealed to many of the sectarian groups that populated the nineteenth-century religious landscape.[30] Communitarians, Transcendentalists, spiritualists, and wealthy dilettantes such as Henry James, Sr., were alike encouraged by his expansive doctrines. John Humphrey Noyes of the Oneida Community perhaps best explained the reasons for Swedenborgianism's appeal to such diverse religious and intellectual dispositions:

> The Bible and revivals had made men hungry for something more than social reconstruction. Swedenborg's offer of a new heaven as well as a new earth, met the demand magnificently. . . . The scientific were charmed, because he was primarily a man of science, and seemed to reduce the world to scientific order. The mystics were charmed because he led them boldly into all the mysteries of intuition and invisible worlds.[31]

The key to Swedenborg's system, and the reason it was simultaneously scientific and metaphysical, was his doctrine of "correspondence." As Ralph Waldo Emerson explained it, the Swedenborgian notion of correspondence represents the "fine secret that little explains large, and large, little. . . . Nature iterates her means perpetually on successive planes." The doctrine of correspondence was not simply a method for understanding the relationship between physical laws and their metaphysical correlates; it was also, and far more importantly, a doctrine of causality. When inner harmony or resonance between realms is established, energy and guiding wisdom from the higher plane can flow into and causally influence the lower plane. Swedenborg was proclaiming that men and women are inwardly constructed so as to be able to receive "psychic influx" from higher planes of reality.

Swedenborg's doctrines gave the nineteenth century its most vivid articulation of a form of piety in which "harmony," rather than contrition or repentance, is the sine qua non of the regenerated life. In historian Sydney Ahlstrom's words, harmonial religion "encompasses those forms of piety and belief in which spiritual composure, physical health, and even economic well-being are understood to flow from a person's rapport with the cosmos."[32] The deity—here conceived as an indwelling cosmic force—is approached not via petitionary prayer or acts of worship, but through a series of inner adjustments. As the barriers separating the finite personality from the "divinity which flows through all things" are gradually penetrated, vitality spontaneously manifests itself in every dimension of personal life.

The harmonial piety so eloquently depicted in both Mesmer's and Swedenborg's writings gave practitioners of unorthodox medicine a metaphysical rationale for the efficacy of their various therapeutic practices. Whitney Cross has aptly summarized the reasons mesmerism and Swedenborgianism established themselves in the American metaphysical imagination to a greater extent than their doctrines probably warranted:

> Before they [nineteenth century Americans] ever heard of Mesmer or Swedenborg, they expected new scientific discoveries to confirm the broad patterns of revelation as they understood them: to give mankind ever-more-revealing glimpses of the preordained divine plan for humanity and the universe. They expected all such knowledge would demonstrate the superiority of ideal over physical or material force, and that it would prove the relationship of man's soul to the infinite spiritual power.[33]

The Swedenborgian world view depicted interaction between the physical and metaphysical orders of reality as a lawful occurrence.

It only remained for adherents of various medical and religious sects to elaborate the means whereby this influx takes place. Thus it was that Swedenborg's American followers gave scrupulous attention to every word of his essay "On the Intercourse Between the Soul and the Body Which is Supposed to Take Place Either by Physical Influx or by Pre-Established Harmony." Most seemed to favor the idea of physical influx. For example, Emerson spoke for the Transcendentalist movement when he concluded that the mind is "an organ recipient of life from God."[34] An 1838 edition of American Swedenborgianism's principal journal, the *New Jerusalem Magazine,* clumsily suggested that "life from God flows-in into man through the soul, and through this into the mind, that is, into the reflections and thoughts of the mind, and from these into the sense, speech and actions of the body."[35]

The combined influence of mesmerism and Swedenborgianism in providing Americans with a way to attribute mental and physical events to metaphysical causes can be seen in Dr. George Bush's 1847 volume, *Mesmer and Swedenborg.* Claiming to have studied most of the two thousand works already published on the subject of animal magnetism, Bush concluded that "when taken together, the investigations of the mesmeric state point to an entirely new class of facts in psychology." And, more to the point, this new class of facts gave empirical support to the Swedenborgian system by proving "the grand principle that man is a spirit as to his interiors and that his spiritual nature in the body often manifests itself according to the laws which govern it out of the body."[36] Bush further reasoned that "the indubitable facts of mesmerism are affording to the many senses of man a demonstration which cannot be resisted, that Swedenborg has told the truth of the other life."[37]

The reports of entranced subjects could safely be considered descriptions of a higher metaphysical plane. Bush himself experimented with mesmerism and found clear evidence of the existence of extrasensory perception, telepathy, and clairvoyance. Many of his subjects reported experiencing periods of mystical rapture as they came under the influence of this numinous state of consciousness. Some even told of seeing "mental atmospheres" composed of ultrafine rays of light surrounding people's heads. Surely animal magnetism must be the medium of psychic influx postulated by Swedenborgian metaphysics all along.

The fusion of mesmerism and Swedenborgianism enabled Bush to link matter, mind, and spirit. The study of the mesmeric state and its revelation of our inward capacity to receive psychic influxes, he claimed, added new scientific information concerning the human constitution "just at that point where anthropology weds itself to Theology."[38] He concluded that "On the whole it must, we think, be admitted that the phenomena of mesmerism taken in conjunction with the developments of Swedenborg, open a new chapter in the philosophy of mind and in man's relations to a higher sphere."[39] And it was precisely these developments that would inject a metaphysically charged vocabulary into the lexicons of many unorthodox American medical philosophies.

The Metaphysical Connection

The contributions of mesmerism and Swedenborgianism to nineteenth-century religious and medical sectarianism go well beyond the measure of their formal memberships; shared reading lists, parallel lecture circuits, joint memberships, and historical patterns of cross-fertilization are all greater indices of sustained traditions in unchurched religious thought. Thus, while relatively few Americans proclaimed exclusive allegiance to these movements, thousands found in them the intellectual categories to identify a "spiritual" or "metaphysical" dimension to life.

Of the unorthodox healing systems we have examined thus far, Thomsonianism was the least influenced by the "metaphysical connection" that mesmerism and Swedenborgianism forged between physical healing and higher spiritual agencies. Thomsonianism presented a clear-cut reliance on the pharmaceutical properties of natural herbs and educed little in the way of a novel world view from its therapeutic activities. Graham's Christian-based dietary reforms were also originally sealed off from contact with heretical cosmologies. Graham was a subscriber to the "ascetic" model of Protestant thought, which posits a wide gulf between the realm of the supernatural and the earthly sphere that is optimally to be controlled by the disciplined human will. Ellen White was likewise a hawkish defender of Protestant orthodoxy and its suspicion of cosmologies that picture the natural order of things as susceptible to invisible influences. Like Graham, she was heir to the ascetic style of American Protestantism and grafted all healing concepts onto a fierce biblical fundamentalism. She wrote at length about the "danger in speculative knowledge" and charged that "One of the greatest evils that attends the quest for knowledge, the investigation of science, is the disposition to exalt human reasoning above its true value and its proper sphere. Many attempt to judge of the Creator and His works by their own imperfect knowledge of science."[40] Especially to be vigilant against were contemporary pantheistic conceptions which "if followed to their logical conclusions sweep away the whole Christian economy."[41]

As it turned out, some of Ellen White's followers strayed from the orthodox tenets of Seventh Day Adventist faith. The San in Battle Creek drew a great many of the period's metaphysical seekers such as mind-curists and sundry spiritualists. They came to the San despite Ellen White's biblical theology, and their influence apparently turned some individuals in new intellectual directions. John Harvey Kellogg himself was sufficiently swayed by the pantheistic cosmologies circulating at the San to find in them a way to reconcile his religious beliefs with scientific evolutionary thought. He eventually went so far as to identify instinct as the voice of God and to write that

God is *in* nature. . . . God actually entered into the product of his creative skill, so that it might not only outwardly reflect the divine conception, but that it might think divinely, and act divinely.[42]

Kellogg's insinuation that matter and spirit might be interpenetrating dimensions of a single lawful reality was a heresy that earned him disfranchisement from the Adventist church. Yet his slight leaning toward harmonial piety was mild when compared to the ways in which C. W. Post assimilated contemporary metaphysical notions into the dietary movement. Post proclaimed that "the white light of the higher intelligence . . . psychic sense, Soul, Life, or Divine Mind, whichever term seems best," is the true source of human well-being.[43] Diet is at best a secondary means of inducing the psychic influences from our higher self to enter into and exert their life-giving properties on our conscious life. Strongly influenced by the mind-cure movement and its reliance upon mesmerist psychology, Post taught that "the real man . . . lies upon a plane above the plane of matter" and that to achieve vibrant living we must learn to make inner contact with this higher dimension of selfhood.[44]

Hydropathy was far more amenable to metaphysical alliances. In 1840, Dr. Russell Trall began to formally instruct new hydropathic practitioners on hydropathy's connections with mesmerism. Among the original faculty in Trall's hydropathic college was Lorenzo Fowler, who constituted something of a living symbol of eclectic thought. Under Fowler's tutelage, practitioners of hydropathy learned to view their healing art as intricately interwoven with such causes as temperance, phrenology, and mesmerism. Another interesting spokesperson for the cause, Mary Gove Nichols, first connected hydropathy with Grahamism before adding mesmerism, free love, and spiritualism. It is, then, not at all surprising that a journal by the name of *The Magnetic and Cold Water Guide* would emerge and include the following testimonial by an Ohio physician:

> Physiology, Phrenology, and Magnetism are the keys that are unlocking the great mysteries of nature and mind, and letting us in, as it were, to the inner temple, where the sunbeams of light and truth are filling the minds and understandings of all the truly devout worshippers of the Eternal principles which govern all things.[45]

Homoeopathy provides the clearest example of the metaphysical dimensions that mesmerism and Swedenborgianism infused into nineteenth-century healing movements. Hahnemann himself had advocated mesmerism as a means of balancing the vital power throughout the body and as a clue to the lawful interconnection between things physical and spiritual. The physical manipulations and mental focusing taught by the mesmerists revealed to him how vital power could flow from a spiritual source into matter and vice versa. Mesmerism afforded homoeopaths a metaphor or conceptual model for affirming a lawful relationship between matter and spirit. That this link proved to be the fundamental attraction of both movements is indicated by John Gray's early history of homoeopathy in the United States. Recollecting the fascinating lessons he had learned from Hans Gram, Gray specifically mentioned Gram's interest in mesmerism and kindred systems and remarked that

In each of these directions Gram led the way to a wider and deeper knowledge of the relations between soul and body, the human and divine, the transitory and the permanent, than can be entertained by purely materialistic researchers.[46]

Homoeopathy had a similar affinity with Swedenborgianism. As Joseph Kett has pointed out, this affinity is to be explained not so much by the number of homoeopaths who formally embraced Swedenborgianism as by the similarity of their visions of an ordered and predictable universe in which matter and spirit were perfectly synthesized.[47] Thus, Transcendentalists such as Theodore Parker, Bronson Alcott, and Elizabeth Palmer Peabody saw homoeopathy as a vital aspect of their Swedenborgian-inspired mystical world view. Likewise, prominent homoeopaths found in Transcendentalism and Swedenborgianism ready-made systems for articulating their intuitive sense of the physical body as but an outer covering of some inner spiritual energy. Dr. William Wesselhoeft and Dr. William Henry Halcombe were among those homoeopathic physicians who found in Swedenborgianism the crucial link between their scientific commitments and their faith in the primacy of spirit over matter.

A final observation is necessary concerning the way in which mesmerism and Swedenborgianism helped provide metaphysical dimensions for both nineteenth-century healing systems and their twentieth-century legatees. Both of these metaphysical movements were prime factors in the emergence of spiritualism as a distinct tradition of unchurched American religiosity. The gaudy seances and shoddy deceptions for which spiritualism is best known have tended to obscure the aesthetic and harmonial spirituality that permeated the movement in its early stages. Andrew Jackson Davis, the leading spokesperson for spiritualism in the nineteenth century, was an apprentice cobbler in 1843 when the famed mesmerist J. Stanley Grimes passed through his hometown of Poughkeepsie. During a lecture-demonstration, Grimes randomly selected the young Davis for a volunteer subject. Davis turned out to be an adept trance subject and was soon performing such standard mesmeric feats as reading from books while blindfolded and reporting clairvoyant travels to distant locales. After several months of repeated journeys into the inner recesses of his mind, Davis suddenly realized that the self-induced mesmeric trance state was one in which "mighty and sacred truths spontaneously gushed up from the depths of my spirit."[48] Davis insisted moreover that these truths were being communicated to him by departed spirits. Not the least of these discarnate entities was Emanuel Swedenborg, who from his vantage point in heaven now had even more lessons to teach.

Davis soon enticed friends to record the metaphysical lessons delivered through him by his contacts in the spirit world. In his major work, *The Harmonial Philosophy,* Davis and his spirit tutors wedded mesmerist psychology to Swedenborgian metaphysics. The text explains that human consciousness is arranged along a continuum, ranging from "rudimental" sensory awareness all the way to the "spiritual state," in which we may experience "a high reality, an expansion of the mind's energies, a subjugation of material to spiritual, of body to soul."[49] Healing became for Davis, as for other prominent "trance channelers" even to this day, a natural extension of a harmonial philosophy centered upon the practical benefits to be derived from becoming attuned to a higher reality. The healing practices of most early spiritualists were almost wholly imitations of those of their mesmeric predecessors and colleagues. Explaining illness as the consequence of an obstruction of the free flow of "spirit" or "vital fluid" in the body, they emphasized the use of hand gestures, or passes, to restore harmony to the body's system. Of central importance is the fact that the founders of chiropractic medicine, D. D. Palmer, and of osteopathic medicine, Andrew Taylor Still, picked up the root metaphors and fundamental techniques of their medical philosophies from mesmerist and spiritualist sources.

Over time, spiritualism gravitated toward the staging of showy seances that offered a paying clientele ostensible evidence that their departed loved ones still "existed" in another realm. As a consequence, those interested in the reconciliation of religion and science shifted their energies elsewhere. In his *In Search of White Crows,* R. Laurence Moore shows how twentieth-century interest in parapsychology and psychical research grew directly out of the same cultural forces that had earlier given rise to spiritualism.[50] The important point is that to this day mesmerist and Swedenborgian metaphysical teachings still abound in the writings and activities of those involved with parapsychology. New Age trance channeling, Eckankar, the Association for Research and Enlightenment, crystal healing, and attempts to link Eastern meditational practices with contemporary American concerns all draw upon a similar cluster of metaphysical conceptions. As we shall see, American culture continues to find metaphysical connections among philosophies of quite diverse origins; the motivating impulse for much of this metaphysical eclecticism appears to be the ongoing interest in unorthodox healing practices.

The Legacy of Mind Over Matter

During his proselytizing tour through New England in 1838, the mesmerist Charles Poyen stopped in Belfast, Maine. Attending his lecture-demonstrations was a young clockmaker who was destined to become the most successful "mental healer" in the United States. Phineas Parkhurst Quimby (1802–1866) was inspired by Poyen's astonishing exhibition to begin investigating the science of animal magnetism on his own. With the help of a particularly adept trance subject by the name of Lucius Burkmar, Quimby soon established his own healing practice. Quimby would put Lucius into the mesmeric state and direct him to use his clairvoyant powers to diagnose a person's illness and then to prescribe an appropriate medicinal remedy. On some occasions Quimby dispensed with Lucius's assistance and instead made the classic mesmeric passes over his patients' heads in an effort to recharge their systems directly with animal magnetism. Whichever the method, Quimby believed that the resultant healings were "the result of animal magnetism, and that electricity had more or less to do with it."[51]

With the passage of time Quimby became increasingly skeptical that animal magnetism alone could be responsible for all of his therapeutic successes. It dawned upon him that Lucius might not be diagnosing the patients' ailments at all, but that, more likely, his assistant was merely using his deep rapport with patients to learn what they already believed to be the cause of their troubles. His "accurate" diagnoses so utterly astonished patients that they put their full confidence in his curative powers. Thus, the herbal remedies Lucius prescribed worked more upon the patients' beliefs about their problems than upon the actual physical disorder. Most of the remedies were innocuous substances that proved equally effective on a number of ailments. On one occasion Quimby actually substituted a less expensive substance for the costly one Lucius had suggested—and the patient recovered just the same!

Many mesmerists had deduced that the patients' beliefs and expectations were at least partially responsible for their rapid recoveries. But Quimby arrived at the more radical conclusion that the illnesses were caused by their ideas or beliefs in the first place. He declared that our minds are the sum total of our beliefs, and that if a person is "deceived into a belief that he has, or is liable to have a disease, the belief is catching and the effects follow from it."[52] Quimby was thus forging a connection between mesmerism-born metaphysical notions of healing and modern psychosomatic medicine. He clarified this connection by specifically identifying faulty ideas—not magnetic fluids—as the root cause of both physical and emotional disorders. In Quimby's words, "all sickness is in the mind or belief . . . to cure the disease is to correct the error, destroy the cause, and the effect will cease."[53]

It is important to note that Quimby's theory of illness was not the mentalistic or purely psychosomatic explanation for which many of his interpreters have mistaken it. He saw the patient's belief or attitude as only an intervening variable. Quimby held that the real source of health was the magnetic fluid, or vital force, flowing into the human nervous system through some deeper level of the mind. Beliefs function like control valves or floodgates—they serve to connect or disconnect the conscious mind and its unconscious depths. "Disease," Quimby insisted, "is the effect of a wrong direction given to the mind."[54] When persons identify themselves solely in terms of outer conditions, they place their minds at the mercy of noxious external stimuli; and as long as the mind is reacting to sensations received through the physical senses, it is unreceptive to the inflow of magnetic forces and therefore depletes the body of its proactive energies. The result is disease.

According to Quimby, health can be achieved only by permanently banishing self-defeating attitudes. It follows that "the theory of correcting diseases is the introduction to life."[55] Quimby thought that if he could but illustrate to his patients "that a man's happiness is in his belief, and his misery is the effect of his belief, then I have done what never has been done before. Establish this and man rises to a higher state of wisdom, not of this world, but of that World of Science . . . the Wisdom of Science is Life eternal."[56]

Quimby's gospel of mind cure had a beautiful simplicity. Right beliefs channel health, happiness, and wisdom out of the cosmic ethers and into the individual's psyche. If we can control our beliefs, we will control the shunting valve that connects us to psychological and physiological vitality. Quimby counseled that the secret to happiness of every kind is to identify oneself in terms of internal reference points. The human nervous system cannot rely solely upon the capricious messages supplied by the physical senses without eventually becoming embroiled in fear, worry, and finally disease. Human misery, then, is the necessary consequence of allowing other persons and outer events to supply us with our sense of self-worth. In Quimby's words, "disease is something made by belief or forced upon us by our parents or public opinion. . . . Now if you can face the error and argue it down you can cure the sick."[57]

Quimby's theories amounted to a translation of the metaphysical categories of mesmerism and Swedenborgianism into a practical philosophy of life. "There are," he declared, "two sciences, one of this world, and the other of a spiritual world, or two effects produced upon the mind by two directions."[58] Quimby seemed to be saying that each of us has a higher and lower nature and that it is within our own power to determine which of the two predominates. He taught his patients that by making appropriate adjustments in the microcosm of the psyche they could establish rapport with the very powers that activate the macrocosm.

Quimby's teachings lived on through the work of his patients. One, Mary Baker Eddy, founded one of the five largest religious denominations to have emerged in American history (Ellen White founded one of the other five). She arrived at Quimby's doorstep in 1862 a helpless physical and mental wreck. The mesmeric healer cured her afflicted body and, in the process, filled her receptive mind with new ideas. Once healed, Mrs. Eddy resolved that she, too, would take up a career in mental healing. Her first public lecture, "P. P. Quimby's Spiritual Science Healing Disease as Opposed to Deism or Rochester-Rapping Spiritualism," made her the first spokeswoman for the philosophy of mind cure. Soon after Quimby's death she transformed the lessons she had learned from him into the foundations of her own Christian Science. Until her death in 1910, Mrs. Eddy worked incessantly at giving literary, theological, and institutional embodiment to the science of mental healing.[59] Her Church of Christ, Scientist, was self-consciously founded as "a church designed to commemorate the word and works of our Master, which should reinstate primitive Christianity and its lost element of healing."[60] Mary Baker Eddy's principal text, *Science and Health with Key to the Scriptures,* made clear her intention to shift the science of healing away from mesmerist categories to ones that bore more resemblance to Christian scripture. In brief, her Christian Science theology asserts that God created all that is, and all that God created is good. Mrs. Eddy followed this line of reasoning to the conclusion that such things as sickness, pain, or evil possess no positive ontological status. They are only the delusional appearances created by an erring, mortal mind. The healing ministry in which Christian Scientists engage is dedicated to the task of assisting individuals in keeping their minds and mental attitudes centered solely on the higher laws of God's spiritual presence. To help people overcome the errors of their mortal minds, Mrs. Eddy established churches nationwide and certified a small army of Christian Science "practitioners" to assist sick individuals by teaching them how they might elevate their mental and emotional lives to a higher spiritual level. Although no formal membership statistics are available, Mrs. Eddy claimed that *Science and Health* had sold more than 400,000 copies by 1900, and the Christian Science denomination is now entering its second century of witnessing to the conviction that the mind has access to a higher spiritual reality that is the source of health and wholeness.

The healing activities of institutionalized religion lie beyond the scope of this book. However, the fact that two of America's five native-born religious traditions emerged with explicit connections to unorthodox healing movements underscores how fully religion and medicine are linked in our cultural heritage. We might also note that the other three native-born religious groups, the Mormons, Jehovah's Witnesses, and various Pentecostal groups, have all had strong interest in religious healing (although, like the Seventh Day Adventists, their healing interests have been overtly connected with biblical rather than metaphysical conceptions of causality).

After Mary Baker Eddy, the second most notable of Quimby's students was a former Methodist Episcopal minister and ardent Swedenborgian by the name of Warren Felt Evans.[61] Evans followed in Quimby's footsteps by opening a healing office of his own in Boston, where for the next twenty years he spearheaded what is variously referred to as the Mind Cure or New Thought movement. Evans, a gifted healer in the Quimby tradition, brought mind-cure ideas to the attention of the nation's large middle class with his pen. By 1875 his *The Mental Cure* (1869) and *Mental Medicine* (1871) had gone through seven and fifteen editions, respectively. In these and numerous other books, with titles like *The Divine Law of Cure, Esoteric Christianity and Mental Therapeutics,* and *The Primitive Mind Cure,* Evans expounded the doctrine that through contact with the deepest recesses of our unconscious minds we can avail ourselves of a divine healing energy.

Evans proclaimed that through their discovery of the higher reaches of the human psyche, the mesmerists and Swedenborgians had recovered the kerygma of the early Christian church. The attainment of mental states in which we are receptive to subtle spiritual influences was for Evans a sacramental experience. He wrote that by learning to cultivate meditative states of consciousness we can all learn to "come into direct and immediate communication with God [so] that His creative energy shall be added to our cognitive and volitional power."[62]

Another New Thought author, Ralph Waldo Trine, provided perhaps the clearest exposition of the movement's harmonial piety:

> In just the degree that we come into a conscious realization of our oneness with the Infinite Life, and open ourselves to the Divine inflow, do we actualize in ourselves the qualities and powers of the Infinite Life, do we make ourselves channels through which the Infinite Intelligence and Power can work. In just the degree in which you realize your oneness with the Infinite Spirit, you will exchange dis-ease for ease, inharmony for harmony, suffering and pain for abounding health and strength.[63]

"As a man thinketh, so is he" was no mere aphorism for the New Thoughters; it was metaphysical law. Mesmerism and Swedenborgianism had laid down the foundations for a cosmology in which mind controls our access to higher causal energies. Thus, Trine could assert that "in the degree that thought is spiritualized, does it become more subtle and powerful . . . this spiritualizing is in accordance with law and is within the power of all."[64] For the New

Thoughters, then, a very real metaphysical power was envisioned when they boasted of "the power of positive thinking." They taught that preoccupation with outer conditions blinds the individual to the higher causal principles governing the universe. It is far more beneficial to spend a few moments alone in silence for the purpose of activating the powers available through the unconscious mind. For just beneath the threshold of waking consciousness resides what Evans termed "a battery and reservoir of magnetic life and vital force" ready to replenish the exhausted nervous system and restore us to a condition of vitality.[65]

The harmonial philosophy exemplified by New Thought has become a ubiquitous element of twentieth-century American religious thought. As Sydney Ahlstrom notes, it is "a vast and highly diffuse religious impulse that cuts across all the normal lines of religious division. It often shapes the inner meaning of the church life to which people formally commit themselves."[66] To appreciate the popular extension of this metaphysical vision, which so readily links contemplative spirituality with schemes for achieving personal success or self-actualization, one need only turn to Norman Vincent Peale's phenomenally popular *The Power of Positive Thinking*. Peale has infected millions of readers with the patently harmonial conviction that "by channeling spiritual power through your thoughts . . . you can have peace of mind, improved health, and a never-ceasing flow of energy."[67]

The concept of a metaphysical linking of the individual's inner mind with a higher cosmic source of spiritual power pointedly addressed the societal dis-ease that accompanied the dawn of modern American culture. Urbanization, industrialization, immigration, and the splintering of any theological consensus around which national life might revolve all jarred the American psyche loose from traditional sources of stability. Whether psychosomatic illness actually increased around the turn of the century is difficult to ascertain. It is, however, safe to assume that Americans' awareness of the mental/cultural origin of so many of their ailments increased dramatically. The often cited writings of Dr. George Beard, a New York neurologist, provide a helpful insight into Americans' earliest efforts to make sense of a world that put increasing strain on our inner or psychological life. Writing in the 1870s and 1880s, Beard was convinced that the rapid rate of change in modern life was robbing individuals of their mental energy.[68] Railway travel, the periodical press, the telegraph, religious liberties, the intellectual activity of women, sectarian religious movements, loud noises, the specialization of labor, social conventions that suppress emotional expression, and the chaotic flux of new ideas were all sapping Americans of their mental strength. The human brain just wasn't equipped to handle so much stimuli and, as a consequence, the American populace had become beset by "nervous exhaustion." The symptoms were many: headaches, insomnia, inebriety, cerebral irritation, emotional distress, premature baldness, hopelessness, fear of being alone, fear of society, fear of fears.

Beard spoke for the entire regular medical profession when he admitted that there was little or nothing physicians could do for these problems. The materialistic basis of his own medical theory led him to the conclusion that any substantial improvements would have to await the future evolutionary development of sturdier neural equipment. In the meantime his contemporaries would just have to learn to cope with diminished inner resources.

Beard's fatalistic prognosis for nervous exhaustion implicitly indicted American culture for an inefficient channeling of the human energies at its disposal. The high incidence of stress-related illness attested to the rigorous demands which a pluralistic society places upon a person's efforts to be inner-directed. Individuals were constantly being forced back upon their own inner resources. Confronted with difficult choices in nearly every area of their lives, many at last fell prey to their own indecisiveness. Their illnesses testified to an agonizing paradox: afflictor and afflicted were one and the same. Outer symptoms mirrored inner conflict. Worse yet, there appeared no way out of the syndrome of nervous exhaustion. Diligence and redoubled effort could only overtax, not replenish, precious human energies. By definition, the debilitated individual lacked the inner resources to bring about a full recovery. Help would have to come from without. But where were these extrapersonal energies to be found? Who would point the way?

The churches were of little help. Intellectual secularism and social pluralism combined to undermine the single most effective healing ritual at their disposal—revivalism. Revivalism had flourished in a comparatively unsophisticated social and intellectual environment. Inner renewal from contact with the Holy Spirit was thought to lead automatically to one or another version of Calvinist piety and membership in a local church. But in the late 1800s Protestant churches lacked the social resources to carry out their former role to bring about personal and cultural renewal. Many suddenly found themselves occupying a "downtown" location. Their memberships were no longer isomorphic with geographical districts. The churches' responsibilities for ministering to the needs of an urban population were as amorphous as their demographic boundaries. Over what domain were the churches to exercise their guidance? To whom should their members direct mutual edification or fraternal correction?

Culture lag had set into church life, creating what intellectual historian Arthur Schlesinger deems "the critical period" in American religious thought. Church ministry had failed "to adjust to the unprecedented conditions created by rapid urban and industrial growth. American Protestantism, the product of a rural, middle class society, faced a range of problems for which it had neither the experience nor the aptitude."[69] The nation's "official" religion, like its "official" medicine, had little to offer those afflicted with nervous exhaustion. A cultural niche was thus opening up in which metaphysically inclined medical systems might flourish, and flourish they have.

The metaphysical healing vision spawned by mesmerism and Swedenborgianism continues even to this day to provide the underlying metaphors and imagery for many alternative healing philosophies. Holistic healing groups, psychic healers, New Age trance channelers, Therapeutic Touch practitioners, and even Alcoholics Anonymous have drawn heavily upon this legacy of belief in the mind's capacity to draw upon higher healing energies. And, too, belief in the power of physical manipulation to realign the body with a higher spiritual power provided the founding vision of two of the most popular of the twentieth century's healing systems, the chiropractic and osteopathic systems of medicine.

4

At the Fringes of Orthodoxy: Chiropractic and Osteopathic Medicine

IN THE LATE nineteenth and early twentieth century, regular physicians redoubled their efforts to rid the medical scene of their irregular counterparts. The regular physicians demarcated the boundaries of orthodoxy through such activities as forming state and local medical societies, lobbying the legislature to protect public well-being through rigid licensing regulations, and—above all—continuing to pressure hospitals to restrict their internships and staff to graduates of recognized medical schools. The New York Academy of Medicine, for example, explicitly excluded from eligibility "all homoeopathic, hydropathic, chronothermal and botanic physicians, and also all mesmeric and clairvoyant pretenders to the healing art, and all others who at any time or on any pretext claim peculiar merits for their mixed practices not founded on the best system of physiology and pathology, as taught in the best schools in Europe and America."[1] The American Medical Association gradually rose above the state and local societies to become the dominant professional organization for orthodox physicians. Henceforth, all other contenders for a share of the nation's medical market would find their unorthodox status clearly and repeatedly defined for them by a formidable adversary.

At the turn of the century, however, the AMA was to find at its fringes two worthy opponents. These unorthodox systems were both rooted in a mesmerism-based metaphysical view of the ulti-

66

mate cause of healing, and both were to endure in the face of the orthodox system's repeated efforts to banish them from cultural respectability. Chiropractic and osteopathic medicine are for this reason paradigmatic examples of the paths metaphysical healing systems would have to take in the twentieth century if they insisted upon openly competing with the AMA for access to the nation's medical marketplace. Although remarkably similar in their founding ideologies, chiropractic and osteopathic medicine subsequently steered quite different courses in their quests for professional recognition and broad-based public support. Each succeeded in carving out for itself a viable niche in the American medical environment. There are currently over 19,000 chiropractic physicians in the United States treating at least three million patients annually.[2] Osteopathic physicians number more than 24,000 and treat twenty million persons per year.[3] And thus, although the founding philosophies of both chiropractic and osteopathy are at considerable variance with medical orthodoxy, they have fully established themselves in the wider institutional context of American health care.

Unlike the twentieth-century healing movements we will study in Chapter 5, both chiropractic and osteopathic medicine have muted their metaphysical overtones. This is particularly true of osteopathy, which in its eagerness for peaceful coexistence with the AMA was fairly quick to drop its mesmeric origins and metaphors. Osteopathy was rewarded with easier access to the hospital and insurance industries, whose doors are well guarded by the accredited sentinels of orthodoxy. Chiropractic medicine has also made considerable progress toward public esteem and full eligibility for government-funded health care programs. It, too, has in large part abandoned metaphysical terminology in favor of increasingly precise specifications of the physical causes of musculoskeletal distress. Importantly, however, both chiropractic and osteopathy have continued to utilize a healing vocabulary of harmonial metaphors (albeit reduced from the level of metaphysical abstraction to their lowest common denominator of physiology). And both have continued to differentiate their theoretical orientation from regular medicine by affirming the innate sanctity of the human body as well as the therapeutic importance of the "laying on of hands." Chiropractic and osteopathic medicine have thus in many ways attenuated, but without fully severing connections with, enduring elements in

America's unchurched religious thought. Even into the 1970s and 1980s chiropractic and osteopathy in varying degrees have continued to draw upon the harmonial metaphors when expressing their theoretical foundations. As one recent popular tract announces, chiropractic is a New Age philosophy that recognizes "that the universe is perfectly organized and that, as extensions of that universal intelligence, we also have an unlimited potential for life and health. . . . In order to express more of your potential, you need only keep the channels of that expression open."[4]

The Healing Hands of D. D. Palmer

Born in 1845 to a shoemaker and his wife, Daniel David Palmer set out, at the age of twenty, to seek his fortune in the burgeoning Midwest. After brief stops in Illinois, Daniel appeared to be settling into a stable life as a grocer and fish peddler in the town of What Cheer, Iowa. His interest in the philosophical and metaphysical issues of his day, however, destined him for a life quite different from that of the typical Midwestern grocer. Almost wholly lacking in formal education, Palmer is nevertheless reputed to have read widely and seemed particularly drawn to what one biographer refers to as "radical ideas." One of these radical ideas was spiritualism. Daniel associated with a good many spiritualists from whom he picked up a number of metaphysical terms and metaphors for humanity's participation in a higher order of things. Even well into his chiropractic days he simply took for granted that "we are surrounded with an aura" and that we are intimately connected with nonmaterial forces and energies.[5] One of Palmer's spiritualist acquaintances is said to have told him of a vision of a sign that read "Dr. Palmer" and that Daniel would one day become a well-known lecturer on a "revolutionary" method of healing disease.[6]

A major step toward the fulfillment of this prophecy occurred when Daniel David Palmer, by this time styling himself D. D. Palmer, crossed paths with a mesmeric healer by the name of Paul Carter. Carter was operating a successful magnetic healing practice in nearby Ottumwa, Iowa, and gradually tutored the inquisitive grocer in the art of imparting magnetic healing energy to diseased persons. Carter was one of many Midwestern magnetic healers who went beyond the mesmeric technique of making passes with their hands over the patients' heads and bodies and actually rubbed or even slapped their bodies. He is reported to have told Palmer that "by rubbing and slapping the entire body of a sick patient, I imparted my magnetism. It cured the sick."[7] Palmer's interest was aroused and he procured several books on mesmeric healing that were to remain central texts in his personal library for the rest of his life.[8] He soon after remembered an incident from his past in which he had cured his mother of intense pain by simply placing his hand on her head. He took this not only as confirmation of Carter's theories but also as proof that he, too, was especially gifted at the art of harnessing and transmitting magnetic healing energy.

D. D. first opened his own magnetic healing office in Burlington, Iowa, and subsequently moved to Davenport. He immediately had a sign painted for the outside of his office which read "Dr. Palmer." For the next nine years he engaged in what appears to have been a thriving healing practice. Seeing as many as ninety patients in a day, he was credited with curing tumors, cancers, rheumatism, neuralgia, sprains, heart disease, stomach ailments, and "female weakness."[9] He later added a "magnetic infirmary" that provided room and board to patients who required prolonged magnetic treatments. His income steadily increased until he was earning over $4,000 per year on the average from his medical practice.

Magnetic healing not only proved lucrative for D. D. Palmer, but also fit nicely with his particular religiosity. D. D. had always been an avid reader of the Bible, books on spiritualism, and literature covering a wide variety of esoteric philosophies. He consequently found in magnetic healing a perfect vehicle for advancing his own theory of humanity's moral and spiritual constitution. Magnetic healing provided him with a means of developing (or at least convincing others that he possessed) an array of intuitive or nonrational sensibilities. There are numerous anecdotes of Palmer displaying a remarkable capacity for precognition and clairvoyance. There are also reports that, much in the manner of other successful mesmeric healers such as P. P. Quimby, he was able to enter into an intense sympathetic rapport with his patients and actually take on their exact pains and symptoms.[10] Finally, magnetic healing prompted him to give sustained attention to a comprehensive theory of the cause and treatment of disease. Already during his magnetic healing days he was speculating that the flow of animal magnetism throughout the body may become blocked by injuries to or other obstructions along the spine. These speculations soon gave rise to a novel healing theory.

Near Palmer's office in Davenport worked a janitor by the name of Harvey Lillard who had been deaf for seventeen years. Although the historical documents do not reveal how Palmer was able to converse at length with Lillard, they do tell us that he asked Lillard what had caused his deafness and thus learned that it dated back to an incident during which he had exerted himself while in a stooped-over position and had felt something give way in his back. Lillard reported that he had instantly become deaf and had never regained his hearing ability. Palmer placed Lillard face-down on a couch and moved his hands up and down Lillard's spine. He felt an unusual lump at one vertebra and applied pressure with his hands. Palmer felt the vertebra move back into place and, lo and behold, Lillard could hear perfectly. Palmer writes that "Shortly after this relief from deafness, I had a case of heart trouble which was not improving. I examined the spine and found a displaced vertebra pressing against the nerves which innervate the heart. I adjusted the vertebra and gave immediate relief."[11]

Palmer recognized that he was on the verge of a significant medical discovery. He reasoned that the vital energy flowing from the brain to the various organs of the body is occasionally blocked by misaligned spinal vertebrae, and concluded that this blockage is the direct cause of disease. Healing consists in exerting manual pressure on the misplaced vertebrae and forcing them back into their proper places, thereby restoring the flow of vital force throughout the body. Palmer began sharing his discovery with neighbors and friends. An ordained Presbyterian minister, the Rev. Samuel Weed, suggested that he call his new medical philosophy "chiropractic" from the Greek words *cheiro* ('hand') and *prakitos* ('done or performed'). By the late 1890s, possibly at the suggestion of his son B. J., D. D. Palmer transformed his magnetic infirmary into The Palmer Infirmary and Chiropractic School and soon graduated its first class of students, who began spreading the newly discovered philosophy of healing.

It was not until 1910 that D. D. Palmer issued a full-length exposition of the philosophy of chiropractic. By this date, however, schools of chiropractic medicine had already proliferated throughout the country and many chiropractors were being trained in chiropractic technique with little heed to the founder's philosophical vision.[12] And, too, by this time D. D.'s son had taken over management of the Palmer School and its publications, including B. J.'s own 1906 volume *The Philosophy of Chiropractic*. It is D. D.'s book, *The Chiropractor's Adjuster,* however, that most fully expounds the world view and conceptions of causality that distinguished the chiropractic system in its early years. According to the elder Palmer, the fundamental principle of chiropractic was the acknowledgement that physical life is an expression of a divine or metaphysical reality. The concepts of cause and effect used in allopathic medicine fall short of accounting for the power that has brought life into existence. A truly scientific approach to the human system must therefore begin with an understanding of the ultimate cause of health and well-being.

> What is that which is present in the living body and absent in the dead? It is not inherent; it is not in any of the organs which are essential to life. An intelligent force which I saw fit to name *Innate,* usually known as Spirit, creates and continues life when vital organs are in a condition to be acted upon by it. That intelligent life-force uses the material of the universe just in proportion as it is in condition to be utilized.[13]

Pushing this line of reasoning one step further, D. D. wished to make it clear that Innate, as exists within the individual human being, is in fact "a segment of that Intelligence which fills the universe." He wrote, "Innate is a part of the Creator. Innate spirit is a part of Universal Intelligence, individualized and personified."[14] The concept of Innate permitted Palmer to fuse his spiritualist and mesmerist background with something along the lines of a philosophy of vitalism.[15] In his view Universal Intelligence, the god of the various world religions, is the fundamental force that has brought the physical universe into existence. The purpose of creation is to enable Universal Intelligence to express itself through the processes of evolution and development. It is worth quoting Palmer at length:

> Life is evolutionary in its development. The mineral, vegetable and animal kingdoms are looking forward and upward, seeking a more refined

and better method of expression. Growth, unfoldment is seen every-where. Each individualized portion of matter is but an epitome of the universe, each growing and developing toward a higher sphere of action; intelligence expressing itself thru matter. . . . The Universal Intelligence collectively or individualized, desires to express itself in the best manner possible. It has been struggling for countless ages to improve upon itself—to express itself intelligently and physically higher in the scale of evolution. Man's aspirations should be to advance to a superior level, to make himself better, physically, mentally and spiritually.[16]

Palmer was envisioning an immanent divine force progressively actualizing itself through the evolutionary process. This monistic and emanationist cosmology was not unique to Palmer or to chiro-practic; it also appeared in much of the mesmerist, spiritualist, and Theosophical literature with which Palmer was familiar and from which he self-consciously borrowed.[17] Palmer's claim to originality lies in his interest in discovering the precise physiological routes through which the individualized segment of divine spirit, Innate, directs the life process within the individual. Palmer asserted that Innate generates life impulses through the medium of the brain, which in turn transmits them along nerve pathways to their differ-ent peripheral endings. Contemporary chiropractors have largely abandoned Palmer's metaphysical theories for a material-cause ex-planation of chiropractic adjusting practices. Palmer, however, in-sisted that nerve impulses have neither a physical nature nor a physical origin. "The apparent origin is in the brain . . . the real origin is back of and behind the brain. . . . 'Life force.' "[18]

Palmer deduced that the nervous system is the key to the proper flow of Innate through the body and that, for this reason, the cor-rect alignment of vertebrae along the spinal column is so critical to physical health. Displacements of the vertebrae, called subluxations by Palmer, pinch the flow of the Innate-generated nerve impulses and sever various bodily organs from the ultimate source of health-ful activity. As the Palmer School of Chiropractic Medicine's official publication, *The Chiropractor,* put it, "We are well when Innate Intelligence has unhindered freedom to act thru the physical brain, nerves and tissues. . . . Diseases are caused by a LACK OF CUR-RENT OF INNATE MENTAL IMPULSES."[19] It follows that chiro-practic medicine "is defined as being the science of adjusting, by hand, any or all luxations of the 300 articular joints of the human body, more especially the 52 articulations of the spinal column, for the purpose of freeing any or all impinged nerves, which cause deranged functions."[20]

The beauty of Palmer's chiropractic philosophy was that, much like Mesmer's theory of animal magnetism, it educed but a single cause of all disease. "All diseases," he asserted, "are but the result of deranged nerves. Ninety-five percent of those are caused by vertebral luxations which impinge the nerves."[21] Palmer's emphasis upon a single cause of all human illness defined what was soon referred to as the "straight" chiropractic philosophy. The single-cause theory of disease became the touchstone of chiropractic orthodoxy and marked the line of dissent for those chiropractors who broke with Palmer and became known as "mixers" for their postulation of multiple causes of disease and their applications of therapeutic practices other than manual adjustment of the spine. The sheer simplicity of Palmer's single-cause theory of disease served another important function for the spread of chiropractic philosophy. It created the aura of the "one-ideaism" that Whitney Cross has observed in the ultraist religious temperament.[22] American religious history is rife with examples of individuals whose progressive-minded approach to spirituality caused them to become attached to ideas well outside the confines of orthodox Christianity. Much like the homoeopaths, hydropathists, mesmerists, and Swedenborgians before him, D. D. Palmer saw in his metaphysical system an all-embracing key to understanding humanity's relationship to God. The doctrine of Innate reduced the abstract theological notion that God had entered into a covenant with humanity to precise physiological laws of cause and effect. The enduring American belief that God has established lawful means whereby humanity might assume its proper role in the providential workings of both nature and history could now be expressed in terms of manual adjustments to the spine.

Palmer and many of the early converts to the chiropractic cause understood the movement's potential for explaining humanity's physical, moral, and spiritual components as a tightly woven unity. To account for our all-too-obvious failure to achieve this unity in our day-to-day lives, Palmer posited a specific—potentially correctable—duality in the human condition. He taught that Innate Intelligence itself is unerring and consists of an eternal spiritual nature that continues to grow and develop even after it sheds the physical body. The Innate is also known as nature, intuition, instinct, and subconscious mind, and is to be contrasted with what Palmer called Educated Intelligence. Educated Intelligence consists of physical life as perceived by the five senses. Educated Intelligence is the identity bestowed upon the self through socialization processes; it consequently gives its allegiance to the world of sense and reason rather than that of intuition and inner guidance. Educated Intelligence is thus responsible for our tragic tendency to live out of harmony with the guiding resources of Innate. As Palmer put it, "Innate would run functions physiologically, while Educated with a perverted mind would make them pathological."[23]

Chiropractic philosophy and techniques were perfectly suited to the total regeneration of the human condition as Palmer understood it. The basic teachings and spinal adjustments were embraced as scientific principles for realigning our moral and intellectual natures with the indwelling Innate. Palmer displayed an understandably messianic zeal for the role he believed chiropractic was destined to play in humanity's spiritual evolution:

> Knowing that our physical health and the intellectual progress of Innate (the personified portion of Universal Intelligence) depend upon the proper alignment of the skeletal frame, prenatal as well as postnatal, we feel it is our right and bounden duty to replace any displaced bones, so that the physical and spiritual may enjoy health, happiness and the full fruition of earthly lives.[24]

To D. D. Palmer, then, chiropractic was a systematic philosophy designed to make "this stage of existence much more efficient in its preparation for the next step—the life beyond."[25]

B. J. Palmer and the Subsequent Growth of Chiropractic

Few father-and-son relationships exhibit the drama and intrigue rivaling that between D. D. and B. J. Palmer. B. J. (1881–1961) claimed that his father denied him love and affection throughout his childhood, citing such cruelties as forbidding him to eat desserts, making him eat with the hired help rather than at the family dinner table, and beating him for sneaking food out of the icebox. D. D. was no less willing to denounce his kin and on one occasion filed legal charges against his son for deliberately running into him with a car. Despite their personal differences, however, they were of a single mind in their basic understandings of chiropractic philosophy. By 1906, D. D. had run up a sizable debt, and B. J. agreed to buy the Palmer School of Chiropractic Medicine from his father for $2,196.79 and a few odd books and spinal fragments. Thus, although D. D. was responsible for the discovery of chiropractic medicine, it was B. J. who developed it into a major force in the American medical marketplace.

B. J. Palmer is perhaps best remembered for his flamboyant personality and somewhat vulgar approach toward turning chiropractic into a profitable profession. His entrepreneurial style struck many as downright tawdry and has prompted contemporary leaders of chiropractic medicine to distance themselves and their profession from his memory. During his career B. J. sanctioned the awarding of mail order degrees, was uninterested in the educational backgrounds of his students and faculty, and was quoted as making crass remarks to the effect that a principal reason for entering the chiropractic profession was to garner high fees from the consumer public. He died a multimillionaire and in fact fully succeeded in bootstrapping chiropractic medicine into a position of widespread public acceptance, even if it remained an object of scorn for the majority of physicians.

B. J. was adamant that chiropractic medicine should not stray from its philosophical foundations.[26] He continually reiterated the philosophy of Innate and for over fifty years imparted to his students and faculty the view that the universe is governed by Universal Intelligence. B. J. taught that what chiropractic calls Universal Intelligence has been known, albeit less scientifically, by the world's great religions and given such names as God, Jehovah, Buddha, and the Great Spirit. He expanded on his father's view that divine spirit is present within every human being in the form of Innate Intelligence. It is, of course, Innate that directs the brain to generate the vital energy needed to enable the body to participate fully and healthfully in the evolutionary scheme of life. It follows that there exists a single cause of disease: the impediment of the free flow of vital force along the spinal column.

Disease per se, from the medical point of view, is a multiplicity of things. The latest Dungleson's Medical Dictionary lists approximately 25,000 diseases. If it is true that there are 25,000 diseases, then ultimately we would have to have 25,000 specifics, because the disease becomes an entity. But disease is not an entity. Disease is not a thing. Now, dis-ease— hyphenating the word to put a new interpretation upon it— . . . is a condition that matter finds itself in. . . . It is interference with the supply of mental impulse that is back of every dis-ease, behind every condition of any and every kind, matter, quantity, character, type, classification or diagnosis.[27]

B. J.'s insistence on a single cause of disease disposed him to deny the need for medical terminology, diagnoses, or etiological explanations of disease. The "one-ideaism" of chiropractic's discoverer and its developer fated the movement to internal schisms and eventual dissolution into irreconcilable factions of "straights" and "mixers." Julius Dintenfass, in his *Chiropractic: A Modern Way to Health,* undoubtedly speaks for the majority of contemporary chiropractors when he says, "Today's chiropractor is well aware that there is no single cause of disease. . . . Modern chiropractic recognizes that although the nervous system participates in numerous disease mechanisms, it never assumes that this is the only source of disease."[28] Even among contemporary "straights" there is pronounced indifference to the movement's founding philosophy. The vast majority of modern chiropractors are instead committed to defining their profession's distinctive medical outlook in terms of the interaction of muscular and skeletal systems and the scientific mechanisms of motion. The metaphysical terminology used by the Palmers is regarded as an embarrassing anachronism that hinders the full integration of chiropractic into the modern health care system.[29] Yet many chiropractors still adhere to the distinctive causal claim advanced by the Palmers, as is evident in A. E. Homewood's chiropractic textbook published in 1962, which states, "The doctor of chiropractic is well aware of the presence of bacteria and concedes that these minute organisms play a role in many diseases. He would, however, emphatically deny that micro-organisms are THE cause of the diseases with which they are associated."[30]

B. J. Palmer was just as relentless in pushing to their logical conclusion the religious claims implicit in chiropractic's founding vision as he was regarding its scientific claims. Several of his publications, most notably *The Bigness of the Fellow Within, Reincarnation,* and *Do Chiropractor's Pray?,* attempt to convince his readers that acceptance of chiropractic's extra-Christian elements is itself an act of spiritual heroics. The spirituality to which Palmer exhorts us repeats chapter and verse the "alternative" religious voice that Robert Ellwood and others have detected in American metaphysical tradition.[31] First, B. J. displays a tendency to discover in Eastern religious thought an authenticity ostensibly lacking in the biblical tradition of the West. Second, he calls on us to abandon our allegiances to institutions, historic traditions, and devotional objects in favor of inner reliance. He informs us that an objective survey of history reveals that "the great men of all times, the men who have done things, have been either rank theological-Biblical-infidels or agnostics."[32] Chiropractic philosophy proves the irrelevance of the Bible and traditional forms of prayer and worship. The "higher power" attested to by the world's religions resides within, not without. Hence there is no necessity for prayer. "Everything that man could ask or pray for he has within. . . . The Chiropractor removes the obstruction, adjusts the cause, and there are going to be effects."[33] True spirituality consists in coming into conscious alignment with the omniscient and omnipotent causal energies of Innate. The esoteric lens of chiropractic insight reveals that it was Jesus's inner reliance on Innate that supplied him with the power to perform healing miracles.[34] It was B. J.'s ambition that greater things than these, chiropractors shall do also.

The emergence and dissemination of chiropractic philosophy represents a structural replay of the sectarian patterns so prominent in American religious history. Although its spirituality is drawn from noninstitutional sources chiropractic nonetheless evidences many features traditionally associated with such native-born American sectarian religious groups as Christian Science, Seventh Day Adventism, the Mormons, Pentecostalism, and the Jehovah's Witnesses. Historians and sociologists have discerned at least four recurring themes or patterns that distinguish the formation of groups whose spiritual commitments place them outside the mainstream of American Protestantism. First, sectarian movements typically tend to emphasize one or two doctrines which they feel are neglected or ignored by orthodoxy. Consider, for example, how Christian Scientists emphasize the healing power of Christian commitment and Seventh Day Adventists emphasize the imminent return of Christ in ways that make these doctrines the key to "true" Christianity. Exclusive emphasis upon one or two elements of a larger body of doctrine alters the nature of belief so drastically that adherents finally find themselves outside the larger tradition from which they have emerged. The Palmers' adherence to the "single-cause" theory of disease played a similarly instrumental role in relegating chiropractic to the fringes of both medical and religious orthodoxy. Second, American sectarian movements tend to emerge around the charismatic leadership of an individual recognized as in some way blessed with an inner spiritual authority. D. D. Palmer, no less than Joseph Smith, Ellen White, or Mary Baker Eddy, was understood to embody a higher spiritual power. He and his son attracted adulatory disciples eager to be enlightened about the path one must follow to achieve inner reconciliation with Innate.[35]

A third characteristic of sect formation is that, unlike established denominations whose members are generally born into and raised with their doctrinal convictions, sects must at least initially rely upon the conversion of adult members. Empirical data indicate that chiropractors make their career choices later than physicians, dentists, or nurses; almost half are unaware of chiropractic medicine until the age of twenty.[36] Those who make their career choice early in life are likely to have experienced a "critical incident" in which chiropractic treatment "miraculously" cured a relative or family friend after medical and osteopathic treatment had failed. Their career choice, then, seems to stem from a convictional experience in which the "higher" truths of chiropractic medicine have demonstrated themselves in such a way as to conquer any previous indifference or skepticism. The relatively higher proportion of "conversion experiences" appears to account for the fact that chiropractors list humanitarian concerns and a belief in the efficacy of their distinctive medical practices as chief reasons for their career choice.[37]

A fourth and somewhat controversial dimension of sect formation is a sect's tendency to draw its constituency from among those who are in some respect at the margins of mainstream society. Christian Science, for example, drew the majority of its members from women, who were unlikely to have had access to positions of cultural power or prestige in late nineteenth-century America; additionally, it appears that women suffered first and worst from the stresses of modern civilization and were thus predisposed to find something of existential relevance in Mary Baker Eddy's healing message. Jehovah's Witnesses and Pentecostals draw heavily from the lower economic classes, who find in their promise of an imminent perfect world a rejuvenating religious commitment. It is possible that chiropractic too draws a disproportionate share of its constituency from the lower half of the socioeconomic stratum.[38] Its male patients may include more laborers, farmers, and salesmen, who would be prone to the musculoskeletal problems for which chiropractic techniques appear best suited. And, too, the comparatively lower fees charged by chiropractors could make them an attractive alternative to M.D.s among the economically disadvantaged. What is more certain is that many of the patients who utilize chiropractic services understand themselves to be at the margins of the concern and interest of M.D.s. Medical doctors are notoriously untrained for, and consequently unsympathetic to, many human ailments of musculoskeletal origin. They often make light of their patients' pain and simply attempt to reassure them by telling them that "nothing is wrong" or that it is "just their nerves." Patients experiencing real pain naturally feel disenfranchised from a medical community whose underlying conceptual framework is blind to the reality of their situation. Gregory Firman and Michael Goldstein perceptively observe:

> The chiropractor, in such situations, fills the patient's needs by validating the patient's beliefs that some definable organic pathosis exists, by empathizing with the patient's idea of how serious, painful, or disabling the condition is, and by impressing upon the patient that the chiropractor will cure the disease by direct intervention.[39]

It appears, then, that chiropractic emerged out of a metaphysical milieu distinctive to nineteenth-century American religious culture and has developed in ways that display at least some of the prototypical characteristics of the nation's sectarian heritage. It is important to remember, however, that chiropractic from the outset aspired to public recognition on the grounds of scientific, not scriptural, authority. The continued disputation and schismatic confrontations endemic to sectarian movements embroiled chiropractic more in matters of practice than in philosophy or doctrine. The concept of Innate has time and again been singled out by chiropractic's detractors as an untestable, and therefore unscientific, theory. Chiropractic physicians have consequently tended to relegate the Palmers' writings to dusty archives and have instead concentrated on demonstrating the therapeutic effectiveness of their techniques. For their part, chiropractic patients are understandably concerned with the relief of pain, not metaphysical abstractions. It is hard to escape the conclusion that chiropractic's public acceptance, professional recognition, and access to government-funded programs has been in direct proportion to the muting of its metaphysical origins.[40]

This gradual secularization of chiropractic, however, has been far from complete. Never has chiropractic lost sight of its major philosophical difference from the allopathic model of medicine: belief in the body's own health-bestowing powers. This, of course, implicitly invokes belief in the causal efficacy of natural forces that are in some fundamental way ontologically "higher" than medicines or surgical techniques. Thorp McClusky's *Your Health and Chiropractic* and Julius Dintenfass's *Chiropractic: A Modern Way to Health* are among the popular works that appeared in the 1960s and 1970s seeking to convince Americans of chiropractic's scientific respectability. Although both texts minimize references to Palmer's Innate, they nonetheless herald the profound healing powers of which chiropractic techniques can avail us.[41] McClusky deftly aligns Palmer's discovery of Innate Intelligence with the benefits of positive thinking. Calling Palmer "ahead of his time," McClusky quotes a Dr. Frank Crane to impress upon his readers the higher power energized by chiropractic technique:

> The smartest man in the world is the Man Inside. By the Man Inside I mean that Other Man within each of us that does most of the things we give ourselves credit for doing. You may refer to him as Nature or the Subconscious Self, or think of him as merely a Force or a Natural Law or, if you are religiously inclined, you may use the term God.[42]

A chiropractic journal entitled *Abundant Living* proclaimed that chiropractic philosophy can open people to a more vibrant mental and emotional existence. Dr. John Stoke edited this journal from 1923 to 1976 to provide "chiropractic educational material distributed in the interest of public health." Filled with short articles extolling the benefits of positive thinking and expanded awareness of "inner space," *Abundant Living* disseminated the conviction that "Chiropractic opens the door to health and a more Abundant Life because its basic principle is the key that turns the lock to the source of supply—the Kingdom Within."[43]

Although chiropractic philosophy has deliberately been muted by its practitioners in their quest for enhanced professional status, for many Americans it continues to be a source of understanding of their relationship to the ultimate agent of health and well-being. Chiropractic physician and former Dean of Philosophy of Sherman College of Chiropractic G. F. Riekman perfectly summarizes chiropractic's continued presence as a "New Age philosophy, science, and art":

> The chiropractic philosophy is based on the deductive principle that the Universe is perfectly organized, and that we are all extensions of this principle, designed to express life (health) and the universal laws. Since vertebral subluxations (spinal-nerve interference) are the grossest interference with the expression of life, the practice of chiropractic is designed to analyze and correct these subluxations, so that the organism will be free to evolve and express life to its fullest natural potential.[44]

Andrew Taylor Still and the Discovery of Osteopathy

Andrew Taylor Still (1828–1917) was born in Virginia, the son of a Methodist minister. His family eventually migrated in order to bring the gospel to the developing Midwest, and as a consequence he grew up knowing many of the hardships of frontier life. Still's formal education was mainly restricted to intermittent tutoring. He did, however, learn a great deal from his father, who, like many clergy in early America, supplemented his ministry by practicing as a self-taught physician. This combination of gospel-preaching and healing may have played a role in determining Andrew's own eventual medical path. As Norman Gevitz points out, Still grew up in a religious milieu of frequent revival meetings during which the Holy

Spirit was thought to descend and, in the twinkling of an eye, wholly transform the physical and spiritual lives of those in attendance.[45] On numerous occasions Andrew would have witnessed the spontaneous eruption of frenzied states during which the flow of Holy Spirit caused a person's whole frame to twist, jerk, and contort en route to a state of peace and well-being. At the very least this must have provided an explicit model for envisioning the causal role a nonmaterial agent plays in healing body and soul.

While helping his father treat local Indian tribes for various diseases, including pneumonia and cholera, Andrew Taylor Still resolved upon a career in medicine and began an apprenticeship under his father. He learned rudimentary physiology and diagnosis, was trained to compound and administer drugs, and was taught to perform minor surgical procedures. Still's early medical practice was more or less that of the regular physicians and he relied upon the common therapeutic arsenal of purgatives and emetics such as castor oil, calomel, quinine, and lobelia.

Andrew soon became dissatisfied with the capricious and unreliable benefits to be had from the tools of materia medica. Forced to sit helplessly by as three of his own children died of spinal meningitis, Andrew resolved to penetrate nature's secrets to discover the key to physical health. In his autobiography he writes that his anguish led him to the conviction that "God was not a guessing God, but a God of truth. . . . And all His works, spiritual and material, are harmonious."[46] We do not know all of the sources from which Still learned the lawful harmonies of divine action. It is certain, however, that spiritualism and the healing philosophies of individuals such as Andrew Jackson Davis figured heavily in Still's developing metaphysic. It is not entirely clear how fully Still absorbed spiritualist doctrines. We do know that he read and was conversant with the spiritualist journal *The Banner of Light* and its numerous articles concerning both spiritualist and mesmerist healing.

In 1874 Still made clear to the citizens of Baldwin, Kansas, that he had abandoned the theories and drug-reliant techniques of regular medicine. Up to this point Still was apparently an upstanding member of the community, as is evidenced by the fact that he was elected to the Kansas state legislature. Still reports, however, that "when I said, 'God has no use for drugs in disease and I can prove it by his works'; when I said I could twist a man one way and cure flux, fever, colds, and the diseases of the climate; shake a child and stop scarlet fever . . . and cure whooping-cough in three days by a wring of its neck, and so on, all my good character was gone at once."[47] His new theory of twisting, shaking, and wringing was met with such scorn and derision that he finally moved away to Kirksville, Missouri, a city of about 1800 people. In Kirksville, Still set up a medical practice and advertised himself as "A. T. STILL, MAGNETIC HEALER." For the next few years he made his living as a mesmerist healer traveling about the small towns of northeastern Missouri and plying his new trade of drugless medicine. Not a great deal is known of his magnetic-healing years, but the mesmeric model was to figure significantly in the final version of his medical philosophy—osteopathy. Among the convictions which were to carry over from his magnetic-healing career into osteopathy were the belief that health represents the harmonious and undisturbed flow of fluid; that manual manipulation can remove any blockage, restoring the free flow of this fluid; and that behind the various apparent physical causes of disease lies the one true ultimate cause, the impeded flow of what Still later called "the highest known order of force (electricity)."

Still developed an interest in bonesetting during the late 1870s, while working as a magnetic healer. Traditionally low in the hierarchy of American medical practitioners, bonesetters were nonetheless an established part of the nation's medical system and performed many of the functions we now associate with orthopedics. Bonesetting in the nineteenth century also extended to the art of exerting manual pressure upon painful areas of the back. Understanding these techniques as a logical extension of his magnetic gestures, Still was soon touting himself as both a magnetic doctor and a "lightning bonesetter." His autobiography tells the story of an Irish woman who came to him with pain under her shoulder blade. Diagnosing her problem as asthma, Still "found she had a section of the upper vertebrae out of line, and stopping the pain I set the spine and a few ribs."[48] This manipulation of the vertebrae proved effective in other patients, too. Soon the "lightning bonesetter" claimed successful cure of heart disease, rheumatism, headaches, and lumbago. Still successfully healed the son of a U.S. senator whose heart ailment had been deemed by regular physicians as beyond hope of cure. Word of Still's remarkable healing practice spread, and its founder dignified his discovery by combining the Greek words *osteon* ('bone') and *pathos* ('suffering') into the newly termed science of osteopathy.

According to Still, osteopathy "is God's law." It is the only science "that analyzes man and finds that he partakes of Divine intelligence. . . . [since] God manifests Himself in matter, motion, and mind."[49] While Still did not envision the kind of influx that American Transcendentalists, Swedenborgians, and most American mesmerists did, throughout his life he referred to a nonmaterial agency, or electricity, in the human system whereby God grants to His creation the capacity for life. As he put it, "All must have, and cannot act without the highest known order of force (electricity), which submits to the voluntary the involuntary commands of life and mind, by which worlds are driven and beings move."[50] From this religious principle he extrapolated his theory of disease causation and, by further inference, his therapeutic doctrine.

> Think of yourself as an electric battery. Electricity seems to have the power to explode or distribute oxygen, from which we receive the vitalizing benefits. When it plays freely all through your system, you feel well. Shut it off in one place and congestion may result; in this case a medical doctor, by dosing you with drugs, would increase this congestion until it resulted in decay. . . . Not so with an Osteopath. He removes the obstruction, lets the life-giving current have full play, and the man is restored to health.[51]

For Still there was but one cause of disease. The many diseases known by regular physicians "are only effects." "All diseases," he wrote, "are mere effects, the cause being a partial or complete failure of the nerves to properly conduct the fluids of life."[52] The osteopath heals not by intervening in natural processes, but by releasing the divine intelligence that is manifest within the physical order. The therapeutic role of the osteopathic physician, according to Still, is that he "keeps life in motion."[53]

By 1892 Still's formulation of the philosophy and techniques of osteopathy was sufficiently advanced to enable him to open the American School of Osteopathy in Kirksville. Charging $500 for a seven-month course of instruction, Still was poised to disseminate his healing discovery.

The "Materialization" of Osteopathy

For Still, studying osteopathy was tantamount to initiation into a mystical sect. The human system, he averred, is the expression of divine principle. "Ten thousand rooms of this temple have never been explored by any human intelligence; neither can it be [explored] without a perfect knowledge of anatomy and an acquaintance of the machinery of life."[54] Physiology was for Still what states of consciousness would be for holistic healers in the 1970s and 1980s; the conduit through which a higher order of life might enter, and subsequently express itself in, the human system. In Still's words, "The human body is a machine run by the unseen force called life, and that it may be run harmoniously it is necessary that there be liberty of blood, nerves, and arteries from the generating-point to its destination."[55] Osteopathy was a kind of practical handmaiden to theology. Small wonder Still was less interested in teaching dry anatomy lessons than in waxing eloquent about how "every advance step taken in Osteopathy leads one to greater veneration of the divine Ruler of the Universe."[56] One of Still's followers observed:

> He rose to the lofty heights of his conceptions of life, health, disease and medicine by the purest of intuition. He wiped the slate of knowledge, as it were, of much if not most of the accepted, accredited teachings of the day, not only in the field of medicine, but also in science, religion, ethics, politics, and endeavored to begin his thinking upon any and every subject with the new data of pure forms, built out of his imagination, with little regard or discomfort if his excursions took him sheer in the face of every accepted belief and profession.[57]

Obviously Still's doctrinal intuitions could not by themselves have established the scientific foundations upon which osteopathy was to build. It was by fortunate chance that a Scottish physician by the name of Dr. William Smith happened to be traveling through Kirksville and hear of the fledgling osteopathic system. Smith called upon Still and became convinced that osteopathy had considerable merit. He agreed to become an instructor in the newly founded American School of Osteopathy and soon began to exert a great deal of influence upon the hiring of faculty, development of curriculum, and evolution of osteopathic theory. Under Smith's leadership, the Kirksville faculty soon came to include a number of professors highly trained in basic science and medical practice. Still objected to the increasing "medicalization" of his osteopathic system, but he never seriously intervened in the new directions that osteopathy was taking. One reason was that Still had attempted to get a bill passed in the Missouri legislature granting osteopathy full licensing privileges, only to have it vetoed by the governor on the grounds that the American School of Osteopathy did not teach the full range of courses found in established medical schools. The Kirksville faculty responded by developing an array of courses in anatomy and physiology. Shortly thereafter, a bill was passed granting licensure for osteopathic physicians.

From the first proposal to include surgery and obstetrics in the osteopathic curriculum, it was evident to all that osteopathy was fated to leave its founder's religiously charged philosophy behind and enter the mainstream of twentieth-century medical and pharmaceutic practice. Still, who had denounced the use of drugs with all the theological vehemence of a Samuel Thompson, at first resisted. But reports of committees of osteopathic physicians concluding that surgery and pharmaceutics can more swiftly accomplish osteopathy's therapeutic goals, coupled with the pressures to earn full licensing privileges in the various state legislatures, made osteopathy's acceptance of allopathic techniques inevitable. A compromise was soon reached which enabled the germ theory of disease, something still not unequivocally accepted by chiropractic, to be seen as compatible with osteopathy's vision of the "electric" force of life. Germs, it was reasoned, are doubtless the precipitating cause of disease and as such ought to be therapeutically combatted. However, spinal displacements, or "lesions," as they were called, are the *predisposing* cause of germ susceptibility. In this way osteopathy's distinctive (or at least historic) interest in spinal manipulation was reaffirmed as an important aspect of preventive medicine even as it was subordinated as a characteristic mode of treatment.

In all of this, Still's original theory of the ontological source of healthful functioning was progressively abandoned in favor of the material-cause explanations underlying medical orthodoxy. Thus, when a meaningful rapprochement between the American Medical Association and the American Osteopathic Association (AOA) began in the 1950s, the AMA's study committee was able to conclude that "modern osteopathic education teaches the acceptance and recognition of all etiological factors and all pathological manifestations of disease as well as the utilization of all diagnostic and therapeutic procedures taught in schools of medicine."[58] The AMA and AOA now cooperate in almost all matters of access to hospital resources, residency programs, internships, and the like. In fact, the "materialization" of osteopathy has gone so far that one of its current principal difficulties is "an identity problem" in differentiating itself from practices traditionally associated with the AMA.[59]

The origins and subsequent history of osteopathy naturally invite comparison with chiropractic. There is, for example, strong evidence suggesting that Palmer borrowed freely from Still's teachings in the development of his own system. Palmer lived near Kirksville, and several Missouri chiropractors reported seeing Palmer's name written in Still's guest book in the early 1890s.[60] Osteopathic historian E. R. Booth has produced evidence that a trained osteopathic physician by the name of Obie Struther personally taught Palmer the techniques of spinal manipulation developed by Still.[61] Beyond these direct connections, both Still and Palmer were well acquainted with spiritualist and mesmerist healing philosophies. Unlike Palmer, however, Still never defined the "electrical energy" underlying physical health in as explicitly metaphysical terms as did Palmer with his theory of Innate. Still's Methodist background seems to have prevented him from finally disposing of a transcendent God in favor of the overtly pantheistic imagery Palmer's Universal Intelligence and Innate. Still's religious discourse was also a bit more rambling and inconsistent, which allowed his followers to read increasingly material meanings into his theories of medical etiology. And whereas D. D. and B. J. Palmer were adamant about their rightful roles as preservers of chiropractic doctrine, Still appeared content to turn over the instruction of osteopathy to a university-educated faculty.

Yet osteopathy, no less than chiropractic, is a fascinating chapter in the "sectarian" meanderings of Americans' unchurched religious thought. Osteopathy, too, has found in nature the workings of an infinite force and provided Americans with an array of manipulative sacraments for availing themselves of its guiding powers. For all his physiological references to nerve forces and bodily fluids, Still never equivocated concerning the "ultimate" causal force operative in the human system. "To obtain good results," he wrote, "we must blend ourselves with and travel in harmony with Nature's truths."[62]

We must arrange our bodies in such true lines that ample Nature can select and associate, by its definite measures and weights and its keen power of choice of kinds, that which can make all the fluids needed for our bodily uses, from the crude blood to the active flames of life, as they are seen when marshalled for duty, obeying the edicts of the mind of the Infinite.[63]

It is clear that many have found in Still's philosophy the "aesthetic Spirituality" that envisions an indwelling divinity as forming humanity's higher self. Early editions of the *Journal of Osteopathy* referred repeatedly to osteopathy's discovery of the interconnection between the human physiological system and the activity of divine spirit; often, the human mind was identified as the agent of interconnection in a manner not unlike that described by P. P. Quimby or Mary Baker Eddy. According to one essay, "God and man are one and yet two: one in possessing the same nature. Man is infinite in his nature but finite in expressing it."[64] The implication, of course, was that this "finite" barrier is largely psychological and self-imposed, and that through the study of osteopathy we can more completely connect ourselves to the healthful currents emanating from their divine source.[65] Osteopaths insisted time and again that they healed no one; it was nature that provided the causal forces for healing. In the very first issue of the *Journal of Osteopathy* Still admonished his readers to "Remember that all power is powerless except the unerring Deity of your being, to whose unchangeable laws you must conform if you hope to win the battle of your life."[66] Still's disciples for the most part interpreted this "Deity of your being" in ways that need not entail belief in the influx of higher energies into the human system. Others, however, picked up on the mesmeric imagery Still was wont to use and reached more daring metaphysical conclusions. An unsigned 1897 article from the *Journal of Osteopathy* suggested that the healing property unleashed by osteopathic techniques "may be the working of a divine presiding mind set in closest vicinage to nature, by which the tides of life, as they ebb and flow within the body, are vivified and purified, even as the tides of the ocean are made periodically fluent and confluent by the invisible attraction of the moon."[67]

Osteopathy could not help but flame the visionary powers of many who sought to encompass the whole of humanity's being within a single theoretical system. An ordained Presbyterian minister from Hamilton, Ohio, by the name of Mason Pressley became enamored of Still's holistic philosophical scheme and abandoned his pulpit for what he called "the ministries of Osteopathy." Having completed the course work at Kirksville, he soon became a regular contributor to the movement's principal publications. Pressley's new gospel came straight from the teachings of Andrew Taylor Still, whom he credited with having built a philosophy that "shall embrace the entire world of thought and of things."

> For man is the embodyment [*sic*] of the contents of universal life. From the lowest element of the inorganic, to the highest of the organic—yes not even excepting God Himself as an infinite and pure spirit, man ranges; and this great trinity of elements is so related and correlated, that it is impossible to separate them in clear and logical thought; and, therefore, you have had the courage to embrace them all in your scheme.[68]

Not everyone acquainted with osteopathic philosophy has been moved to embrace a theology predicated upon humanity's embodiment of divine spirit. Even in the early years, when Still kept the religious underpinnings of osteopathy prominent, the movement's general spiritual tone was closer to Thomsonianism or to the Christian health philosophies of an Ellen White or Sylvester Graham. An ascetic spirituality was invoked whereby humanity's religious duty is to be obedient to lawful structures imparted to nature by a transcendent deity at the time of creation. In this way a drugless reliance upon God's ways could be considered a form of religious piety while not asking persons to abandon their commonsense "materialism" concerning the physical world. Belief in a God who transcends the world of matter makes it easier to view nature scientifically. The practical consequence was that osteopathy could progressively embrace the therapeutic techniques of materia medica without painful struggles of conscience. This is in sharp contrast to chiropractic, which for two generations had to wrestle with the Palmers' sacred texts and unambiguous attribution of causal power to Innate. The Palmers' writings forced those chiropractors who were more scientifically minded to identify themselves as sectarian (i.e., "mixers"). Andrew Still, on the other hand, conveniently refrained from interfering significantly with the therapeutic directions taken by the first generation of osteopaths. And, for their part, Still's disciples were very well aware that their paying clientele were interested in relief from material pains, not in metaphysical insights at variance with their midwestern Christian heritage. Osteopaths went to considerable lengths to disassociate themselves from the spiritualist and mesmerist philosophies that had been so congenial to the movement's founder.[69]

Chiropractic and osteopathic healing are remarkable instances of the intersection of American religious and medical thought. The unorthodox visions of the founders have for the most part been relegated to the pages of history and are pointedly neglected by the newest generation of practitioners who are content to trade earlier philosophical distinctions for contemporary professional recognition within the ranks of orthodoxy. All sects face the problem of instilling in successive generations the ardent conviction of those who were part of the movement's charismatic beginnings. For institutionalized religions, sacred writings and the role model supplied by the founder ordinarily provide both a sense of tradition and the seeds from which conservatism and reactionary attitudes will sprout. Chiropractic and osteopathy, however, were launched into cultural waters where authority derived from empirical (i.e., clinical and scientific) rather than revealed forms of knowledge. Financial support was to come from clients paying for material relief, not from the donations of persons wishing to dabble in metaphysical theory. These two movements were thus almost fated to be assimilated by modern secular culture rather than remaining its loyal opposition. This is not to suggest that the commitment to nonmaterial views of disease causation have ever wholly been lost in these traditions. And, in fact, a modest revival of their distinctive roots occurred in the 1960s and 1970s as American consumers of medical systems once again began to voice their enthusiasm for "holistic" approaches to the healing enterprise.

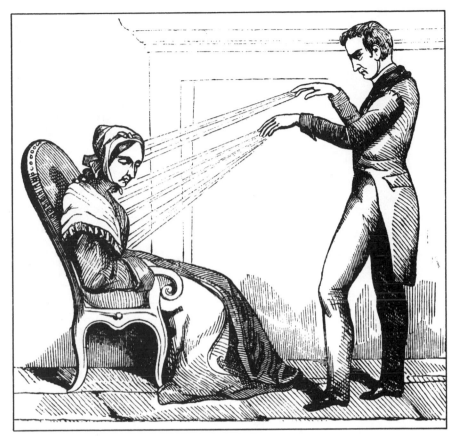

Woodcut of a mesmeric healer, about 1840. Courtesy of the Wellcome Institute.

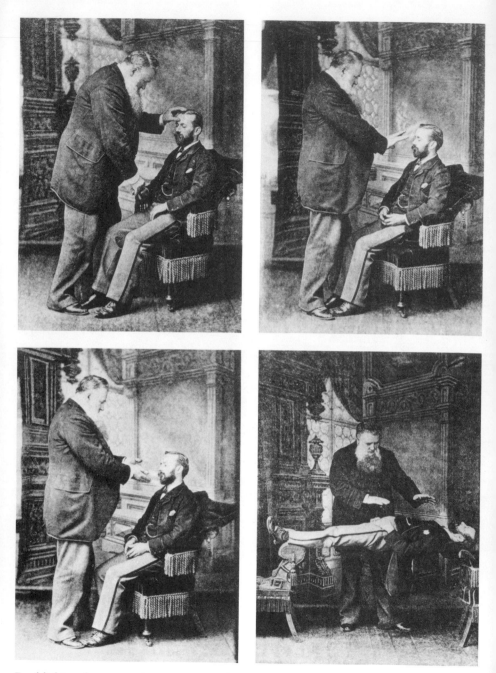

Establishing the mesmeric trance state. Courtesy of the Wellcome Institute.

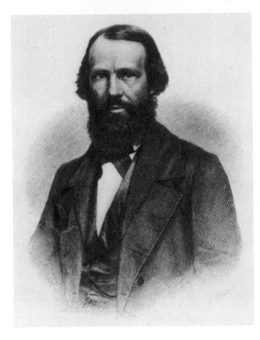

Dr. Russell Trall. From Trall, *The Pathology of the Reproductive Organs* (Boston: B. Leverett Emerson, 1862).

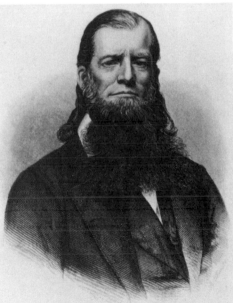

Dr. James Caleb Jackson. From Jackson, *The Sexual Organism* (Boston: B. Leverett Emerson, 1982).

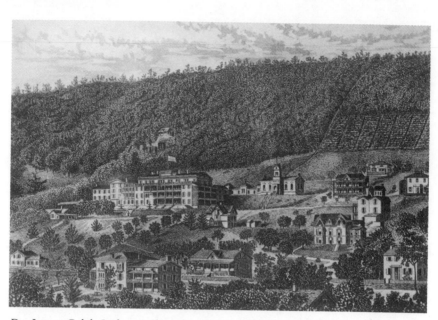

Dr. James Caleb Jackson's famed health retreat, "Our Home on the Hillside," Dansville, New York, as it appeared in the 1860s.

Russell Trall's Hygeian Home and Hygeio-Therapeutic College at Florence Heights, New Jersey. From J. D. Scott, *Historical Atlas of Burlington County, New Jersey* (Philadelphia, 1876).

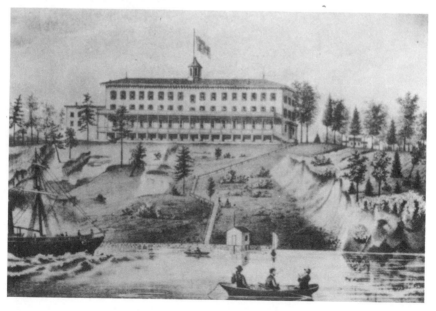

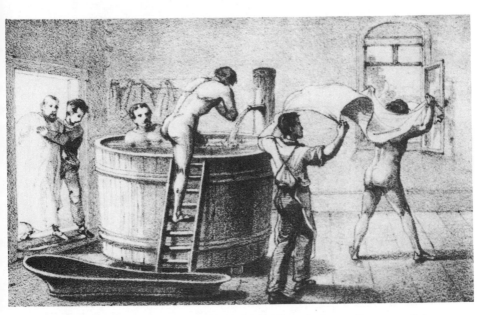

Illustration of the full-bath and air-bath hydropathic techniques. Courtesy of the Wellcome Institute.

Illustration of the shower and body-binding hydropathic techniques. Courtesy of the Wellcome Institute.

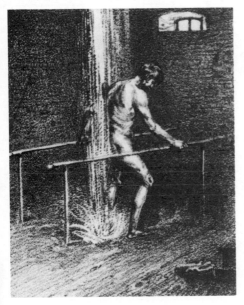
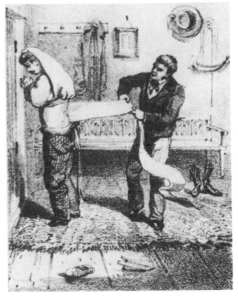

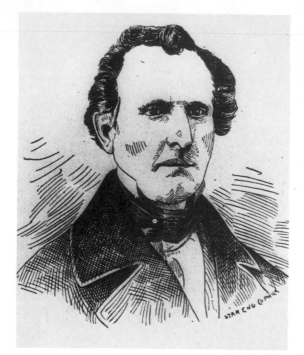

Sylvester Graham. From Graham, *Lectures on the Science of Human Life* (New York: Fowler and Wells, 1858).

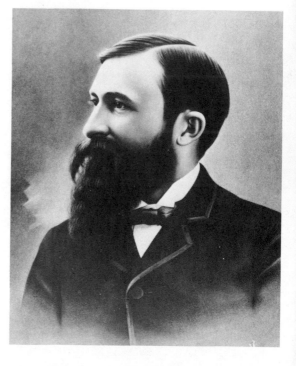

J. H. Kellogg. From Kellogg, *Plain Facts for Old and Young* (Burlington, Iowa: I. F. Segner, 1882).

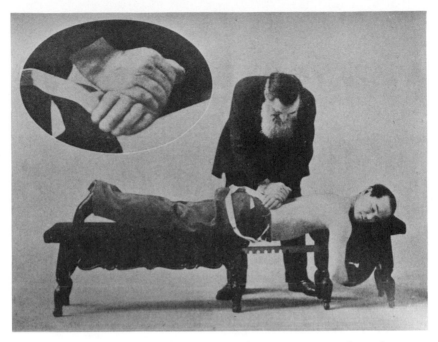

D. D. Palmer demonstrating chiropractic technique. Courtesy of David D. Palmer Health Sciences Library, Palmer College of Chiropractic.

The American School of Osteopathy, Kirksville, Missouri, 1898. Courtesy of A. T. Still Memorial Library, Kirksville College of Osteopathic Medicine.

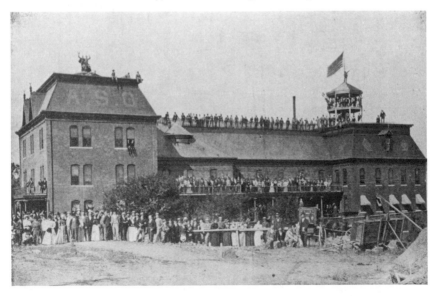

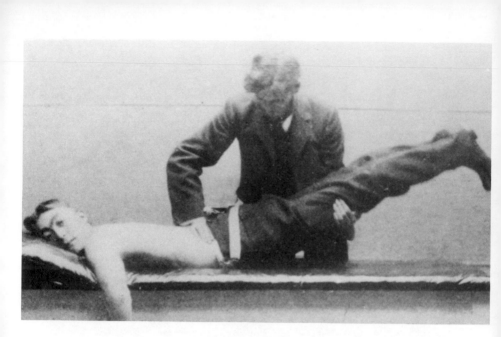

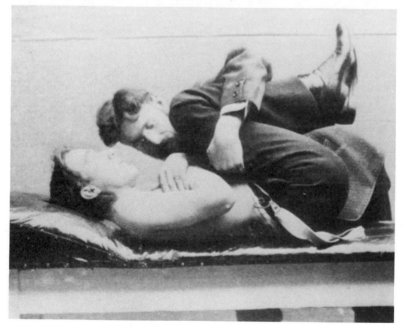

An early osteopathic physician demonstrating manipulative techniques. From Dr. Dain Tasker, *Principles of Osteopathy* (Los Angeles: Baumhgardt, 1919). Courtesy of A. T. Still Memorial Library, Kirksville College of Osteopathic Medicine.

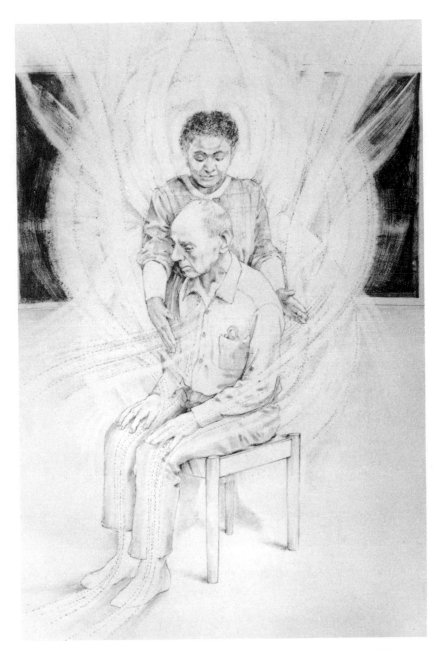

An artist's illustration of Therapeutic Touch. Reprinted from Janet Macrae, *The Therapeutic Touch* (New York: Alfred A. Knopf, 1987), with permission of Michael Sellon, artist.

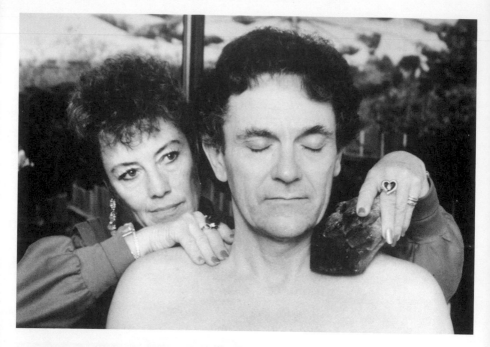

(*Above*) A California crystal therapist treats bronchitis with an amethyst crystal. Alan D. Levenson/*Time* Magazine, reprinted with permission.

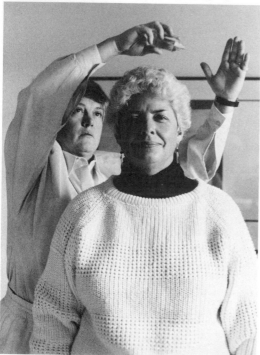

(*Left*) An Indianapolis crystal practitioner demonstrating the Vogel-cut crystal techniques. Courtesy of Linda Laing and Cynthia Rumbaugh, photographer.

5

The Contemporary Scene: Images of the "Higher Self" in Holistic and Psychic Healing Movements

UNORTHODOX HEALING SYSTEMS have proven remarkably suggestive to the American religious imagination. This is not simply a quirk of history, a sort of prescientific gullibility that disappeared under the pressures of modernity. The 1960s, 1970s, and 1980s have witnessed an astonishing resurgence of healing systems that overtly embrace a metaphysical notion of causality. And while the continued presence of these metaphysical healing systems may reflect a certain credulity characteristic of American culture, it should more properly be called extra-, rather than pre-, scientific. What strikes even the casual observer is the extent to which these movements draw their adherents from the ranks of the middle and upper classes, precisely those who must be counted among the culturally and educationally "sophisticated." These alternative healing systems appear to be expressions of an unsatisfied spiritual hunger rather than signs of desperation among the poor or ill-educated. It is for this reason that these nontraditional healing groups are such promising candidates for a study of Americans' unchurched religious life.

The Holistic Health Movement

The holistic healing movement that gathered momentum throughout the late 1970s is rife with symbols evoking an explicitly religious interpretation of the healing process. The basic premise of holistic approaches to healing is relatively straightforward and at first glance appears to be little more than the rhetoric of a generation of Americans eager to rehumanize their technological society: "Every human being is a unique, wholistic, interdependent relationship of body, mind, emotions and spirit."[1] This is, however, far from an innocuous truism. The introduction of the term "spirit" alongside "body," "mind," and "emotions" carries with it a bold metaphysical interpretation of reality. It entails commitment to a belief in the interpenetration of physical and nonphysical spheres of causality to a degree that is inherently incompatible with the naturalistic framework of our modern scientific heritage.

A helpful introduction to the general principles underlying holistic conceptions of medicine is Herbert Otto's and James Knight's edited volume *Dimensions in Wholistic Healing: New Frontiers in the Treatment of the Whole Person*. This introductory text explains that holistic healing places "reliance on treatment modalities that foster the self-regenerative and self-reparative processes of natural healing."[2] Implicit in this description is confidence in the beneficence of nature and respect for the fundamental dignity and sovereignty of the individual, both core conceptions of unorthodox American medicine. The holistic variation on these themes, however, emphasizes the psychological components of cure. Increased awareness of psychosomatic illness, as well as the general "psychologizing" of American culture, has disposed the popular reading public toward acceptance of attitudinal/psychological factors in the healing process. Otto and Knight all but neglect the curative role played by material-cause modalities such as pharmaceutics and surgery. Instead, they tout the value of teaching the patient to accept responsibility for his or her own well-being. The ill, they note, generally have difficulty coping with their condition and are in desperate need of love, care, and understanding. It is therefore imperative that healing personnel give "abundantly of their warmth, empathy and understanding and [furnish] the type of emotional nurturance particularly needed at a time of illness."[3]

Knight and Otto draw attention to the interpersonal environment and its effect upon healing and health. They counsel that a holistic understanding of healing makes optimum use of the "dynamic and therapeutic forces inherent in group interaction." Their medical advice centers on how healers can relate to individuals in ways that enhance the patient's self-image and mobilize natural self-regenerative tendencies. But Knight's and Otto's conception of healing becomes most differentiated from orthodox medical practice in their insistence that the "larger environment" that humans inhabit includes an inner continuity with energies that are spiritual and divine. Like most holistic healers, they set forth this claim rather cautiously. Echoing the aesthetic spiritual tradition of Ralph Waldo Emerson and William James, they describe holistic medicine as predicated upon the recognition that every human being has vast untapped potential, resources, and powers. Significantly, however, these resources and powers are not self-contained within the physical or psychological system. Rather, "everyone is part of a larger system." Holistic healing must utilize the patient's spiritual resources to help "open the pathways or flows and harmonics necessary to unfold the channels of the self within the body and the self within the world, the Universe, and God."[4] What began as a rather mild acknowledgment of the body's self-recuperative potential slides imperceptibly into a metaphysical doctrine in which the physical system is seen as receptive to the sanative energies flowing into it from without.

Kenneth Pelletier's *Holistic Medicine* is another text representative of the world view promulgated under the banner of holistic healing. Like nearly all of the movement's spokespersons, Pelletier introduces holistic concepts as an outgrowth of recent research in the field of psychosomatic illness. The discovery that an individual's mental and emotional states can directly affect physiological processes has convinced Pelletier and others that reliance on "material" factors is inadequate. He writes, "A fundamental philosophical revision is taking place in our paradigm of medicine. Central to this revision is the concept that all stages of disease are psychosomatic in etiology, direction, and the healing process."[5] At first glance, Pelletier appears to be introducing the causal role played by psychological and attitudinal factors in physical healing. On closer examination, however, it becomes evident that psychosomatic interaction alone hardly requires the fundamental revision in concepts of causation that he has in mind. His further elucidation of the direction he believes the revisions in medical science ought to take reveals the degree to which the holistic movement is guided by religious faith, not medical fact. His "new paradigm" is clearly less concerned with introducing the concept of the causal role of mind in our perception of matter than with infusing the notion of spirit into both. Pelletier points us toward the Chinese yin/yang philosophy, which asserts that all physiological processes are governed by a spiritual agency that emanates from the divine (Tao). He also endorses the general drift of Fritjof Capra's *The Tao of Physics*. Capra's book is cited by many advocates of holistic healing because it argues that the only philosophical frameworks compatible with post-Einsteinian physics are the Eastern mystical traditions, which deny any sharp distinction between spirit and matter and portray God as a spiritual energy continuously exerting causal influences within the physical universe. Especially revealing in this regard is Pelletier's anecdotal illustration of this new view of healing. He tells how a Zen practitioner healed herself of diabetes and cardiac irregularities by tuning within and opening "a tiny hole of light" through which spirit entered and enveloped her whole being with light.[6]

The holistic emphasis on viewing humans in terms of body, mind, and spirit has fostered what often appear to be deliberately vague references to nonphysical energies. Consider, for example, the writing of Norman Cousins. A former editor of and frequent contributor to the *Saturday Review*, Cousins confronted a serious illness for which medical physicians had given him a rather bleak prognosis. His best-selling book, *Anatomy of an Illness*, has become a classic indictment of the medical profession and its needlessly materialistic views of the healing process. Cousins recounts his own decision to will himself back to health through a deliberate regimen of optimistic and cheerful thinking. His account of his remarkable recovery brought a great deal of popular attention to the role of attitudinal factors in both creating and curing physical disease. Yet lurking in Cousins's descriptions of the curative powers of the mind are oblique references to a "higher" force. In *Anatomy of an Illness* he writes:

> I have learned never to underestimate the capacity of the human mind and body to regenerate—even when the prospects seem most wretched. The life-force may be the least understood force on earth. William James said that human beings tend to live too far within self-imposed limits. It is possible that these limits recede when we respect more fully the natural drive of the human mind and body toward perfectibility and regeneration.[7]

The invocation of William James is especially revealing in light of James's unquestioned role as the legitimator of all things metaphysical in American religious and intellectual thought. In both his classic *The Varieties of Religious Experience* and *A Pluralistic Universe* James clearly locates the source of humanity's "higher" energies in a metaphysical dimension of experience just beyond that detected by the rational intellect.[8] James's major legacy to American religious thought is his emphatic belief in humanity's capacity to open up to a higher spiritual power that enters our lives through the deep recesses of our unconscious minds. Cousins makes this implication more explicit in a later text entitled *Human Options,* when he writes that "the human brain is a mirror to infinity. . . . no one knows what great leaps of achievement may be within the reach of the species once the full potentiality of the mind is developed. As we create an ever-higher sense of our cosmic consciousness, we become aware of our ever-higher possibilities and challenges."[9]

Consider, too, a journal for nursing and community health professionals entitled *Health Values: Achieving High-Level Wellness.* The inaugural issue defined the concept of "high-level wellness" as "the integration of the whole being of the total individual—his body, mind, and spirit."[10] Striving to make it clear that spirit was to be understood as something over and beyond mental attitudes, the journal states that the highest levels of human well-being require the activation of an "energy force field" emanating from our "inner world." Thus, although psychological variables such as our general disposition or commitment to sound values affect the degree to which this energy flows from the "inner world" into our psychological system, high-level wellness in the final analysis depends upon an extrapsychological activating energy. The journal advises us to learn to open up to this inner world so that we may have "communion with the universal."[11] We are further told that making this inner connection with the universal awakens an unerring source of moral guidance and personal creativity.

Implicit in the holistic healing movement's faith in the sanative power of extraphysical and extrapsychological energies is its reverence for altered states of consciousness. The well-known physician Bernard Siegel is fairly typical in this regard. Incorporating the holistic approach into his medical practice, Siegel has cancer patients read books on meditation and psychic phenomena so that they can learn practical techniques for tapping into higher healing energies. Describing the "theophysics" he believes will emerge in the scientific world in the near future, Siegel states:

> If you consider God, and you can use this label scientifically as an intelligent, loving light, then that energy is available to all of us. We are part of it, we have a collective unconscious. . . . if you get people to open to this energy, anything can be healed.[12]

The Institute for the Study of Humanistic Medicine in San Francisco published a volume intended to introduce medical professionals to the fundamental postulates of the holistic approach to medicine. The institute's central message is that all interaction between a physician and a patient should be based upon the premise that "a person is more than his body."[13] To activate the therapeutic properties of the "more than body" aspects of a patient, the institute advises physicians to utilize empathic listening, massage, and guided daydreaming. The rationale for these procedures is not explicit, but there are many references to the writings of such psychologists as Carl Jung, Rollo May, Erich Fromm, Viktor Frankl, Carl Rogers, Roberto Assagioli, and Abraham Maslow. These psychologists hold in common a belief that the unconscious mind is capable of channeling extramundane energies into the human system; all extol such things as empathic interpersonal relationships and altered states of consciousness as the royal road to higher spiritual realms.[14] The fact is that these so-called humanistic methods and techniques are not really humanistic at all, but frankly religious.

A final theme of the holistic health movement is its fascination with Eastern religious thought. What Eastern philosophies provide adherents of sundry American healing systems is legitimation of their belief in the existence of "subtle energies" and the efficacy of certain meditational states of consciousness in opening individuals to wide ranges of experience unattainable through reason or sensory awareness alone. Particularly intriguing to advocates of the holistic movement is the Hindu doctrine of the ultimate unity of the Atman (individual psyche) and Brahman (god or divine energy). The idea that, at its deepest levels, the human self has a point of continuous interconnection with divine spirit suggests that "miraculous" changes in our inner life are in fact explainable by the higher laws of our being. The many volumes that appeared in the late 1970s to inform Americans about the various systems of holistic healing all included encyclopedic descriptions of Eastern systems for meditation and inner purification. *The Holistic Health Handbook, A Visual Encyclopedia of Unconventional Medicine,* and *Wholistic Dimensions in Healing* all sought to acquaint their readers with "a variety of representative systems for healing the whole person and awakening the spirit within."[15] Among those Eastern religio-medical systems described in these volumes are Tai Chi, Yoga, Ayurvedic literature, Shiatsu, and Chinese acupuncture (including background information on the concept of the Tao).

Too much attention to the historical and theological accuracy of these uses of Eastern religious thought can become a hindrance to comprehension of their American manifestations. In his study of unconventional American spirituality, Robert Ellwood cautions that Americans' use of Eastern symbols is better approached through what he calls "the American emergent and excursus heritage from Emerson, Thoreau, Whitman, the Shakers and Spiritualists, to the cults of the depression era, or to the 'beatniks' and the 'hippies.' "[16] At the popular level, Eastern religious thought is invariably interpreted as consonant with a number of convictions endemic to America's unchurched metaphysical tradition: an emanationist view of creation, coinherence of the physical and spiritual realms of life, the progressive or evolutionary character of an immanent divine force, and the primacy of certain altered states of consciousness for attuning humans to this divinely guided evolutionary flow. In fact, the holistic healing literature generally does not distinguish among these diverse Eastern traditions and tends to assume that their primary teachings are essentially identical with the parapsychological beliefs associated with Kirlian photography or out-of-the-body experiences. As one text phrases it, the common thread running through these various metaphysical systems is thought to be the belief that "we are all affected by the universal Life Energy."[17]

Therapeutic Touch and Alcoholics Anonymous

Two striking examples of Americans' involvement with holistically oriented healing movements can be seen in the more than five thousand nurses who have studied Dolores Krieger's Therapeutic Touch and the millions of citizens from every walk of life whose lives have been regenerated through Alcoholics Anonymous.

Dolores Krieger, a nursing instructor at New York University, developed a healing technique predicated upon the existence of a universal energy underlying all life processes. Saying that the Western scientific tradition in which she was trained "does not understand energy within the same context as does the Eastern world," Krieger has described her healing discovery using terminology borrowed from Hindu, Buddhist, and Taoist religious traditions.[18] Her study of the healing techniques employed in yoga, Tibetan mysticism, and Chinese acupuncture has led her to identify the subtle energy that permeates the universe with what the Hindu tradition calls *prana*. Krieger states that *prana* is the metaphysical agent responsible for all life processes and is thus the ultimate power behind every form of healing regardless of the particular rationale or techniques a physician might employ. Every living organism, she writes, is an open system and has continuous access to *prana*. So long as an individual retains contact with this vital energy he or she remains healthy; illness ensues when some area of the body develops a deficit of *prana*. "The act of healing, then, would entail the channeling of this energy flow by the healer for the well-being of the sick individual."[19]

Recapitulating Franz Anton Mesmer's science of animal magnetism in nearly every detail, Krieger has devised a system of practices for nurses to use in their efforts to "channel" *prana* into patients. She explains that in order to heal someone, we must first become inwardly receptive to the flow of this spiritual energy into our own system before it can be transmitted to the patient. Healers must learn to purify and open up their own internal *chakras,* or spiritual energy centers, through which *prana* enters into the human nervous system. To do this we must acquire a whole new set of mental and spiritual habits, which will facilitate our entry into meditative, receptive states of consciousness. Once nurses learn to increase their ability to capacitate this life-enhancing power, they are then in a position to channel it to their patients through an elaborate ritual of touching. Much as mesmerists made their passes and D. D. Palmer and Andrew Taylor Still made their adjustments, nurses trained in Therapeutic Touch restore the free flow of vital force within a patient's system. According to Krieger, during the healing process both patient and healer experience tingling sensations, pulsations of energy, and a radiation of heat—all tangible evidence of the activation of *prana*.

Krieger is not simply introducing nurses to new techniques that will supplement the impersonal and overly materialistic therapies associated with medical science. She is promulgating a new world view in which the physical is understood to be enveloped by a metaphysical agent undetected by the senses. Instruction in Therapeutic Touch, she says, "is an experience in interiority. . . . [It] presents you with a rich lode of circumstances through which you can explore and grapple with the farther reaches of the psyche."[20] Opening oneself to the nonmaterial energy underlying physical existence is a "symbolic experience" and initiates an "archetypal journey" that will initiate newcomers to the metaphorical language of the psyche.[21]

• Alcoholics Anonymous (AA) is one of the most interesting examples of Americans' faith in the power of spiritual factors to cure disorders of the mind and body. Founded in the 1930s, Alcoholics Anonymous now has well over one million members with about 35,000 groups meeting weekly in over ninety different countries. Any group that helps individuals mend their broken lives and discover the secrets of personal happiness has natural affinities with religion. In the case of Alcoholics Anonymous this transformative experience is overtly attributed to a supernatural cause. The group's standard reference manual reports that members typically discover that "in order to recover they must acquire an immediate and overwhelming 'God-consciousness' followed at once by a vast change in feeling and outlook."[22] This belief in the therapeutic efficacy of "God-consciousness" is couched in terms that disassociate AA from America's churched traditions and link it with the metaphysical currents set loose in American cultural thought by William James.

In his history of Alcoholics Anonymous, entitled *Not-God*, Ernest Kurtz convincingly argues that AA represents a paradigmatic instance of twentieth-century American spirituality.[23] The principal founder of the movement, Bill Wilson (or simply Bill W., as he is customarily referred to within the movement), was himself an alcoholic who became acutely aware of his inability to overcome his addiction. Finally, in a moment of desperation, Bill W. found himself crying out, "If there is a God, let Him show Himself! I am ready to do anything, anything!"

> Suddenly the room lit up with a great white light. I was caught up into an ecstasy which there are no words to describe. It seemed to me, in the mind's eye, that I was on a mountain and that a wind not of air but of spirit was blowing. And then it burst upon me that I was a free man. Slowly the ecstasy subsided. I lay on the bed, but now for a time I was in another world, a new world of consciousness. All about me and through me there was a wonderful feeling of Presence, and I thought to myself, "So this is the God of the preachers!" A great peace stole over me and I thought, "No matter how wrong things seem to be, they are all right. Things are all right with God and His world."[24]

Alcoholics Anonymous drew both substance and style from the evangelical piety of America's Puritan origins. Recovery from addiction, like salvation, must begin with our personal recognition that we are not in control of our lives. Wholeness is something that is received, not commanded. Improvements of any kind can proceed only upon our prior recognition that we are not-God, but are rather limited in both power and significance. Yet it is this very acknowledgment of our limitation as not-God that makes possible our connection with the Fulfilling Other. Bill W. borrowed further from the evangelical tradition when he organized AA into small groups centered on the weekly rituals of new converts personally describing their previous unworthiness and consequent discovery of a higher power. Moreover, the mutual edification and fraternal correction so characteristic of Protestant pietism played a significant role in Bill W.'s fundamental conception of AA as a group of drunks talking over a cup of coffee.

Despite AA's appropriation of evangelical themes, Bill W. was extremely wary of religion per se. He was particularly suspicious of the moralism associated with biblical religion. Knowing that many alcoholics were painfully aware of their inability to live up to moral absolutes, he rejected traditional religious dogma and transplanted the dynamics of personal regeneration to a metaphysical basis more in keeping with the liberal and pragmatic tendencies in modern American intellectual thought.

A major influence on early AA thinking was the psychologist Carl

Gustav Jung. Jung had treated Rowland H., another pioneer of AA, for alcoholism and in the process profoundly impressed upon him the impossibility of recovery by either medical or psychological treatment. According to Jung, the alcoholic suffered from personality disorders so profound as to be curable only through a spiritual or religious experience. Jung had rejected his Christian heritage because he believed it had become lifeless and no longer spoke to our inner experience. He instead spoke of God as an inwardly available power or impulse toward self-unification. It was from Jung that AA borrowed its religious insight that the self must first give way or become deflated before the regenerative process can begin. Jung's argument was not so much theological as practical. For him it was simply the case that the personality structures that compose the primary identity or persona of most individuals are too rationalistic and egocentric to permit higher influences to enter into and spiritualize the entire personality. Thus, although AA insisted upon the alcoholic's "deflation at depth," it was motivated not by belief in human depravity before a transcendent deity but by an insight into the individual's own role in making "God-consciousness" possible.

The real inspiration behind Bill W.'s emergent spirituality, however, was William James. It was from James that AA inherited a mode of religiosity that was at once uniquely American and uniquely modern. Shortly after his recovery, Bill W. came upon James's monumental *The Varieties of Religious Experience* and found in it just the formulation of the spiritual life that would enable AA to attract the nonreligious while preserving the founder's original insight:

> Spiritual experiences, James thought, could have objective reality; almost like gifts from the blue, they could transform people. Some were sudden brilliant illuminations; others came on very gradually. Some flowed out of religious channels; others did not. But nearly all had the great common denominators of pain, suffering, calamity. Complete hopelessness and deflation at depth were almost always required to make the recipient ready. The significance of all this burst upon me. *Deflation at depth*—yes, that was *it*. Exactly that had happened to me.[25]

James never used the phrase "deflation at depth." Nor indeed did he say that the self must first become hopeless before it could be transformed through contact with a higher power. Yet James's psychological investigations of religious experience were significant for the realization of Bill W.'s ambition to espouse a nondoctrinal spirituality. James had accumulated a wealth of evidence to support his claim that, under certain conditions, transmundane energies can enter into human consciousness and exert regenerative influences available in no other way. This psychological "fact" allowed James to retain belief in religious or supernatural events while repudiating biblical religion as a form of mythological expression no longer tenable in an age of science. James called his own system of beliefs a piecemeal or crass form of supernaturalism. By this he meant that a fully empirical examination of human experience can establish the fact that higher energies do occasionally enter into and become an actual force in our world.

William James believed that his psychological investigation of religious experience established solid empirical foundation lacking in traditional theology. Because he believed that the "truth" of religion lies in experience and not in abstract doctrine, he maintained that all religious beliefs must be tentatively held and continuously revised in light of one's own and others' experiences. James imparted to modern religious thought its characteristic open-mindedness and acceptance of the culturally conditioned character of all religious doctrine. Religion of this kind can make allowances for personal differences. It can also be co-scientific because it is anchored in personal experience rather than ancient scriptural texts or rationalistic theology. In this way, James provided Bill W. and other modern Americans with a mode of spirituality that was at once deeply personal, optimistic, progressivist, and couched in the essentially therapeutic language of self-transcendence and self-actualization.

Bill W.'s suggestion that William James was "a founder of Alcoholics Anonymous" is thus not entirely an exaggeration. For it was James who gave to AA a language and metaphysical rationale that would give it a right to the typical claim of being "spiritual rather than religious." Although AA has over the years moved from what Ernest Kurtz calls "the possibly mysterious to the sheerly vivid," it has nevertheless retained a distinctively spiritual flavor. For example, the group's self-help manual *Twelve Steps and Twelve Traditions* continues to warn against relying on willpower or one's own natural resources. The key to personal regeneration is attainment of the "feeling of being at one with God and man."[26] The unique blend of mysticism and pragmatism found in such prototypically American religious thinkers as William James and Ralph Waldo Emerson is carried on in AA's insistence that true self-reliance is possible only once we have experientially connected ourselves with the Other: "The more we become willing to depend upon a higher power, the more independent we actually are."[27] AA's mystical, nonscriptural approach to spiritual regeneration makes its doctrines anathema to most of America's religious establishment; its denunciation of both material and psychological/attitudinal factors in favor of an overtly metaphysical view of healing makes it anathema to the American medical establishment. But its open-minded and eclectic sense of the presence of spiritual forces in the determination of human well-being makes it one of the most powerful mediators of wholeness in America today.

Psychic Healing

Another wing of contemporary American metaphysical healing is "psychic healing." The term covers a vast array of practices in which the healer employs some kind of parapsychological faculty to initiate the healing process. Psychic healing thus belongs to the category of what are called "psi phenomena." Psi phenomena are defined as events that defy explanation according to the canons of scientific theory, such as alleged instances of telepathy, clairvoyance, telekinesis, or the transmission of nonphysical energies from a healer to a patient. Nearly every form of unorthodox medicine espousing a metaphysical concept of healing has at least some psychic overtone (e.g., Therapeutic Touch's transmission of *prana* or Alcoholics Anonymous's advocacy of meditation so as to enable a higher power to enter into the finite personality). Ultimately, the difference between psychic healing and some of the metaphysically oriented holistic healing groups is only a matter of tone or emphasis. While holistic healing groups are trying to broaden conventional medical theory to include a role for spiritual factors, psychic healing groups are primarily concerned with establishing the lawful activity of an extrasensory reality.

Perhaps the most studied of recent American psychic healers are

Olga and Ambrose Worrall. The Worralls have treated thousands of patients in a manner strongly resembling that of the nineteenth-century mesmeric healers. Like most psychic healers, the Worralls believe that all illness is "functional" rather than "organic" in that it is the result of persons having fallen out of harmony with the wider, nonphysical environment that surrounds them. Ambrose explains:

> I believe there exists a field of energy, akin to life itself, around and about us. We draw our daily supply of energy from this inexhaustible store-house. When we insulate ourselves by wrong thinking or wrong living from this source of supply we become sick. . . . We are like batteries that need recharging.[28]

The Worralls explain that the spiritual healer "is a person who is spiritually, psychically, and biologically adaptable as a conductor between the source of supply and the patient. Under the proper conditions, healing energy will flow from the source through the healer to the patient."[29] Patients who receive the Worralls' laying-on-of-hands treatment report sensations of heat, tingling, and vibra-tory motion. Their testimonies thus corroborate the contention that the Worralls are capable of imparting a mysterious spiritual energy into their systems. Importantly, the Worralls also claim that their ability to diagnose and treat diseases is augmented by clairvoyant vision as well as the ability to communicate with departed spirits. Psi phenomena, they say, are lawful processes within a properly scientific world view.

The Worralls insist that their healing and parapsychological ac-tivities are compatible with Christianity and are, in fact, the means whereby Jesus engaged in his healing work. The energy they chan-nel into a patient stems from God, the universal source of all intelli-gence and power.[30] Although religious belief on the part of the patient is not necessary for healing to take place, the healing process is said to bring the microparticles of the patient's body back into a harmonious relationship with the "universal field of energy." This, it would seem, is the psi equivalent of a personal reconciliation with God.

Other works on psychic healing also insist that paranormal heal-ing does not require the patient's adherence to credal religion. The majority nevertheless believe that psi phenomena are expressions of divine law. For example, in his *A Complete Course in Parapsychology,* Paul Krafchik says that psychic healing "is spiritual, but not in a religious sense." He believes that the divine is omnipresent in the universe in the form of "auric radiations" that surround every living thing and provide the medium through which all psi phenomena— including healing—transpire.[31] Defining God as an impersonal energy enables psychic researchers such as Krafchik and the Worralls to maintain a loosely Christian faith despite their rejection of the need for a scripturally based religious philosophy. And, significantly, they fervently contend that their "discovery" of the lawful activity of auric radiations is perfectly compatible with modern science. Occasional references to scientific theory and the use of scientific-sounding neologisms give the impression that although psychic healing is perhaps not yet a part of science, it is nonetheless a logical extrapolation of known laws and principles.

What often draws practitioners of unorthodox medicine to the defense of psi phenomena is their concern to explicate a theory of reality that gives credence to the transpersonal states of consciousness in which body, mind, and spirit are integrated. A good example of this can be seen in the saga of Irving Oyle, who left his Long Island medical practice for California, where he blossomed into one of the preeminent spokespersons for New Age medicine. Oyle's metaphysical pilgrimage began with his repudiation of "orthodox Cartesian materialists" and their tendency to view healing "as nothing but mindless behavior of insensate atoms."[32] His own experiences with holistic healing led him to embrace a world view in which atoms themselves in some way participate in a higher order of things. He reasoned that "our new medical model must be built on a firm foundation. The theories of Einstein, Teilhard de Chardin and Jung seem like sturdy pillars. In Einstein's cosmos, matter dissolves into energy, energy into shifting configurations of something unknown. Is this something a complementary aspect of the body?"[33]

Oyle's conviction that matter dissolves into energy and energy into the unknown led him to espouse a medical theory grounded on metaphysical eclecticism. His writings draw on Tibetan-Buddhist lore, C. G. Jung, Alan Watts, and the so-called new physics, to buttress his belief that the human body is an "energy packet consisting of wave phenomena."[34] Oyle reasons that disease reflects a disorganization of the body's energy waves. The task of the healer is to help patients open their unconscious minds so that they can draw upon a higher energy (which he variously refers to as *ch'i* or *prana*) capable of restoring order to the bodily system. Our unconscious minds, Oyle notes, are directly connected to the psi field. It therefore follows that insofar as we can learn to shift our consciousness away from the overly rational ego state, "all the energy in the universe which is not in our consciousness can communicate with us."[35]

Yet another example of how the psychic aspect of unorthodox healing stimulates Americans' metaphysical imaginations is found in the career of Edgar Cayce.[36] Cayce gained nationwide renown in the early part of this century by both diagnosing illness and prescribing dietary remedies while in a deep hypnoticlike trance. Cayce explained that while in the entranced condition his subconscious mind could utilize the powers of telepathy and clairvoyance to glean information from the subconscious minds of individuals who had turned to him for medical help. Ill-educated and with no medical training whatsoever, Cayce nonetheless succeeded in healing hundreds of individuals suffering from a wide variety of physical ailments. Upon his death, his son Hugh Linn Cayce helped organize the Association for Research and Enlightenment (ARE), which to this day serves as a clearinghouse for a wide variety of metaphysical and occult interests. Organized into study groups and exposed to volumes of Cayce's trance-bound messages from the universal mind, the 160,000 annual subscribers to ARE literature are instructed in dietary practices, karmic laws governing reincarnation, metaphysical dream interpretation, and spiritual secrets known in ancient Egypt and the lost civilization of Atlantis.[37]

Those who become involved in psychic healing do so out of a sense of religious calling. Their healing powers come to them as gifts and beckon them to become emissaries for a higher spiritual reality. Stanley Krippner and Alberto Villoldo studied three North American psychic healers and noted how all three use their healing powers to convince people of the reality of higher worlds. Dona Pachita of Mexico City, for example, one night dreamed about

a "spirit guide." This "spirit" told her that she would develop as an instrument of the Divine Will. Different "spirits" would come to her, in her dreams as well as when she was awake, to teach her about medicinal plants and herbs, about "spiritual purification," and about "magnetic passes" used in healing.[38]

Dona Pachita's healing activities thus become a testimonial to the world of spirits and the fact that these spirits take an active interest in human affairs. Rolling Thunder, a Native American healer also studied by Krippner and Villoldo, is likewise an ambassador for the spirit realm and a vocal advocate of such related psi phenomena as spirit mediumship and astral projection. Rolling Thunder subordinates psychic phenomena to the importance of surrendering our ego and thereby discovering our rightful place in the greater scheme of things. Rolling Thunder teaches those who come to him for healing that "each of us has a mission to fulfill in life. People should find out what work is meant for them."[39] Much as Jesus's ministry employed healing miracles to demonstrate the reality of his claims concerning the divine, American psychic healers appear at least as interested in spiritual edification as they are in physical healing.[40]

Of final note is the fact that transpersonal psychologist Lawrence LeShan made psychic healing the capstone of his widely read *The Medium, the Mystic, and the Physicist,* a theoretical work on the paranormal. In this book LeShan argues that mediums, mystics, and post-Einsteinian physicists all maintain that there is much more to our universe than the space-time "reality" traditionally acknowledged by our sciences. LeShan takes all of this as testimony to the existence of a "Clairvoyant Reality" that in some way coinheres with—even as it transcends—the world of physical causation. In this Clairvoyant Reality such phenomena as telepathy, precognition, and clairvoyance are fully lawful events. LeShan maintains that psychic healing is empirical proof of the existence and usefulness of this Clairvoyant Reality. He set about studying the various types and forms of psychic healing and eventually concluded that they all fall into one of two basic types. In "Type 1" healing, the healer enters an altered state of consciousness in which he or she feels him/herself and the patient merging into a single entity. Essential to this type of psychic healing is the healer's ability to use some technique (prayer, meditation, drugs, etc.) to enter personally into the Clairvoyant Reality and at the same time establish an empathic bond with the patient. According to LeShan, this creates a psychic field in which the patient is "completely enfolded and included in the cosmos with his 'being,' his 'uniqueness,' his 'individuality' enhanced."[41] By incorporating the patient psychically into the Clairvoyant Reality the healer creates an "ideal organismic situation" in which self-repair and self-recuperation systems operate at a level close to their maximum potential. Psychic healing is thus a byproduct of the patient's participation in Clairvoyant Reality. LeShan's "Type 2" healing is essentially the mesmeric model, in which the healer attempts to transmit some kind of healing energy to the patient. Type 2 healing entails the healer's active efforts first to capacitate and then transmit a subtle energy to a patient, who is otherwise unaffected by the process. Whichever the healing type, LeShan suggests that psychic healing brings to the most vivid of realizations the dictum of all great religions that "God is Love":

> The recurring theme "God is Love" appears to mean exactly what it says; that there is a force, an energy, that binds the cosmos together and moves always in the direction of its harmonious action and the fruition of the separate connected parts. In man, this force emerges and expresses itself as love, and this is the "spark of the divine" in all of us. . . . It seems to me that the challenge to science, to man, to the human experiment is, finally and irrevocably, whether or not man can accept that he is a part of the energy of the universe and can only function harmoniously within it through his capacity to love—infinitely.[42]

New Age and Crystal Healing

The cultural climate that favored holistic and psychic healing has also proved to be hospitable to the blossoming of a number of New Age religious movements. "New Age religion" is a convenient term for the newly resurfacing metaphysical currents set loose a century ago by the mesmerists, Swedenborgians, and spiritualists. It embraces everything from organized movements such as Unity, Divine Science, or Eckankar to popular interest in Richard Bach's bestseller *Jonathan Livingston Seagull*. Contemporary Americans, it seems, are still fascinated by descriptions of the existence of a suprafine ether that pervades the universe, our possession of a subtle etheric or astral body, and the imminent possibility of connecting with higher cosmic planes. No less attractive is the claim—made popular in the nineteenth century by Madame Blavatsky, Annie

Besant, and other Theosophists—that a host of ascended master teachers exist in the spirit world and are transmitting revelations to the human race through persons who can enter into a mediumistic trance. Part and parcel of these occult supernaturalisms is the prototypically American confidence in the practical benefits to be had from religious experience. Steeped in the New Thought's rhetoric of the power of positive thinking, New Age piety thrives on the avowedly therapeutic and self-actualizing nature of the spiritual power available through our unconscious minds. The New Age of which they speak is not to be inaugurated by the physical return of Christ from beyond. It is, rather, the utopian state even now taking shape in the progressive unfolding of the "Christ consciousness" within.

Interest in trance mediumship and the channeling of metaphysical teachings ostensibly sent to us from ascended masters seems to have mushroomed in recent years. Throughout the 1960s New Age devotees found inspiration in the works of Edgar Cayce and Stewart Edward White's recordings from the spirit world, entitled *The Betty Book* and *The Unobstructed Universe*. In the 1970s Elizabeth Clare Prophet channeled messages from ascended masters and disseminated them through her Church Universal and Triumphant, while Jane Roberts' *The Seth Materials* introduced thousands to the language of astral bodies and the human capacity to become receptive to nonphysical energies.[43] So-called trance channelers proliferated throughout the 1980s and have gained a measure of acceptance among middle- and upper-class Americans. The prototype of this phenomenon is the housewife J. Z. Knight's ministry on behalf of a spirit named Ramtha. Ramtha is said to be a member of an unseen brotherhood of spirit teachers (a group to which Jesus belongs) who are "now preparing mankind for a grand project":

> It is time for man to realize his divinity and immortality. . . . There is coming a day very soon when great knowledge will be brought to this plane by wonderful entities who are your beloved brothers. No longer will there be the aging and death of the body, but continuous life.[44]

Delivered by the voice of the entranced Mrs. Knight, Ramtha tells those preparing for the New Age to discover the "God within you." The "God within" is a far cry from the remote Being depicted by the majority of America's churches. It is to be thought of as "the isness of All That Is" and exhibits a decidedly Buddhist and Taoist coloring. Such a god, we are told, is available to us for personal development and self-healing.

One of those attracted to Ramtha's message of the "God within" and its implications for spiritual healing, as described in her much-publicized book and TV miniseries *Out on a Limb,* is actress Shirley MacLaine, who started under the tutelage of trance channeler Kevin Ryerson. Ryerson himself is a longtime disciple of the American occult tradition who studied at the Edgar Cayce Institute in Virginia Beach. Ryerson discovered while meditating that entities from the astral plane could take hold of his physical body and use it to send messages to humanity. The spirit who channels messages through Ryerson's vocal chords has apparently selected Shirley MacLaine as his special publicity agent. MacLaine's celebrity status has enabled her to reach millions with her new-found faith in such things as reincarnation, the lost civilization of Atlantis, and the spiritual ecstasy to be had in out-of-the-body experiences. The consciousness-expanding techniques taught to MacLaine by Ryerson and others enabled her to see "the most beautiful white light above me. I can't describe how that light felt. It was warm and loving and real. It was real and it was God or something."[45] Having felt herself "vibrating with a strange magnetic energy," MacLaine is convinced that we possess a higher spiritual nature:

> The higher unlimited superconsciousness can best be defined as one's eternal soul—the soul that is the real "you.". . . It is also the energy that interfaces with the energy which we refer to as God. It knows and resonates to God because it is a part of God. . . . The great spiritual masters such as Christ and Buddha were totally in touch with their higher unlimited selves and were therefore capable of accomplishing whatever they desired.[46]

Shirley MacLaine's personal spiritual quest has prompted her to travel across the country conducting weekend seminars and teaching Americans to make inner contact with their higher selves. The focus of her efforts in recent years has been on the healing powers such spiritual advancement makes possible. She now teaches that we can all learn to heal ourselves simply by visualizing colors. Each color has the power to set loose higher vibrations in our consciousness that can heal ailments of various parts of the body: blue for problems in the throat, orange for the liver, green for the heart, yellow for the solar plexus, and so on.

"Color healing" goes to the very heart of New Age faith in the multidimensional nature of the universe. According to New Age theology, the entire cosmos is but a manifestation of the "pure white light" of divine spirit. Every plane of reality—mineral, vegetable, animal, mental, astral, among others—expresses this same source of light at a different rate of vibration. As for humans, the white light of divine spirit "enters the consciousness of the soul through the aura, and is diffused into seven component colors. Each color infuses the appropriate soul center (*chakra*) with power and vitality."[47]

> When white light flows harmoniously into the interior centers (the *chakras*), our condition becomes healthy and more harmonious. When there is some obstruction in the *chakra*, blocks are formed, and these blocks prevent energy from flowing freely, and the body is unable to heal itself.[48]

The "science of color" reflects the New Age appropriation of Eastern metaphysical beliefs concerning the existence of seven distinct spiritual centers, or *chakras*, in the human body. Each *chakra* receives and transmits throughout the body one of the seven color rays into which white light is refracted as it enters the human plane. Red, orange, yellow, green, blue, indigo, and violet thus correspond to the seven *chakras* located along the spinal column. Any technique that can aid us in activating the proper flow of light through our various *chakras* can thereby stimulate the healing process.

The principles of New Age color healing also apply to the healing uses of rock crystals and other precious gems. Belief in the healing properties of crystals can be found in nearly all shamanic traditions, including those of Native Americans. Western interest in the occult powers of crystals, however, dates back to Baron Charles von Reichenbach's studies in the 1840s and 1850s. Reichenbach took up the scientific study of Mesmer's theory of animal magnetism and refined it into his own concept of "odic force." Early in his investigations he noted that crystals seemed to activate this vital force just as effectively as magnets had for Mesmer. His experiments convinced him that when passed over a patient's body, quartz crystals had an "exciting power on nerves" and were capable of restoring the free flow of odic force throughout the body.[49]

Crystal healing has become something of a rite of passage through which many modern Americans have entered into the spiritual path charted by New Age principles. Enthusiasts claim that because rock crystal is almost entirely devoid of color, it is an almost perfect capacitator and refractor of divine "white light." A healer known as Daya Sarai Chocron explains:

> The quartz crystal acts as a catalyst, a conductor of energy. It is both a receiver (or receptor) and a transmitter. It is a protective ally that balances and harmonizes the aura, giving it equilibrium. Crystals attune themselves automatically to human vibrations because of their affinity with the human spirit, creating spiritual links when they are worn or held.[50]

Although uniform in their praise for the healing power of rock crystals, healers often equivocate about the reason for their therapeutic potency. Korra Deaver observes on the one hand that "crystal is able to tap the energies of the universe."[51] Yet in other contexts she notes that "the healing qualities of the crystal seem to be mainly an amplification of the energies of the one working with the stone."[52] The confusion as to whether these energies are personal or extrapersonal in origin is possibly due only to semantic difficulties in the New Age lexicon. Crystal healers employ a fairly intricate vocabulary—largely of Theosophical and mesmeric parentage—which describes the interpenetration of the different bodies we inhabit. The metaphysical world view underlying crystal healing takes it for granted that we exist simultaneously in the physical, etheric, and astral planes. The healing power of crystals is due to their unique ability to harmonize the physical body with the etheric fields from which spiritual energy ultimately emanates.

> Crystals act as transformers and harmonizers of energy. Illness in the physical body is a reflection of disruption or disharmony of energies in the etheric bodies, and healing takes place when harmony is restored to the subtler bodies. The crystal acts as a focus of healing energy and healing intent, and thereby produces the appropriate energy.[53]

Crystal healing is undertaken with the same kind of reverence and mystery as a shamanic ritual.[54] Meticulous attention is given to every stage of preparation. This begins with careful selection of the precise gemstone or crystal that would most enhance one's own personal "vibrations." Introductory manuals in the art of crystal healing are explicit about the importance of selecting a stone with the appropriate psychic qualities:

> Kirlian photographs of various crystals show that the energy emanations are all different. Individual crystals produce identical patterns each time they are photographed—but each crystal has its own energy signature. The best results are obtained when your own energies and that of the crystal are harmonious.[55]

After an appropriate stone has been selected, the healer must intensify her or his commitment to self-purification. Healers must learn to center themselves inwardly and to purify their psyches of "lower" desires and emotions. Breathing exercises, relaxation techniques, meditation, and the repetition of spiritual affirmations are all recommended as techniques for properly centering oneself. American crystal healers call attention to the affinity of their use of crystals with the ancient art of using crystal balls for divination. "Crystal gazing," as it is called, is described as "the science of inhibiting normal outward consciousness by intense concentration on a polished sphere. When the five senses are thus drastically subdued, the psychic receptors can function without interference."[56] The usefulness of crystals as an aid in developing inner receptivity contributes further to their importance in New Age spirituality. Chocron confidently proclaims that "We are now living in an era of great cleansing and purifying for everyone. . . . The crystals and stones are the catalysts that bring about the purification."[57] Many books describe the use of crystals as a tool for amplifying the transformations of consciousness sought in meditation. We are told to hold a crystal in our hand, close our eyes, and repeat over and over such phrases as "I am the Light of God," "I am filled with the Light of the Christ," and "I am a radiant Being of Light temporarily using a physical body."[58] The crystal is said to amplify the energies these affirmations set in motion and help strengthen these qualities within us.

As crystal healer Katrina Raphael writes:

Crystal healings are designed to allow the recipient to consciously access depths of being previously unavailable, and draw upon personal resources to answer all questions and heal any wound. . . . The person who is receiving the crystal healing has the unique opportunity to contact the very essence of being.[59]

Kora Deaver emphasizes the healer's need to put the ego aside in order to become a purer channel and cautions that "the strong energy vibrations which emanate from [the crown *chakra*] could be of a disruptive nature if one has not overcome the personal will, for when this chakra is opened, it must be made available to that which comes from the Highest Self, or the Soul, with the will quiescent and waiting to follow the Higher Guidance."[60] Crystal healing, then, is both a spiritual path and a spiritual discipline in its own right. Hence Deaver counsels that "even if the breakthrough is only in your own understanding of yourself-as-a-soul, as a Cosmic Being, your efforts will not have been in vain."[61]

Metaphysical Healing and Contemporary American Religous Thought

The survey of unorthodox healing groups in this chapter barely scratches the surface of contemporary American interest in nonmedical systems of healing and health. There are, for example, a number of herbal or vitamin therapies that closely mirror Thomsonianism in their translation of ascetic Protestantism's concern for righteous living into a kind of hygienic piety. Understanding that God has imparted to nature a design of perfection, herbal and vitamin therapies provide specific instructions concerning our covenantal obligation to accord ourselves with nature's "higher law."[62] And, too, a number of Afro-American healing traditions have emerged, both in Florida and in major urban areas in the North, introducing a host of supernaturalisms into their followers' conceptions of human well-being. The use of amulets, Voodoo rituals, curses, exorcism, and psychopompic excursions to the spirit realm all find their way into discrete American subcultures, particularly those whose members have recently immigrated from the Caribbean.[63]

Although the groups examined here do not illustrate the whole of

Americans' interest in alternative methods of cure, they nonetheless focus attention on an enduring mode of American spirituality. Unlike herbal or vitamin therapies, these metaphysical groups adhere to a decidedly supernaturalist view of reality. They are not simply referring to a different set of material factors dismissed as ephemeral by the medical establishment, but rather are witnessing to the existential significance of religious receptivity. And, unlike the Afro-American traditions that flourish largely among the recently immigrated and educationally impoverished, they represent not cultural disenfranchisement from scientific and religious orthodoxy in this country but self-conscious repudiation of orthodoxy's fundamental premises. What is most significant about the healing groups we have been considering is the fact that they flourish among those for whom bold Enlightenment rationalism and Judeo-Christian faith are viable hypotheses in the quest for physical and mental wholeness. Their members have, however, found the positivism born of our Enlightenment heritage too confining. Scientific rationality has failed to sustain their optimism or to further their capacity to experience life's ecstasies. Intellectual sophistication has made biblical religion even more problematic. Scriptural doctrine stikes many as hopelessly premodern, eroded by the progressive onslaught of discoveries made in evolutionary science, the study of comparative religion, the higher criticism of biblical texts, and social-scientific critiques of religion's role in fostering psychological and sociocultural stagnancy.

Contemporary interest in holistic and psychic healing can be traced to more sources than just the historical legacy of nineteenth-century metaphysical movements. One must also acknowledge the role of what historian William McLoughlin calls the "Fourth Great Awakening" in American cultural life.[64] McLoughlin draws our attention to the ways in which social, political, and even environmental events during the 1960s sent millions of Americans searching for more relevant or more functionally useful ways of understanding their world. Jarring disjunctions appeared between norms and experience, between old beliefs and new realities, and between dying and emerging patterns of personal behavior. The earliest hints of these cultural rumblings can be seen in the appearance of the so-called Beat Generation in the late 1950s. Writers such as Allen Ginsberg, Alan Watts, Gary Snyder, and Jack Kerouac focused attention on the alienation Americans experienced with regard to scientific and religious authority. Their call for a counterculture echoed a widespread dissatisfaction with the narrow-mindedness of biblical religion and the spiritual bankruptcy of scientific positivism. In the late 1960s and 1970s Americans in increasing numbers seriously experimented with Oriental philosophies, psychedelic drugs, and sundry transpersonal psychologies, all in an attempt to find for themselves what Emerson once described as "an original relationship to the Universe." And while their quest for attunement to nature's higher reaches sometimes smacked of narcissism and hedonism it far more often bespoke a spiritual hunger for wholeness and union with a transcendent Other.

In periods of cultural renewal, the pendulum of religious belief almost invariably swings away from God's transcendence to notions of divine immanence. In the urgency of "wholeness hunger," the spiritual and physical worlds seem to intermingle, making it possible to locate God as easily in a rock crystal or subtle bodily energy as in a church. A commitment to theological immanence adds excitement to the religious quest; it implies that the only barrier between us and a higher power is self-imposed and accidental and can be obliterated by a single chiropractic adjustment, the wave of a crystal, or a nurse's therapeutic touch. It is striking how closely these healing groups resemble McLoughlin's description of the theological reorientation emerging in those who, while deeply religious, are irretrievably outside the churched traditions. This reorientation, he writes, is still taking shape but will most likely include

> a new sense of the mystical unity of all mankind and of the vital power of harmony between man and nature. The godhead will be defined in less dualistic terms, and its power will be understood less in terms of an absolutist, sin-hating, death-dealing "Almighty Father in Heaven" and more in terms of a life-supporting, nurturing, empathetic, easygoing parental (Motherly as well as Fatherly) image.[65]

The healing groups we have been examining are in their own right significant manifestations of contemporary American religious thought. The fact that they rarely identify themselves as religious should not blind us to their full complicity in proselytizing for an alternative theological vision. As Robert Ellwood has pointed out, unconventional spirituality rarely assumes forms that compete directly with established religious institutions. What Ellwood calls "emergent and excursus religion" avoids such competition by taking either more diffuse (e.g., offering little more than workshops, pamphlets, or ad hoc appointments) or more intensive (e.g., communes, radical reprogramming efforts) forms than the normative. An emergent mode of spirituality, Ellwood writes,

> does not set up altar against altar, or doctrine against doctrine, in opposition to the Judeo-Christian establishment, so much as present itself as *dealing with aspects of life* other than established religion, and with teachings which, rightly understood, only complement the received confessions. These movements are ostensibly noncompetitive with the great denominations, even as they survive on religious interests and needs aroused—but perhaps not met—by them.[66]

A final understanding of metaphysically oriented healing systems thus requires examination of how they "deal with aspects of life other than" those addressed by either established medicine or established religions. We must therefore turn to an assessment of how these groups function as therapeutic agents and, in the process, initiate Americans into the experiential foundations of religion.

6

Healing as an Initiatory Rite

THE VERY PRESENCE of metaphysical healing groups in contemporary American culture raises a number of questions about the relationship between religion and healing in an age whose conceptions of medicine have undergone considerable secularization. It remains for us to consider just how these unorthodox systems turn healing into a religious ritual and thereby set a curative process in motion. We shall do so by examining how these metaphysical healing groups utilize the resources of religion to stimulate their adherents' psychosomatic well-being. Insofar as these groups succeed in their task of making religion relevant to the salvation (i.e., healing or making whole) of multiple aspects of human existence, it may be argued that they provide a form of spirituality that successfully addresses the needs of many contemporary Americans.

The persistence of metaphysical healing groups in American society appears at first glance to run contrary to widely accepted theories concerning the gradual secularization of Western culture. The term "secularization" refers to the gradual decline of religion as a consequence of the growth of scientific knowledge and the continued diversification of social and ethnic groups in the Occident. There are at least four different ways in which the secularization process is thought to have altered both the nature and function of religion in modern life.[1] The first of these is the overall decline of religious institutions; that is, religious institutions and doctrines

118

that previously exercised great authority over Western culture have over time lost a great deal of their prestige and sociopolitical influence. The second aspect of secularization is reflected in modern religion's tendency to focus more on the enhancement of everyday life than on matters pertaining to the afterlife. Third, and perhaps most important for our study, the term "secularization" draws attention to the increasing privatization of religion. As religion has become disengaged from the public domain, it has become increasingly associated with the personal sphere of life. A fourth significance of secularization discussed in social-scientific literature is the gradual desacralization of Western world views. Secularization theory tells us that as the natural and social sciences have become increasingly sophisticated in their delineation of the causal forces that govern human well-being, religious beliefs have been relegated to the margins of cultural respectability.

The first three implications of secularization—the decline of religion's influence on the public domain, the conformity of religion with worldly pursuits, and the privatization of religion—are straightforward and relatively uncontroversial descriptions of historical trends. However, the alleged desacralization of the Western perception of the world may be more a reflection of the ideological stance of certain modern intellectuals than an actual social reality. As evidenced by the groups we have been exploring, the general process of secularization has not so much eradicated as relocated humanity's attestations to the causal presence of an extramundane reality in our lives. It is helpful in this context to remind ourselves that experiences of the sacred may be, but equally as well may not be, connected with institutions, scripture, or remembered tradition. The point here is that although the secularization process has indeed served to privatize religion and divorce the doctrines of institutional religion from the realm of public life (including, of course, from the activities of the AMA), it has by no means eliminated the human capacity or tendency to confront the sacred. Robert Ellwood has noted that secularization, by divorcing religious expression from major social structures, simultaneously "liberates religion to exist principally, possibly even to prosper unprecedentedly, within subjectivity and in small groups."[2] As we shall see, metaphysical healing systems are almost perfectly suited to the secular character of our age in that they provide experiential access to the sacred while neatly sidestepping modern disquietude concerning traditional religious authority. In this way they initiate individuals otherwise quite at home in the modern world into a distinctively religious vision of the forces upon which health and happiness depend.

Healing as a Rite of Initiation

As noted above, secularization theory would have us believe that Americans—particularly the educated, book-reading public from whose ranks these healing groups largely draw their clientele—have for the most part a desacralized understanding of the cause-and-effect relationships operating in the physical world. Yet it seems that it is precisely the sacralizing aspects of these systems that are most responsible for their popular appeal. So prominent are the religious overtones of the healing movements that it is tempting to think that they function only secondarily as purveyors of therapeutic techniques; their primary function, in this view, is to enable individuals to achieve what William James called a "firsthand" religious faith. That is, they give to individuals for whom religion has consisted of dull habits and lifeless doctrines handed to them by others both experiences and concepts that turn it into a personally meaningful way of life. And, in fact, the literature produced by metaphysical healing groups is more widespread and more avidly consumed than are their actual healing practices. The ideas they promulgate are apparently perceived as being at least as life-enhancing as their physical techniques. The introductory section of *The Holistic Health Handbook* actually suggests, "Perhaps more important than the techniques is the expansion of consciousness they foster."[3] Studying the principles of holistic health, we are told, can open up a "relationship to inner worlds" and thereby "awaken the spirit within."[4] Similarly, Dolores Krieger informs students of Therapeutic Touch that they have commenced an "archetypal journey." By learning to center themselves through meditation and the reading of Eastern metaphysical texts such as the *I Ching* they will learn that "the feed-back from one's unconscious contents can become a life-long friend and teacher."[5] A couple whose *cat* had been cured by the Worralls could hardly find words to express their gratitude for "the past several years. The most priceless of all, the *beautiful spiritual life* to which you have led us, and a glorious happiness we never deemed possible."[6]

It is evident that newcomers to unorthodox medicine go through cognitive and experiential transformations similar to those Mircea Eliade attributes to participants in the initiatory rites of primitive religions. A member of an American metaphysical healing group is likely to be introduced to doctrines and practices which by their very nature "involve his entire life" and restructure his consciousness so that he becomes "a being open to the life of the spirit."[7] Eliade has shown that nearly all initiatory rites utilize some form of death/rebirth symbolism to help structure a process through which individuals are induced to discard a no longer functional identity and discover a new, "higher" self. The therapeutic context of American metaphysical healing practices supports this same death/rebirth, or regenerative, structure of personal renewal. Metaphysical healers encourage their clients to abandon former identities and world views that have proved literally self-destructive and invite them to inhabit a new world of seemingly unlimited energy and power. And, too, the sensations of heat and tingling vibrations that routinely accompany metaphysical healing are classic features of initiation into religious mysteries.[8] Whether it is called *ch'i,* animal magnetism, *kundalini, num,* ectoplasm, or *prana,* experiential contact with a psychic energy appears to be a cross-cultural rite of initiation into esoteric knowledge of reality's higher laws and forces. Believing that one has become directly connected with the primal reality upon which life is dependent evokes vivid sensations of wonder, ecstasy, and self-transcendence.

Initiation into unorthodox healing systems tends to transform individuals' lives in ways not sanctioned by either conventional science or conventional theology. For example, an early student of chiropractic was moved by her direct communion with Innate to jettison her former religious belief that humans have a soul. Chiropractic had brought her to appreciate the vital difference between believing that one *has* a soul and believing that one *is* a soul. As she put it, it is "not that I have an Innate Intelligence, but that I am Innate Intelligence in this physical shell."[9] An even clearer illustration of unorthodox medicine's capacity to initiate individuals into esoteric belief systems can be found in the case of professional nurses introduced to Therapeutic Touch. No longer agents of a

pharmaceutical technology, these nurses instead learn to understand themselves as "channels." Consider the self-descriptions provided by two of Krieger's students:

> A channel, definitely, for the universal power of wholeness. I am certain
> it is not "I" who do it. . . . see myself as. . .a vehicle through which
> energy can go to the patient in whatever way he or she can use it.[10]

The notion of serving as a channel or vehicle is not without cultural
significance; Krieger was herself introduced to metaphysical healing
by well-known spiritualists and Theosophists. And, too, the decidedly gnostic allusion to the "not-I" (but a higher power that works
through me) expresses a highly mystical religious commitment not
unlike that described by Paul in the early days of Christianity.

As one of Krieger's students expressed it, "using Therapeutic
Touch has changed and continues to change me. . . . [It] requires a
certain philosophy, and this philosophy permeates one's total existence."[11] This "certain philosophy" redefines these nurses' definitions of the conditions affecting human health and well-being.
Understanding a nonphysical energy to be the primary source of
human vitality, these nurses now identify introspective exercises
like meditation as the royal road to abundance of every kind. The
benefits they attribute to their newly acquired philosophy read like
a page from Abraham Maslow's studies of peak experiences: increased independence from the approval of others, increased self-
reliance; the ability to view things in their totality; a more caring
(Bodhisattva-like) attitude toward others; the sense of being an
integral part of the universe; and the abandonment of the "scientific method" as the sole approach to the nature of life. Individuals
trained in nursing science now avidly read books on Yoga meditation, Tibetan mysticism, and the relationship between the "new
physics" and Eastern religious traditions.[12]

The continuing presence of metaphysically charged healing systems in American culture is in no small part due to their ritual
power to lift individuals beyond the everyday world enabling them
to temporarily experience numinous forces and powers. Whether
centered on the act of mesmeric passes or the waving of crystal
rocks, American metaphysical healing systems have made creative
use of ritualistic activity to structure personal encounter with a

higher spiritual power. In this they recapitulate what Arnold van Gennep and Victor Turner have identified as the threefold process whereby rituals assist individuals in regenerating their lives through contact with the sacred.[13] Metaphysical healing, like revitalization rituals generally, (1) removes individuals from their accustomed identities and modes of experience, (2) temporarily induces an altered state of consciousness understood to impart a vivid insight into ontological truths otherwise beyond human comprehension, and (3) returns these experientially reinvigorated persons to everyday reality armed with new insights into the nature of life.

This structural affinity between metaphysical healing activities and religious rituals is without question a crucial factor in their therapeutic success. It is also responsible for their remarkable ability to promulgate religious beliefs that are at considerable variance with those of the established churches. Almost all healing activities, including those of conventional medicine, take place in settings removed from the hustle and bustle of daily existence. The unorthodox systems we have been examining amplify this separation by encouraging specific attitudes or inward dispositions that help destructure the ego-dominated rationality of modern Western life. Patients are encouraged to become silent and receptive in the company of a healer who is understood to be in special rapport with higher cosmic powers. The healer, furthermore, establishes a highly empathetic rapport with the patient and helps break down typical defense systems and "higher order" rational processes that often serve as a barrier against awareness of emotions and other preverbal sensations.

Through this ritualized "death" of the socially defined ego, patients are temporarily freed from the stress of communal life. They are also particularly receptive to a range of emotions and sensations rarely experienced in their normal waking state. In this receptive state adherents of these groups claim to feel an infusion of extramundane energies. In this connection, we might note Victor Turner's observation that religious healing is marked by the presence of powers that are felt "in rituals all over the world to be more than human powers, though they are invoked and channeled by the representatives of the community."[14] Turner further explains that this experience of power, or what he refers to as the experience of spontaneous communitas, "is richly charged with affects, mainly pleasurable ones. . . . Spontaneous communitas has something 'magical' about it. Subjectively there is in it the feeling of endless power."[15]

While in this euphoric condition, initiates believe themselves to be reestablishing inner harmony with the very source of physical and emotional wholeness. The techniques and beliefs to which they have been introduced impress upon them that disease and even moral confusion are but the unfortunate consequence of falling out of rapport with the invisible spiritual workings of the universe. Conversely, health and personal virtue are the automatic reward of living in accordance with the cosmic order. Hence, when individuals return from the therapeutic setting to again take up their social roles and responsibilities, they feel that they have attained a higher level of participation in the divine scheme of things. They are, for this reason, not only healed but raised to a new plane of spiritual awareness. This new perspective on the meaning and purpose of health is, as William Clebsch and Charles Jaekle have shown, the principal characteristic that distinguishes religious from secular healing.[16] It also accounts for the compelling attraction that the cosmological aspects of these healing systems have for their adherents. Proponents of metaphysical healing systems appear particularly drawn to what might be described as evolutionary or emanationist cosmologies; in these cosmologies the very purpose of creation is to enable an immanent divine spirit to manifest itself progressively through the continuous evolution of our personal and collective consciousness. In this world view, the healer becomes a kind of role model or symbol of humanity's capacity to draw upon a higher energy and help channel it toward the amelioration of life on earth. Adherents of these groups are thus enabled to conceptualize a higher meaning and purpose for their individual lives. As channels of an ever-progressive divine spirit, they can now affirm that they participate directly in the unfolding of God's providential powers.

Religion and Healing—The Role of Suggestion

It is not surprising that the scientific and medical communities tend to dismiss unorthodox medicine's alleged successes as either utterly coincidental or caused by some other factor such as suggestion. For example, it can be demonstrated that there is a natural variability in all diseases. Every illness, acute or chronic, goes through periods of escalation and remission. All but the most serious ailments go through a brief series of "ups" and "downs" before the body's natural recuperative powers eventually restore health. Assuming that the practices used by unorthodox medical systems are absolutely harmless, the natural variability of disease alone will prompt patients to credit the unorthodox healers with having caused improvements. After all, if B follows A, it is natural to assume that A and B are linked in some fundamental way. Karl Sabbagh has argued that if a fringe medical practitioner provides treatment of any sort whatsoever to a sick patient, four possible outcomes are possible:

> First, the patient could start to improve. Natural variability will ensure that this possibility is always present. If it happens, it immediately "proves" that the treatment is effective. The second thing that could happen is that the disease remains stable. This *also* "proves" that the treatment is working because it has arrested the disease.... A third possibility is that the patient continues to get worse. However, the practitioner need not be at all put out by this, even if the patient is, because this can be taken to mean that the dosage was inadequate and must be stepped up, or that the treatment hasn't been taken long enough. The fourth, and saddest, outcome is that the patient dies. Even in this case, the good fringe-practitioner need not accept defeat. The death is an indication that the treatment was delayed too long and applied too late.[17]

Typical of the scientific and medical communities' attitude toward religious or metaphysical healers is William Nolen's *Healing: A Doctor in Search of a Miracle*. Nolen studied several unorthodox healers and conducted follow-up interviews with the patients they had allegedly cured. He was unable to find any compelling evidence that these individuals had been healed in any way. In Nolen's professional judgment, the few cases where the patient had made slight recovery could be explained by making a distinction between "organic" and "functional" disease. Whereas the former is wholly physiological in origin, the latter has to do with psychosomatic interaction and could therefore conceivably be alleviated through nonmedical—but perfectly understandable—means. Thus, although unequivocally dismissing even the slightest possibility of the influence of an extramundane healing agent, Nolen nonetheless conceded the possibility that "suggestion" (e.g., aroused hope, confidence in the healer, increased adrenaline flow) may have been of some help to these patients:

> Let me repeat: a charismatic individual—a healer—can sometimes influence a patient and cure symptoms of a functional disease by suggestion, with or without a laying on of hands. Physicians can do the same thing. These cures are not miraculous; they result from corrections by the patient in the function of his autonomic system.[18]

The most noted authorities in the field of transcultural psychiatry likewise imply that the reputed effectiveness of nonmedical healing systems can be reduced to the common denominator of suggestion. Studies by Ari Kiev, Jerome Frank, and E. Fuller Torrey are typical of those social-scientific studies that interpret unorthodox medical systems as inadvertent psychotherapies.[19] And while they grant metaphysical healers a higher success rate than does Nolen, they are no less incredulous concerning the presence of spiritual energies or the ability of these healers to successfully treat organic illness. All three emphasize the healer's ability to "name" the patient's illness in a way that evokes deeply rooted cultural beliefs about the nature and meaning of illness. The healer's seeming expertise concerning the origins of the illness has a natural tendency to elicit the patient's confidence and hope of recovery. As Frank explains:

> The ideology and ritual supply the patient with a conceptual framework for organizing his chaotic, mysterious and vague distress and give him a plan of action, helping him to regain a sense of direction and mastery and to resolve his inner conflicts. . . . Methods of religious healing also have aspects that heighten the patient's sense of self-worth. Performance of the ritual is usually regarded as meritorious in itself.[20]

Meredith McGuire is one of the few scholars to have applied this kind of social-scientific analysis to American metaphysical healing groups.[21] Her studies have focused upon what she calls the "personal empowerment" attested to again and again by the adherents of these movements. She concludes that American unorthodox healing systems employ a "ritual language" that represents and objectifies a higher power believed to be capable of augmenting the individual's internal resources. The ritual language that nonmedical healers use to describe their practices is, McGuire contends, therapeutic in and of itself. It transforms "hope in hope itself" to hope in the efficacy of a strong transcendent power. The ritual language employed by these healers is thereby capable of fostering a vivid sense of hope in an imminent cure. McGuire reasons:

> Increasing evidence in Western medical terms suggests that illnesses previously thought to be biogenic are related to social and psychological states such as stress, conflict, sense of "threat," rapid social change, and sense of powerlessness. . . . If this is the case, it is plausible that non-"scientific" healing methods, such as we are studying, may be able to address problems as well as, if not better than, the dominant scientific medical system. *Believing oneself* to be in touch with a greater power may very well *literally empower* the individual believer to be more effective in daily life or at least to cope more adequately.[22]

Implicit in McGuire's remarks is the assumption that these groups are therapeutic *not* because of the actual existence of the metaphysical agents they invoke, but because of the power of suggestion. She does make an important distinction between simple belief *in* a greater power and belief that one has *experienced* this power ("believing oneself to be in touch with a greater power"), but her analysis does not really make use of this distinction and falls back upon the role of suggestion or sheer credulity. In other words, it is assumed that insofar as a given illness is psychosomatic in origin—and studies reveal that up to eighty percent of all illnesses are—metaphysical healers stand as good a chance of helping their patients as M.D.s.

It should be pointed out that this kind of reasoning amounts to little more than substituting one ideology for another. The academic community's commitment to a world view that recognizes only physiological, environmental, and psychological causes of disease/healing is deftly allowed to subsume the metaphysical healing community's belief in supernatural causes. The implication is that these metaphysical systems ought to be tolerated because their spiritual mumbo jumbo acts as a kind of harmless placebo and seems to help certain nonscientific sorts of persons. Dismissed in this analysis is any consideration of the type of interaction individuals feel themselves to be having with a sacred reality, much less the possibility that this experience—symbolic or otherwise—might have a beneficial effect upon the healing process.

Religion and Healing—The Experience of a Higher Power

Surely the continued presence of metaphysical healing groups among educated, middle-class Americans merits a less reductionistic assessment. More careful consideration should be given to the ways in which felt experiences of the sacred might indeed have the therapeutic value attested to by their enthusiastic adherents. The point I want to pursue is whether religious experience of the sort associated with these groups can be argued to have a therapeutic value distinct from that of other, nonreligious types of suggestion. Academic investigation is unlikely to either prove or disprove the reality of the spiritual agents acclaimed by these groups. It can, however, support an argument for a uniquely and distinctively religious dimension to the healing process. The link between religious experience and healing can, I think, be demonstrated in three steps: (1) by using psychosomatic medical theory to establish the relationship between physical health/illness and distinct psychological conditions; (2) showing how these psychological conditions are related to general personality structures that are uniquely affected by the experience of relationship with a higher power; and (3) demonstrating how metaphysical healing groups make this relationship with a higher power available to modern Americans in ways that can most effectively "heal" the psychological structures underlying health/illness. This argument concerning the therapeutic efficacy of certain types of religious experience makes no attempt to establish the truth of these beliefs. It does, however, lend credence to the notion that these metaphysical healing movements mobilize therapeutic resources that are unlikely to be tapped in nonreligious ways.

Contemporary medical theories recognize stress as an etiological factor in disease.[23] Stress has been implicated in the etiology of gastrointestinal disorders, respiratory disease, cardiovascular disease, hypertension, duodenal ulcer, and even cancer. We know, furthermore, that a variety of psychological conditions are particularly associated with the onset of illness and overall personal disintegration. Among those most relevant to our study are the experience of meaningless-ness, major sociocultural change, poorly channeled aggression, loss of hope, and the emotional impoverishment that comes from the lack of reciprocity or depth in interpersonal relationships.[24]

This is not to say that the exact meaning of the word "stress," much less the neurophysiological mechanisms that translate activi-ties in the social environment into physical disorders, are at all understood. Recent criticisms of the concept of stress as a causal explanation of illness have noted that there is a great deal of confu-sion about what makes a particular event stressful for a given indi-vidual.[25] David Barnard has reviewed these criticisms and shown that, in general, they recommend that the attempt to identify stress-producing characteristics of external events be abandoned in favor of a new focus upon the intrapersonal processes through which individuals respond to such events.[26] Stress is thus to be understood in terms of cognitive activities or psychological dispositions that adversely affect a person's ability to function within his or her environment. We must therefore look to those psychological activi-ties that prevent an individual from maintaining a vigorous relation-ship with his or her environment and thereby produce the meaning-lessness, emotional impoverishment, aggression, and overall sense of futility that medical literature recognizes as associated with the origins of despair and disintegration.

It is precisely here, in the individual's psychological structures for preserving a vigorous orientation to life, that we can discover the therapeutic value of the beliefs and practices of the groups we have been examining. To this end, we must determine the relationship between those psychological structures that promote positive rather than negative psychosomatic interaction and an experience of a higher power. To do this we will turn to a brand of psychoanalytic thought known as object relations theory and its cousin movement, "self psychology." Object relations theory and self psychology are especially helpful tools for elucidating the psychological processes that underly psychosomatic vulnerability (e.g., the conditions of meaninglessness, emotional impoverishment, and poorly channeled aggression) and are effectively addressed by metaphysical healing movements. Both of these psychoanalytic theories are based upon Freud's insight that our early relationships with objects and persons in our immediate environment have lasting psychological influence.

The work of theorists such as Melanie Klein, Otto Kernberg, D. W. Winnicott, and Heinz Kohut has subordinated the importance of instinctual dynamics in favor of the structures whereby an individual relates to others in the context of personal relationships. Beginning with our earliest encounters with a nurturing parent, we are caught between two compelling and to some extent conflicting psychological needs. On the one hand we need to stand out, be separate, and express individuality. On the other hand we have an equally compelling need for merger, for uniting with an idealized image or parent from which we will receive security and a sense of meaningfulness. Throughout the entire course of life we need to address and balance these conflicting needs for a sense of autonomy and for alliance with a higher power.

The way in which we balance these two psychological needs is a function of our development within the medium of personal relationships. Optimal psychological development requires a responsive social environment in which individuals have continuous access to a nurturing parent or suitable culturally valued power in terms of which they can feel their personal worth mirrored. As the psychoanalytic theorist Henry Guntrip has observed, "For good or ill, the universe has begotten us with an absolute need to be able to relate in fully personal terms to an environment that we feel beneficially relates to us."[27] The newborn finds such an environment supplied by the nurturing parent. In the world of the infant, moreover, there is no clear-cut demarcation between the I and the you. The self is merged with the "higher" being of the parent and finds its worth mirrored in his or her affirming presence. This mirrored sense of worth gives rise to a healthy narcissism—that is, the earliest psychological ability to maintain a sense of a prized, cohesive self.

It is inevitable that the child's need for recognition and admiration eventually fails to be met by the valued and esteemed parent upon whom he or she has placed unrealistic demands. The blow to self-esteem produced by the unmet need for recognition and admiration creates frustration and internalized rage and aggression. This blow to self-esteem and the accompanying sense of rage become the core of the pathological distortions of the individual's narcissistic structures. In stark contrast to popular conceptions of narcissism as a condition marked by excessive self-love, it is now understood to be the psychological consequence of an individual's inability to form relationships that will provide recognition and a sense of self-worth. (In other words, narcissism is characterized by too little, not too much, self-esteem.) The core of the narcissistic condition is the formation of psychological barriers to protect the self from further emotional hurt. The individual becomes increasingly incapable of genuine reciprocity in relationships with others. Psychological narcissism is thus characterized by a shallow emotional life and almost total lack of empathy. The narcissistic personality is incapable of intimacy or openness with others. He or she is closed off from the give and take of interpersonal relationships and consequently unable to recognize the needs of others, identify with any consistent set of moral values, or have a realistic sense of his or her own finitude. Importantly, the precarious self-image and self-esteem associated with narcissism create continuous frustration, rage, and aggression that is ordinarily internalized and directed against oneself (circumstances which we have already related to the etiology of psychosomatic illness).

As psychoanalyst Heniz Kohut and cultural theorist Christopher Lasch have pointed out, a fairly large percentage of those living in modern Western societies have at some point in the course of their development suffered a crisis of self-esteem sufficient to make them susceptible to at least some degree of narcissistic disorder.[28] It is important to remember that narcissism is a reflection of the precariousness of sustaining wholesome self-esteem and is thus to some extent characteristic of the human condition. Narcissism (i.e., the need to be acknowledged and prized by an idealized Other) is only a "negative" phenomenon in its pathological distortions. Kohut has emphasized that the narcissistic structures of personality as they develop in our ability to see ourselves mirrored and esteemed by the nurturing parent constitute the developmental foundations of a strong, cohesive self. Because these narcissistic structures underly our ability to view the world in relation to ourselves, they contain the seeds of the "highest" developmental achievements of adult life. Creativity, humor, empathy, genuine object love, and wisdom all require the capacity to engage life in ways that undercut the rigid demarcations between the self and the world and allow a felt sense of continuity with the world. *If* our narcissistic needs are adequately met and channeled, they provide the foundation for the most mature and fulfilling engagements with life based upon what Kohut describes as a felt "sense of supraindividual participation in the world."[29]

This link between the narcissistic structures of personality and a range of emotional conditions associated with health and illness helps to clarify how metaphysical healing groups "literally empower" (to use Meredith McGuire's phrase) their adherents. It would seem that the success and continued popularity of these unorthodox healing systems rest in large part in their ability to engage and transform the narcissistic self. They do this in at least three distinct ways: (1) by helping to heal the psychological conditions that cause many psychosomatic ailments; (2) by alleviating the blow to self-esteem that accompanies nearly all forms of illness; and (3) by addressing the need for wholesome self-esteem even in those who are not ill.

First, it is reasonable to infer that the rage, frustration, and internally directed aggression created by our unmet narcissistic needs are prime causal factors in the etiology of psychosomatic illness and that these illnesses are thus potentially resolvable through the beliefs and techniques of these movements. As Kohut has pointed out, the internalized rage, hostility, aggression, and precarious self-esteem associated with narcissism are all potentially modifiable through empathy in interpersonal relationships. Through relationships that substantiate an individual's self-worth, narcissism can be transformed into the foundations of a self capable of relating to the world in a deep and meaningful way. The healing groups we have examined provide precisely such empathic experiences. Healers in these traditions typically give generously of themselves, providing patients with a significant Other through whom they find their self-worth substantiated. From the early mesmerists through Phineas P. Quimby to contemporary practitioners of Therapeutic Touch, the unorthodox healing tradition has strongly emphasized the importance of an interpersonal environment in which individuals can feel themselves to be prized and cared for as well as sufficiently free of inhibitions to express parts of themselves ordinarily stifled or repressed. To take one contemporary example, Herbert Otto's and James Knight's *Dimensions in Wholistic Healing* reads like a manual for proper parental nurturing of "healthy" narcissism. Holistic healing is said to require the provision of empathy and abundant warmth. The fundamental premise of the healing process is that every human being is part of a larger cosmic energy system and thus has his or her own untapped reservoir of creative potential providing that the proper "pathway" is established to enable harmony or reciprocity between the self and the world without. The interpersonal environment between the healer and patient must be structured in such a way as to create "greater harmony between the person, the self within, and God or the universe without."[30]

The alternative healing groups we have been studying encourage individuals to expand their ontological or metaphysical imaginations. The beliefs and practices of these groups are designed to foster experiential awareness of unseen spiritual agencies. In this way they enable individuals to create a zone of ontological safety serving a purpose very similar to that of what D. W. Winnicott describes as the "transitional objects," with which young children learn to engage life creatively and without feeling continuously threatened. One of the major contributions of object relations theory has been its emphasis upon the fact that psychological health depends not only upon the development of strong, ego-dominated rationality, but also upon an ongoing ability to engage life in nonrational ways such as fantasy and imagination. Fantasy and imagination (as well as those states associated with religious practices of meditation, introspection, prayer, etc.) blur the sharp distinction between internal and external reality and in so doing create a "safety zone" into which an individual may venture, protected from potential psychological wounds. Winnicott has drawn attention to the way in which children respond to the initial crisis of selfhood created by the increasingly absent mother by forming relations with a transitional object such as a teddy bear or imaginary friend. This transitional object permits the child to interact with, and contribute to, an independent reality. The important point here is that this relationship to a nonphysical Other helps the child to avoid the emotional turmoils of a damaged self even while he or she ventures actively into the world. Winnicott further notes that this transitional zone of fantasy and play can continue throughout life and make possible our engagement with the "arts and . . . religion and . . . imaginative living and . . . creative scientific work."[31]

Marie Rizutto has continued this line of thinking and directly connected it to the ongoing psychological importance of God as a transitional object. She has observed how the mental image of God emerges alongside those of imaginary playmates and favorite stuffed animals at a critical juncture in childhood. The formation of a relationship with God, as with other transitional objects, makes it possible to tolerate feelings of inadequacy, shame, frustration, and isolation. Yet, as other transitional objects gradually lose their power to sustain a realistic experience of being related to a valued "higher being," the concept of God continues to maintain what Rizzuto calls its "superior status." The concept of God is psychologically unique. It is experienced as having an ontological reality that can provide the sense of being related to a higher power even amidst the most precarious experiences. For this reason, Rizutto argues, the experienced relationship to God "is not an illusion. It is an integral part of being human, truly human in our capacity to create nonvisible but meaningful realities capable of containing our potential for imaginative expansion beyond the boundaries of our senses."[32] It seems to follow that by providing experiences of relationship with a spiritual agent such as *ch'i* or *prana,* metaphysical healing groups help individuals overcome their destructive narcissistic rage and release this psychological capacity for restoration and expansion.

Second, the onset of illness itself provokes narcissistic rage that subsequently serves as an impediment to recovery until adequately transformed. Illness presents individuals with a severe challenge to their ability to affirm their own significance within the cosmos. As Eisenberg has written (and should apply as equally to women as to his generic male):

> The patient who consults a doctor because he has experienced discomfort or dysfunction seeks more than remission of his symptoms; his quest is for relief from the fears aroused by the disruption in the continuity of his accustomed self. Beset by distress, he searches for an interpretation of the meaning of the misfortune which has befallen him.[33]

Thus, from the outset, the healing relationship is a process in reconstructing a meaning system in which the individual can know him/herself as existing in harmony with those causal forces promoting harmony and well-being. The human experience of disease—as distinct from the disease itself—is fraught with an overriding sense of being out of harmony with the ultimate powers upon which life and well-being depend. It would appear that a renewed sense of accessibility to these ultimate powers could be a necessary, even if not sufficient, cause of healing.

An excellent example of the capacity of metaphysical healers to regenerate their patients' sense of being prized and cohesive individuals is the recovery of actress Jill Ireland from breast cancer. Ireland was severely traumatized by her condition and found her life increasingly chaotic, senseless, and terrifying. She was introduced to a "holistic health practitioner" who taught her to meditate. She also learned to make use of what she describes as the "healing properties of quartz crystals for focusing and energizing my mind and body." Her discovery of nonmaterial healing energies and her newfound interest in meditational practices designed to attune the self to this metaphysical power gradually enabled her to regenerate herself psychologically and to overcome the damaged self-image, sense of meaninglessness, vulnerability, isolation, and internalized aggression born of her illness. Interestingly, among the "gifts" which she attributes to her cure from cancer are: "More confidence"; "More at ease with myself"; "It has helped me to be myself"; "It has brought meditation to my life"; and "It has enriched my relationships with my children and the people close to me."[34]

And, third, the unique capacity of these movements to bring the resources of religion to bear upon the transformation of our narcissistic needs makes them highly attractive and, indeed, empowering even for those who are not physically ill. Metaphysical healers provide a felt sense of relationship to an eminently accessible spiritual power and thereby make possible a religious resolution of the dilemma of narcissism. Their doctrines (myth) and practices (ritual) envision God as sufficiently immanent to permit the merger and yet sufficiently transcendent to constitute the idealized object capable of affirming and bestowing meaning upon the self. The language of *prana,* animal magnetism, Innate, and the like depicts God in ways that mobilize an individual's need to feel united with a higher power while encouraging him or her to accept responsibility for permitting this higher power to work "through" their own actions. Without exception, these groups provide either explicit instructions or at least implicit clues about gaining inner accessibility to a higher spiritual power. Their adherents find themselves related to a transitional object (*prana,* the Innate, etc.) that increases their capacity for empathy and imparts a felt sense of supraindividual participation in the world. Unorthodox healing systems afford individuals the opportunity to ground their self-esteem on the sacred (thereby effecting what Kohut calls the "mirror transference") and develop stronger goals and life-styles (thereby effecting what Kohut calls the "idealizing transference" whereby the patient internalizes values and goals associated with the prized Other). For many modern individuals, initiation into these metaphysical healing systems can thus quite literally open up new worlds and release inherent tendencies toward creativity, wisdom, and empathy for the needs of others.

Unorthodox Medicine and the Accessibility of God

Unorthodox medical systems, by meeting the individual's need for access to and merger with God, address an important aspect of personal life. The psychologist of religion Peter Homans has drawn attention to the fact that the Protestant denominations that have so influenced American religious life emerged in Western culture precisely because of their ability to meet this fundamental "prerequisite" of psychological, physical, and spiritual vitality. His comments bear directly upon the reasons that unorthodox medical groups can function as a kind of cultural successor to classical Protestantism for some modern Americans.

> [Classical Protestantism] created a unique and highly effective solution to the universal psychological needs for idealization and merger. Protestantism synthesized these needs with viable and appropriate cultural objects through its doctrine of the transcendent existence of God, which met the need of the self for idealization, and through the evangelical doctrine of the believer's oneness with Christ—I am in Christ and Christ in me—which nurtured the believer's associated need for merger with a supreme cultural object. In this way Protestant Christianity articulated with the narcissistic needs of its followers.[35]

Homans observes that the capacity to merge psychologically with "a supreme cultural object" is a necessary precondition of a vital spirituality. Yet many individuals in modern Western culture find it increasingly difficult to "idealize" adequately the God of institutional religion and establish any profound psychological connections. Intellectual assent to the "higher" status of God has become all but impossible for many who have been influenced by such developments as the advent of modern science, historical sophistication concerning the origins of early Church doctrine or scripture, and awareness of the cultural relativity of religious "truth." Moreover, modern society is so pluralized that any one religious tradition is limited in its capacity to socialize individuals into a world view that will provide access to, and merger with, an appropriately idealized image of God. Though it is true that the 1970s and 1980s have witnessed a resurgence in the ability of fundamentalist churches to mobilize and energize their adherents, these groups provide a biblically-depicted God who is unlikely to appeal to those whose cognitive rejection of traditional religious faith makes evangelical commitment impossible.

In this context unorthodox medical systems emerge as fascinating examples of the forms of religious belief and practice that can successfully mediate a sense of the sacred to individuals during a period in which institutional religion exerts increasingly less influence on the public realm. As Donald Capps suggests:

> If religion exerts less influence on the social order but retains its influence on personal life, as various secularization theories suggest, this "privatization" of religion provides a favorable context for an increasingly close association of religion and narcissism. . . . A transformed narcissism may provide the foundation not only for psychological well-being but also for such spiritual well-being as can realistically be expected in a secular world.[36]

In his famous essay "The Will To Believe," William James observed that the scientific character of our age tends to make the hypothesis of religion dead, avoidable, and trivial. Religion—the conviction that there is a higher power from which we might receive healing powers—becomes a genuine option only when its claims confront us in such a way as to be of "the forced, living, and momentous kind."[37] Illness almost invariably makes the religious hypothesis both forced and momentous. It is to the credit of these metaphysical healing systems that they have enabled many Americans to perceive the religious hypothesis as a living one. Insofar as growing numbers of modern individuals have difficulty maintaining a vital sense of self-love and suffer from emotional impoverishment, questions concerning the psychological accessibility of God are far more fundamental to the emergence of genuine spirituality than are those of instinctual renunciation and moral obedience.

The existence and continued popularity of unorthodox healing systems appear to testify to the fact that secularization has in no way detracted from Americans' capacity to envision their lives as in some way participating in a sacred reality. Through their myths and rituals, these groups have succeeded in relocating many modern Americans' point of access to the sacred in ways that are well tuned to the psychological and sociological structures of our day. Although undoubtedly destined to remain at the fringes of both American medical and religious orthodoxy, these groups have nonetheless reminded us that the sense of personal relatedness to the sacred is a vital component of personal well-being.

Notes

Chapter 1

1. Shirley MacLaine, *Dancing in the Light* (New York: Bantam Books, 1985), p. 8.

2. Ibid.

3. Jill Ireland, *Life Wish* (Boston: Little, Brown and Co., 1987), p. 77.

4. See the discussion of healing in Gerhard Kittle, *Theological Dictionary of the New Testament* (Grand Rapids, Mich.: William B. Eerdmans Publishing Co., 1978), 3: 194–215; and William Clebsch and Charles Jaekle, *Pastoral Care in Historical Perspective* (New York: Jason Aronson, Inc., 1975).

5. It should be noted that many massage and breathing therapies utilize Eastern notions of a subtle body energy such as *ch'i* or *prana* and thus implicitly invoke world views in which the physical realm of life is ontologically dependent on either sustaining continuous "harmony" with, or periodically receiving "influxes" from, an ultimate metaphysical reality such as Brahman, the Tao, or the Cosmic Body of the Buddha. Thus, systems such as acupuncture, acupressure, and Shiatsu do utilize what this book defines as supernaturalist-cause explanations of healing even though many adherents emphasize their known physiological properties. A discussion of contemporary unorthodox medicine's tendency to rely upon religiously charged conceptions of "healing energy" can be found in David Hufford's "Contemporary Folk Medicine," in Norman Gevitz, ed., *Other Healers: Unorthodox Medicine in America* (Baltimore: The Johns Hopkins University Press, 1988).

6. See the discussion of the formal (as opposed to functional) properties of religious consciousness in Peter Berger, "Some Second Thoughts on Substantive Versus Functional Definitions of Religion," *Journal for the Social Scientific Study of Religion* 13, no. 2 (June 1974): 125–134; and Giles Gunn, *The Interpretation of Otherness* (New York: Oxford University Press, 1979).

7. See Howard Kerr and Charles L. Crow, eds., *The Occult in America: New Historical Perspectives* (Urbana: University of Illinois Press, 1983); and Robert Ellwood, *Alternative Altars* (Chicago: University of Chicago Press, 1979).

8. Robert Ellwood notes that knowing too much about the historical lineage of these groups might well obscure interpretations of the distinctive style in which Americans appropriate their beliefs and teachings. Observing that the harmonial tradition in American thought (dating back at least to Emerson) has profoundly influenced the ways in which Oriental or occult thought is understood in this country, Ellwood goes so far as to suggest that, because American adherents of these groups share common reading lists, any attempt to make hard and fast differentiations among their separate belief systems may well be misguided. See Ellwood, *Alternative Altars*, p. 168.

9. Sydney Ahlstrom, *A Religious History of the American People* (New Haven: Yale University Press, 1972), p. 1019.

10. William James, *The Varieties of Religious Experience* (New York: P. F. Collier, Inc., 1961), p. 110.

11. Ibid., p. 399. See also James, *A Pluralistic Universe* (New York: E. P. Dutton, 1971), p. 266.

12. James, *The Varieties of Religious Experience*, p. 102.

13. *The Holistic Health Handbook* (Berkeley: And/Or Press, 1978), p. 13.

Chapter 2

1. The medical practices of Native Americans were (and in their modern remnants still are) too complex and varied to be conveniently summarized. In general, we might recognize at least two primary forms: (1) the use of "natural" herbs and vegetation as emetics and purgatives and (2) the use of the supernatural by medicine men or shamans who contact the spirit world both to diagnose and prescribe treatment for disease. John Duffy, in the chapter on "the myth of Indian medicine" in his *The Healers: A History of American Medicine* (New York: McGraw-Hill, 1976), is undoubtedly correct in his assessment that North American Indians made few contribu-

tions to the historical development of medicine. Native American medicine is, nonetheless, fascinating and not without considerable spiritual significance. Interested readers might consult Ake Hultkrantz, *The Religions of the American Indians* (Berkeley: University of California Press, 1961); Donald Sandner, *Navaho Symbols of Healing* (New York: Harcourt Brace Jovanovich, 1979); or Virgil Vogel, *American Indian Medicine* (Norman: University of Oklahoma Press, 1970).

2. It is difficult to estimate just how much African religious medical heritage has survived sufficiently intact to have a continuing influence on the healing practices of black Americans. Much of the use of potions, herbal remedies, and occult techniques found today among blacks living in cities such as Miami and New York derive from more recent Caribbean immigration rather than from colonial America. Interested readers might wish to consult Jon Butler's "The Dark Ages of American Occultism, 1760–1848," in Howard Kerr and Charles L. Crow, eds., *The Occult in America: New Historical Perspectives* (Urbana: University of Illinois Press, 1983); George Eaton Simpson, *Black Religions in the New World* (New York: Columbia University Press, 1978); and Albert Raboteau, *Slave Religion: The "Invisible Institution" in the Antebellum South* (New York: Oxford University Press, 1978).

3. This discussion of early nineteenth-century medical theory borrows heavily from Charles Rosenberg's essay "The Therapeutic Revolution: Medicine, Meaning, and Social Change in Nineteenth-Century America," in Charles Rosenberg and Morris Vogel, eds., *The Therapeutic Revolution: Essays in the Social History of American Medicine* (Philadelphia: University of Pennsylvania Press, 1979).

4. Benjamin Rush, cited in Duffy, *The Healers*, p. 99.

5. John Harley Warner, *The Therapeutic Perspective* (Cambridge, Mass.: Harvard University Press, 1986), p. 4.

6. Duffy, *The Healers*, p. 105. John Warner cautions against crediting sectarian movements with effecting changes in the orthodox profession's therapeutic practices. While these groups undoubtedly did cause regular physicians to lessen their reliance on heroic remedies, they also fostered a "dogmatic adherence to tradition" and moved them to "hold all the tighter to the therapies that represented their own professional tradition." See his "Medical Sectarianism, Therapeutic Conflict, and the Shaping of Orthodox Professional Identity in Antebellum American Medicine," in W. F. Bynum and Roy Porter, eds., *Medical Fringe and Medical Orthodoxy, 1750–1850* (Wolfeboro, N.H.: Croom Helm, 1987), pp. 234–260.

7. Many fine works document the institutionalization of American medicine. Among the most widely recognized are Joseph Kett, *The Formation of the American Medical Profession: The Role of Institutions, 1780–*

1860 (New Haven: Yale University Press, 1968); Henry B. Shafer, *The American Medical Profession 1783 to 1850* (New York: Columbia University Press, 1936); Richard Shyrock, *Medical Licensing in America, 1650–1965* (Baltimore: Johns Hopkins University Press, 1967); and Richard Shyrock, *Medicine in America: Historical Essays* (Baltimore: Johns Hopkins University Press, 1967).

8. Cited in William Rothstein's excellent work, *American Physicians in the Nineteenth Century* (Baltimore: Johns Hopkins University Press, 1972), p. 173.

9. Ibid.

10. Ibid., p. 287.

11. Samuel Thomson, *New Guide to Health: or, Botanic Family Physician, Containing a Complete System of Practice, on a Plan Entirely New; with a Description of the Vegetables made use of and Directions for Preparing and Administering Them, to Cure Disease, to which is Prefixed a Narrative of the Life and Medical Discoveries of the Author*, 3rd ed. (Boston: 1832), p. 16.

12. Rothstein, *American Physicians*, p. 128.

13. *Boston Thomsonian Manual* 3 (November 15, 1837): 21.

14. *Thomsonian Botanic Watchman* 1 (October 1834): 140.

15. Samuel Thomson, quoted in James Harvey Young's "American Medical Quackery in the Age of the Common Man," *The Mississippi Valley Historical Review* 47 (1961): 581.

16. A helpful discussion of the feminist appeal of Thomsonian is to be found in Kett, *The Formation of the American Medical Profession*, pp. 117–122.

17. Charles Rosenberg in Rosenberg and Vogel, *The Therapeutic Revolution*, p. 4.

18. William McLoughlin, *Revivals, Awakenings and Reform* (Chicago: University of Chicago Press, 1978).

19. Ibid., p. 103. I took considerable liberty in reducing this passage.

20. Whitney R. Cross, *The Burned-Over District* (New York: Harper and Row, 1965), p. 236.

21. Kett, *The Formation of the American Medical Profession*, p. 129.

22. "Remarks of Mr. Scott in the Senate. . . ," *Trans., Med. Soc. State N.Y.*, 6 (1844–46), p. 73, cited in Kett, *The Formation of the American Medical Profession*, p. 127.

23. *Botanical Medical Record* 12 (1844): 356.

24. *The Boston Thomsonian Medical and Physiological Journal* (April 15, 1846): 219.

25. Samuel Christian Hahnemann, *Organon of the Rational Art of Healing* (New York: E. P. Dutton, 1913), p. 5.

26. Ibid., p. 11.

27. A complete account of homoeopathy's development in the United States can be found in Martin Kaufman's *Homoeopathy in America: The Rise and Fall of a Medical Heresy* (Baltimore: Johns Hopkins Press, 1971).

28. Rothstein, *American Physicans.*

29. Kett, *The Formation of the American Medical Profession,* pp. 139 ff., 155.

30. Edward Bayard, *Homoeopathia and Nature and Allopathia and Art* (New York: 1858), p. 3.

31. Hahnemann, *Organon,* p. 102.

32. Hahnemann, *The Chronic Diseases; Their Specific Nature and Homoeopathic Treatment,* cited in Kaufman, *Homoeopathy in America,* p. 26.

33. John F. Gray, *Early Annals of Homoeopathy in New York* (New York, 1863), cited in Kett, *The Formation of the American Medical Profession,* p. 141.

34. The best works on hydropathy in American are Harry Weiss's and Howard Kimble's *The Great American Water Cure Craze* (Trenton, N.J.: The Past Times Press, 1967) and Marshall Scott Legan's "Hydropathy, or the Water-Cure," in Arthur Wrobel, ed., *Pseudo-Science and Society in Nineteenth-Century America* (Lexington: University of Kentucky Press, 1987), pp. 74–99. For additional historical background in American water-cures, see Carl Bridenbaugh, "Baths and Watering Places of Colonial America," *The William and Mary Quarterly* 3 (1946): 151–181; and Marshall Scott Legan, "Hydropathy in America: A Nineteenth Century Panacea," *Bulletin of the History of Medicine* 45 (1971): 267–280.

35. Joel Shew, *The Water-Cure Manual* (New York: La Morte Barney, 1847), p. 36.

36. See G. H. Taylor's "Philosophy of Water-Cure," in *Water-Cure Journal* 19 (1855): 2.

37. Henry L. Nichols, "A Review of the 'Pathies,' " *Water-Cure Journal* 12 (1851): 26. See also "The Horrors of Allopathy," *ibid.,* p. 138.

38. Unsigned editorial entitled "The Natural State of Man," in *Water-Cure Journal* 12 (1851): 25.

39. Unsigned article in *Water-Cure World* 1 (April 1860): 5. This citation appears in Catherine Albanese's superb essay "Physic and Metaphysic in Nineteenth-Century America: Medical Sectarians and Religious Healing," *Church History* 55 (1986): 489–502.

40. Russell Trall, *Water-Cure Journal* 11 (1851): 13.

41. James C. Jackson, "Considerations for Common Folks—No. 4," *Water-Cure Journal* 10 (1850): 97.

42. Susan Cayleff, *"Wash and Be Healed": The Water-Cure Movement and Women's Health* (Philadelphia: Temple University Press, 1987).

43. Cited in Susan Cayleff's "Gender, Ideology, and the Water-Cure Movement," in Norman Gevitz, ed., *Other Healers: Unorthodox Medicine in America* (Baltimore: The Johns Hopkins University Press, 1988), p. 86.

44. Stephen Nissenbaum, *Sex, Diet, and Debility in Jacksonian America* (Westport, Conn.: Greenwood Press, 1980), p. ix.

45. James C. Whorton, *Crusaders For Fitness: The History of American Health Reformers* (Princeton: Princeton University Press, 1982), p. 40.

46. Sylvester Graham, *Journal of Health* 2 (1830): 164. Citation found in Nissenbaum, *Sex, Diet, and Debility,* p. 80.

47. Sylvester Graham, *Chastity in a Course of Lectures to Young Men* (New York, 1857), p. v.

48. Sylvester Graham, *Lectures on the Science of Human Life,* 2 vols. (Boston, 1839), 1: vi.

49. Ibid., p. 265.

50. *North American Review* 47 (1838), as cited in Kett, *The Formation of the American Medical Profession,* p. 123.

51. An excellent study of the health philosophy at the core of Ellen G. White's ministry is to be found in Ronald L. Numbers, *Prophetess of Health: A Study of Ellen G. White* (New York: Harper and Row, 1976).

52. Ellen G. White, cited in Gerald Carson, *Cornflake Crusade* (New York: Rinehart and Co., 1957), p. 5.

53. Cited in Numbers, *Prophetess,* p. 105.

54. See Arthur Wrobel's introduction to his *Pseudo-Science and Society in Nineteenth-Century America.*

55. Stephen Nissenbaum, *Sex, Diet, and Debility,* pp. 136 ff.

56. Albanese, "Physic and Metaphysic."

57. W. O. Woodbury, "Homoeopathy the Only True Medical Practice," cited in Albanese, "Physic and Metaphysic," p. 493.

Chapter 3

1. A more complete account of Poyen's lecture tour can be found in my *Mesmerism and the American Cure of Souls* (Philadelphia: University of Pennsylvania Press, 1982). This chapter is, in fact, constructed from materials presented in that book. The citation here comes from Poyen's personal account of his efforts on behalf of mesmerism, entitled *Progress of Animal Magnetism in New England* (Boston: Weeks, Jordan, 1837).

2. The best secondary accounts of Mesmer's life and theories are Henri Ellenberger, *The Discovery of the Unconscious* (New York: Basic Books, 1970); Vincent Buranelli, *Franz Anton Mesmer: The Wizard from Vienna* (New York: McCann, Cowan, and Geoghegan, 1975); Margaret Gold-

smith, *Franz Anton Mesmer: The History of an Idea* (London: Barkert, 1934); and Frank Podmore, *From Mesmer to Christian Science* (New York University Books, 1963).

3. Franz Anton Mesmer, quoted in Ellenberger, *The Discovery of the Unconscious*, p. 62.

4. Poyen, *Progress*, p. 35.

5. William Stone, *Letter to Dr. A. Brigham on Animal Magnetism* (New York: George Dearborn, 1837), p. 81.

6. Poyen, *Progress*, p. 55.

7. A Practical Magnetizer [pseud.], *The History and Philosophy of Animal Magnetism and Practical Instructions for the Exercise of Its Power* (Boston: 1843), p. 8.

8. See LaRoy Sunderland, *"Confessions of a Magnetizer" Exposed* (Boston: Redding, 1845), p. 22.

9. A Gentleman of Philadelphia, *The Philosophy of Animal Magnetism Together with the System of Manipulating Adopted to Produce Ecstasy and Somnambulism* (Philadelphia: Merrihew and Dunn, 1837).

10. See Chauncy Townshend, *Facts in Mesmerism* (London: Bailliere Press, 1844).

11. Ibid., p. 222.

12. Sunderland, *"Confessions,"* p. 22.

13. George Bush, *Mesmer and Swedenborg* (New York: John Allen, 1847), p. 160.

14. Joseph Buchanan, *Neurological System of Anthropology* (Cincinnati: 1854), p. 195.

15. Ibid., Appendix I.

16. Ibid.

17. Poyen, *Progress*, p. 88.

18. Ibid.

19. A Gentleman of Philadelphia, *The Philosophy of Animal Magnetism*, p. 68.

20. Ibid., p. 71.

21. A Practical Magnetizer, *The History and Philosophy of Animal Magnetism*, p. 19.

22. John Dods, *The Philosophy of Electrical Psychology* (New York: Fowler and Wells, 1850), p. 57.

23. Charles G. Finney, *Lectures on Revivals*, cited in William McLoughlin, *Revivals, Awakenings, and Reform* (Chicago: University of Chicago Press, 1978), p. 125.

24. Finney, *Lectures*, cited in William McLoughlin, *Modern Revivalism* (New York: Ronald Press, 1959), p. 84.

25. Finney, *Lectures*, cited in McLoughlin, *Revivals*, p. 126.

26. Whitney R. Cross, *The Burned-Over District* (New York: Harper and Row, 1965), p. 183.

27. Ibid.

28. Ibid., p. 175. The quoted material comes from a November 17, 1830, communication to Finney from William Clark, Cooperstown.

29. Theodore Leger, *Animal Magnetism, or Psychodynamy* (New York: D. Appleton, 1846), p. 18.

30. An especially concise account of "the Swedenborgism impulse" can be found in Sydney Ahlstrom, *A Religious History of the American People* (New Haven: Yale University Press, 1972), pp. 483–488.

31. John Humphrey Noyes, *History of American Socialisms*, cited in Cross, *Burned-Over District*, p. 343.

32. Ahlstrom, *A Religious History*, p. 1019.

33. Cross, *Burned-Over District*, p. 342.

34. An excellent discussion of Swedenborg's influence upon Emerson is to be found in Kenneth W. Cameron's *Young Emerson's Transcendental Vision* (Hartford: Transcendental Books, 1971). Quotation is from p. 297 of this work.

35. Cited in ibid., p. 297.

36. Bush, *Mesmer and Swedenborg*, p. 147.

37. Ibid., p. 69.

38. Ibid., p. 15.

39. Ibid., p. 137.

40. Ellen G. White, *The Ministry of Healing* (Mountain View, Cal.: Pacific Press, 1974), p. 287.

41. Ibid., p. 288.

42. John H. Kellogg, *The Living Temple* (Battle Creek: Good Health Pub. Co., 1903), p. 40.

43. C. W. Post, *I Am Well!* (Boston: Lee and Shepard, 1895), p. 4.

44. Ibid., p. 10.

45. *The Magnetic and Cold Water Guide* 1 (June 1846): 8. This citation comes from Catherine Albanese's "Physic and Metaphysic in Nineteenth-Century America: Medical Sectarians and Religious Healing," *Church History* 55 (1986): 489–502.

46. John F. Gray, *Early Annals of Homoeopathy in New York* (New York, 1963), cited in Joseph Kett's *The Formation of the American Medical Profession: The Role of Institutions, 1780–1860* (New Haven: Yale University Press, 1968), p. 141. Kett further documents the connection between mesmerism and homoeopathy on p. 142, n. 24.

47. Kett, *The Formation of the American Medical Profession*, p. 153.

48. Andrew Jackson Davis, *The Great Harmonia* (Boston: Mussey, 1852), p. 47. The interested reader might wish to consult Robert W. Delp's

"Andrew Jackson Davis and Spiritualism," in Arthur Wrobel, ed., *Pseudo-Science and Society in Nineteenth-Century America* (Lexington: University of Kentucky Press, 1987), pp. 100–121.

49. Andrew Jackson Davis, *The Harmonial Philosophy* (London: William Rider, 1957), p. 76.

50. R. Laurence Moore, *In Search of White Crows* (New York: Oxford University Press, 1977).

51. Phineas P. Quimby, *The Quimby Manuscripts* (New York: Thomas Crowell, 1921), p. 30.

52. Ibid.

53. Ibid., p. 180.

54. Ibid., p. 319.

55. Ibid., p. 62.

56. Ibid., p. 243.

57. Ibid., p. 173.

58. Ibid., p. 210.

59. Mary Baker Eddy's indebtedness to Quimby has been the subject of heated debate. Julius Dresser's *The True History of Mental Science* (Boston: Alfred Budge and Sons, 1887) and his son Horatio's *The History of New Thought* (New York: Crowell Company, 1919) marshaled considerable evidence to show that Mrs. Eddy's writings were little more than garbled distortions of Quimby's unpublished manuscripts. Other detractors of Christian Science's foundress include Richard Daken in his *Mrs. Eddy: The Biography of a Virginal Mind* (New York: Charles Scribner's Sons, 1929) and Stefan Zweig in his *Mental Healers: Anton Mesmer, Mary Baker Eddy, and Sigmund Freud* (New York: F. Ungar Publishing Co., 1962). Mary Baker Eddy's most able apologists are Stephen Gottschalk in his *The Emergence of Christian Science in American Life* (Berkeley: University of California Press, 1973) and Robert Peel in his three-volume biography, *Mary Baker Eddy: The Years of Discovery* (New York: Holt, Rinehart and Winston, 1966), *Mary Baker Eddy: The Years of Trial* (New York: Holt, Rinehart and Winston, 1971), and *Mary Baker Eddy: The Years of Authority* (New York: Holt, Rinehart and Winston, 1977).

60. Mary Baker Eddy, *Manual of the Mother Church* (Boston: A. V. Stewart, 1916), p. 17.

61. Accounts of Evans's life and works can be found in Charles Braden, *Spirits in Rebellion* (Dallas: Southern Methodist University Press, 1963); and John F. Teahan, "Warren Felt Evans and Mental Healing: Romantic Idealism and Practical Mysticism in Nineteenth-Century America," *Church History* 48 (March 1979): 63–80.

62. Warren Felt Evans, *Mental Medicine: A Treatise on Medical Psychology* (Boston: H. H. Carter, 1886), p. 266.

63. Ralph Waldo Trine, *In Tune with the Infinite* (New York: Crowell, 1897), p. 16.

64. Ibid., from the preface.

65. Evans, *Mental Medicine*, p. 104.

66. Ahlstrom, *A Religious History*, p. 1019.

67. Norman Vincent Peale, *The Power of Positive Thinking* (New York: Prentice-Hall, 1952), pp. viii, vii.

68. George Beard, *American Nervousness* (New York: G. P. Putnam, 1881). The interested reader might wish to consult John L. Greenway's " 'Nervous Disease' and Electric Medicine," in Arthur Wrobel's *Pseudo-Science and Society in Nineteenth-Century America.*

69. Arthur Schlesinger, "A Critical Period in American Religion, 1875–1900," *Proceedings of the Massachusetts Historical Society* 64 (1930–32): 523–528.

Chapter 4

1. Cited in Philip Van Ingen, *The New York Academy of Medicine: Its First Hundred Years* (New York: 1949), p. 13.

2. Statistics for the number of practicing chiropractic physicians vary from 13,000 to over 25,000 while estimates of their annual patient load vary from three to more than six million.

3. See the *1986–87 Yearbook and Directory of Osteopathic Physicians,* published by the American Osteopathic Association, and Norman Gevitz's *The D.O.'s: Osteopathic Medicine In America* (Baltimore: Johns Hopkins University Press, 1982).

4. G. F. Riekman, D.C., "Chiropractic," in *The Holistic Health Handbook* (Berkeley: And/Or Press, 1978), pp. 171–174.

5. D. D. Palmer, *The Chiropractor's Adjuster* (Portland, Ore.: Portland Printing House, 1910), p. 319. This volume is also known as *Text-Book of the Science, Art and Philosophy of Chiropractic.*

6. See Joseph E. Maynard, *Healing Hands: The Story of the Palmer Family* (Freeport, N.Y.: Jonorm Pub. Co., 1959), p. 10.

7. Ibid., p. 9. It is interesting to note that the renowned mesmerist and mind-curist Warren Felt Evans wrote: "By the friction of the hand along the spinal column an invigorating life-giving influence is imparted to all the organs within the cavity of the trunk." See his *Mental Medicine: A Treatise on Medical Psychology* (Boston: H. H. Carter, 1886), p. 212.

8. The archives of the Palmer College of Chiropractic library contain the collection of books that D. D. had bound together for convenient reference. Among these are J. W. Caldwell's *How to Mesmerize* (Boston,

1883), E. D. Babbit's *Vital Magnetism* (New York, 1801), and James Wilson's *How To Magnetize, or Magnetism and Clairvoyance* (New York, 1886).

9. Vern Gielow, *Old Dad Chiro* (Davenport, Iowa: Bawden Bros., 1981), p. 58.

10. See Maynard, *Healing Hands*, p. 16.

11. D. D. Palmer, *The Chiropractor's Adjuster*, p. 18.

12. Joseph H. Donahue has argued that by 1910, when D. D. Palmer first published an elaborate account of his theory of Innate, he was far removed from the mainstream of chiropractic activity. See his "D. D. Palmer and Innate Intelligence: Development, Division and Derision," *Chiropractic History* 6 (1986): 31–36. Although I think that Donahue, as well as other current historians seeking to show chiropractic's early commitment to scientific research, minimizes the metaphysical dimensions that Palmer had injected into the movement in its early days, he rightly draws attention to the diversity of thought that characterized chiropractic theory from the start.

13. Ibid., p. 35. Emphasis mine.

14. Ibid., p. 491.

15. For a fuller discussion of D. D. Palmer's view of Innate and its roots in both spiritualism and vitalism, see Donahue, "D. D. Palmer and Innate Intelligence"; Joseph Donahue, "D. D. Palmer and the Metaphysical Movement in the Nineteenth Century," *Chiropractic History* 7 (1987): 23–27; and Walter I. Wardwell, "Before the Palmers: An Overview of Chiropractic's Antecedents," *Chiropractic History* 7 (1987): 27–33.

16. D. D. Palmer, *The Chiroractor's Adjustor*, p. 821. Readers interested in the expansionist cosmology and "emergent evolution" themes in early chiropractic might wish to consult A. A. Erz's "The Science of Life and Chiropractic Research," *The Chiropractor* 3 (December 1907): 30–35, and Joy Luban's "Dual Evolution," *The Chiropractor* 5 (March 1909): 67–76.

17. Palmer himself acknowledged, "I saw fit to date the beginning of Chiropractic with the first adjustment (1895), although quite a portion of that which now constitutes Chiropractic I had collected during the previous nine years" (*The Chiropractor's Adjuster*, p. 101).

18. Ibid., p. 52.

19. *The Chiropractor* 5 (1909): Inside front cover. Note: D. D. Palmer severed ties with the Palmer School of Chiropractic medicine and his role as editor of *The Chiropractor* in 1906. This wording is, however, consistent with earlier versions appearing on the inside of the front cover of this journal and more readily lent itself to use in this paragraph.

20. *The Chiropractor* 1 (1905): Inside front cover.

21. Ibid.

22. See Whitney Cross's discussion of ultraism in *The Burned-Over District* (New York: Harper and Row, 1965), pp. 173, 187, 274–277, 342.

23. D. D. Palmer, *The Chiropractor's Adjuster,* p. 497.

24. Ibid., p. 8.

25. Ibid.

26. A discussion of B. J.'s role in developing chiropractic philosophy can be found in a book by his devoted disiple A. August Dye, entitled *The Evolution of Chiropractic* (Philadelphia; A. August Dye, 1939).

27. B. J. Palmer, quoted in Dye, *The Evolution,* p. 31.

28. Julius Dintenfass, *Chiropractic: A Modern Way to Health* (New York: Pyramid Books, 1975), p. 65.

29. See, for example, Peter Bryner's discussion of this issue entitled "Isn't It Time to Abandon Anachronistic Terminology?" in *Journal of the Australian Chiropractor's Association* 17 (June 1987): 53–59.

30. A. E. Homewood, *The Neurodynamics of the Vertebral Subluxation* (Thornwood, Ont.: Chiropractic Publishing, 1962), p. 174.

31. See Robert Ellwood, *Alternative Altars* (Chicago: University of Chicago Press, 1979).

32. B. J. Palmer, *Do Chiropractors Pray?* (Davenport, Iowa: The Palmer School of Chiropractic, 1911), p. 25.

33. Ibid., p. 27.

34. See B. J. Palmer, *The Bigness of the Fellow Within* (Davenport, Iowa: The Palmer School of Chiropractic, 1949), p. 25. See also W. I. Miller's connection of Jesus's healing ministry and chiropractic in his "Chiropractic—Reasons for Its Existence," *The Chiropractor* 4 (August 1908): 11–13.

35. Note, for example, how A. August Dye boasted of having had "the rare fortune of knowing personally the Discoverer" for whom he has a "sincere reverence" (*The Evolution of Chiropractic,* p. 11). Joseph Maynard makes the hagiographic disclaimer that

> B. J. is not a superman. He is not physically "different" from other men. But he is perhaps more practical because he let Innate direct him. . . . He listened to Innate Intelligence. Innate led him to the right action; Innate gave him the right words to say. (*Healing Hands, p. 77*)

36. This literature is surveyed in Gregory Firman and Michael Goldstein, "The Future of Chiropractic: A Psychosocial View," *The New England Journal of Medicine* 293 (September 25, 1975): 639–642. Readers might also wish to consult the responses to this somewhat controversial issue in Volume 294 (February 5, 1976) of the same periodical. Representative studies of chiropractic professional commitment are the Stanford Research Insti-

tute's *Chiropractic in California* (Los Angeles: Haynes Foundation, 1960); Donald Mills, *Study of Chiropractors, Osteopaths and Naturopaths in Canada* (Ottawa: The Queen's Printer, 1966); and Marjorie White and James Skipper, "The Chiropractic Physician: A Study of Career Contingencies," *Journal of Health and Social Behavior* 12 (1971): 300–306.

37. See White and Skipper, "The Chiropractic Physician"; and Walter Wardell, "A Marginal Professional Role: the Chiropractor," in W. Richard Scott and Edmund Volkart, eds., *Medical Care* (New York: John Wiley and Sons, 1966), pp. 51–67.

38. See Firman and Goldstein, "The Future of Chiropractic," p. 640.

39. Ibid.

40. A helpful review of the tension between "cultism and science" in chiropractic history is Russell W. Gibbons's "Chiropractic in America: The Historical Conflicts of Cultism and Science," *Journal of Popular Culture* 10 (1977): 720–731.

41. Dintenfass, *Chiropractic*, and Thorp McClusky, *Your Health and Chiropractic* (New York: Pyramid Books, 1962).

42. McClusky, *Your Health*, p. 48.

43. *Abundant Living* 49 (1973): Back cover.

44. Riekman, "Chiropractic," p. 174.

45. Gevitz, *The D.O.'s*, p. 2. A good deal of the following narrative of osteopathy draws upon Gevitz's work.

46. Andrew Taylor Still, *Autobiography of Andrew T. Still* (Kirksville, Mo.: Published by the author, 1897), p. 99.

47. Ibid., p. 112.

48. Ibid., pp. 115–116.

49. Ibid., pp. 275 and 226.

50. Ibid., p. 235.

51. Ibid., pp. 289–290.

52. Ibid., p. 108.

53. Ibid., p. 275.

54. Ibid., p. 196.

55. Ibid., p. 221.

56. Ibid., p. 309.

57. Henry S. Bunting, "The Real A. T. Still," cited in Gevitz, *The D.O.'s*, p. 20.

58. "Report of the Committee for the Study of Relations between Osteopathy and Medicine, *Journal of the American Medical Association* 152 (1953): 734–739, cited in Gevitz, *The D.O.'s*, p. 109.

59. See Gevitz's discussions "A Question of Identity," "Osteopathy's Lesion," in *The D.O.'s*, pp. 88–98 and 141–144, respectively.

60. Russell Gibbons, "The Evolution of Chiropractic's Medical and So-

cial Protest in America," in Scott Haldeman, ed., *Modern Developments in the Principles and Practice of Chiropractic* (New York: Appleton-Century-Crofts, 1979), p. 13. See also James Brantingham's helpful article "Still and Palmer: The Impact of the First Osteopath and the First Chiropractor," in *Journal of Chiropractic History* 6 (1986): 19–22.

61. E. R. Booth, *History of Osteopathy* (Kirkville, Mo.: Privately published, 1924).

62. Andrew Taylor Still, *The Philosophy and Mechanical Principles of Osteopathy* (Kansas City, Mo.: Hudson-Kimberly, Pub., 1902), p. 17.

63. Ibid., p. 13.

64. L.E.W., "Law, Infinite and Finite," *Journal of Osteopathy* (October 1891): 3.

65. See, for example, Lizzie Walker's "Health: What It Is and How Obtained," *Journal of Osteopathy* 1 (September 1894): 4.

66. *Journal of Osteopathy* (May 1894), p. 1. See also E. E. Tucker's "Osteopathic Campaign," *Journal of Osteopathy* 9 (December 1901): 413–417.

67. "Vis Mediatrix Naturae," *Journal of Osteopathy* 4 (November 1897): 275.

68. *Journal of Osteopathy* 3 (March 1897): 6.

69. In the early years osteopathic physicians were regularly confused with spiritualists, mesmerists, Theosophists, Christian Scientists, and practitioners of Swedish massage. Many took out advertisements in newspapers or printed brochures to distance themselves from their "nonscientific" counterparts at the fringes of medical orthodoxy. Not that these disclaimers always worked. Upon hearing a careful explanation that osteopathy was not identical to Theosophy, a woman from Cleveland, Ohio, is said to have remarked, "Oh, it's all the same thing." See Gevitz, *The D. O.'s,* pp. 35–36.

Chapter 5

1. Mary Belknap, Robert Blau, and Rosaline Grossman, eds., *Case Studies and Methods in Humanistic Medicine* (San Francisco: Institute for the Study of Humanistic Medicine, 1973, 1975), p. 18.

2. Herbert A. Otto and James W. Knight, eds., *Dimensions in Wholistic Healing: New Frontiers In the Treatment of the Whole Person* (Chicago: Nelson-Hall, 1979), p. 3.

3. Ibid., p. 10.

4. Ibid., p. 13.

5. Kenneth Pelletier, *Holistic Medicine* (New York: Delacorte Press, 1979), p. 93.

6. Ibid., p. 94. Fritjof Capra, *The Tao of Physics* (Boulder, Colo.: Shambhala Press, 1975).

7. Norman Cousins, *Anatomy of an Illness* (New York: W. W. Norton, 1979), p. 48.

8. See, for example, *The Varieties of Religious Experience* (New York: P. F. Collier, Inc., 1961), where James writes:

> The whole drift of my education goes to persuade me that the world of our present consciousness is only one out of many worlds of consciousness that exist, and that those other worlds must contain experiences which have a meaning for our life also; and that although in the main their experiences and those of this world keep discrete, yet the two become continuous at certain points, and higher energies filter in. (p. 401)

And in *A Pluralistic Universe* (New York: E. P. Dutton, 1971), James describes the "deeper reaches" of human nature as follows:

> The phenomenon is that of new ranges of life succeeding on our most despairing moments. There are resources in us that naturalism with its literal and legal virtues never recks of, possibilities that take our breath away, of another kind of happiness and power, based on giving up our own will and letting something higher work for us, and these seem to show a world wider than either physics or philistine ethics can imagine. (p. 266)

9. Norman Cousins, *Human Options* (New York: W. W. Norton, 1981), p. 167.

10. Halbert Dunn, "What High-Level Wellness Means," *Health Values: Achieving High-Level Wellness* 1 (1977): 10.

11. Ibid., p. 11.

12. "Interview with Bernard Siegel," in *ReVISION* 7 (Sering, 1984): 92.

13. Belknap, Blau, and Grossman, *Case Studies*, p. 18.

14. See Robert C. Fuller, *Americans and the Unconscious* (New York: Oxford University Press, 1986).

15. *The Holistic Health Handbook* (Berkeley: And-Or Press, 1978), p. 13. See also *A Visual Encyclopedia of Unconventional Medicine* (New York: Crown Publications, 1978) and Leslie Kaslof, ed., *Wholistic Dimensions in Healing* (Garden City, N.Y.: Doubleday & Co., 1978).

16. Robert S. Ellwood, *Alternative Altars* (Chicago: University of Chicago Press, 1979), p. 168.

17. *The Holistic Health Handbook*, p. 17.

18. Dolores Krieger, *The Therapeutic Touch* (Engelwood Cliffs, N.J.: Prentice-Hall, Inc., 1979), p. 11.

19. Ibid., p. 13. Krieger's reference to "channeling" healing energy, or *prana*, clearly indicates that she is speaking of a metaphysical force. What distinguishes gifted healers from other individuals is not their possession of superior amounts of *prana* but their superior "access" to it. Krieger further indi-

cates the extramundane, transpersonal character of *prana* when she states that it is the energy of the medium that makes telepathy possible (p. 70).

20. Ibid., p. 77.

21. Ibid., pp. 77, 80.

22. *Alcoholics Anonymous*, 2d ed. (New York: Alcoholics Anonymous, 1955), p. 569.

23. Ernest Kurtz, *Not-God: A History of Alcoholics Anonymous* (Center City, Mon.: Hazelden Press, 1979).

24. Cited in Kurtz, *Not-God*, pp. 19–20.

25. Ibid., p. 21.

26. *Twelve Steps and Twelve Traditions* (New York: Alcoholics Anonymous, 1952), p. 63.

27. Ibid., p. 37.

28. Ambrose Worrall and Olga Worrall, *The Miracle Healers* (New York: Signet Books, 1969), p. 141.

29. Ibid.

30. Edwina Cerutli discusses the Worralls' Christian faith in her *Olga Worrall: Mystic with the Healing Hands* (New York: Harper and Row, 1975).

31. Paul Krafchik, *A Complete Course in Parapsychology*, 10 vols. (Sherman Oaks, Cal.: American Parapsychological Research Foundation, 1971), 9: 3.

32. Irving Oyle, *The Healing Mind* (Millbrae, Cal.: Celestial Arts Pub. Co., 1979), p. 96.

33. Ibid., p. 44.

34. Ibid.

35. Ibid., p. 83.

36. See Thomas Sugrue, *There Is a River* (New York: Dell Publishing Co., 1979); and Jess Stearn, *Edgar Cayce—the Sleeping Prophet* (New York: Doubleday & Co., 1967).

37. A "Fact Sheet" published by the Association for Research and Enlightenment (Virginia Beach, Va.) states that they have 36,000 members worldwide, there are 160,000 persons on their mailing list, their press sells 283,000 books annually, and that more than twelve million books on Edgar Cayce have been sold to date.

38. Stanley Krippner and Alberto Villoldo, *The Realms of Healing* (Millbrae, Cal.: Celestial Arts, 1976), p. 72.

39. Ibid., p. 69.

40. Krippner's and Villoldo's own assessment of psychic healing reveals the great extent to which the movement is motivated by a spiritual and cognitive malaise: "In summary, it is quite possible that research in paranormal healing will eventually result in a paradigm shift and necessitate a revision of our scientific world-view" (p. 48).

41. Lawrence LeShan, *The Medium, the Mystic, and the Physicist* (New York: Viking Press, 1974), p. 109.

42. Ibid., p. 167.

43. See Stewart Edward White's *The Betty Book* (New York: E. P. Dutton, 1937) and *The Unobstructed Universe* (New York: E. P. Dutton, 1940); Elizabeth Clare Prophet, *The Great White Brotherhood* (Los Angeles: Summit University Press, 1975); and Jane Roberts, *The Seth Material* (Englewood Cliffs, N.J.: Prentice-Hall, 1970).

44. Steven Weinberg, *Ramtha* (Eastbound, Wa.: Sovereignty Press, 1986), p. 2.

45. Shirley MacLaine, *Dancing in the Light* (New York: Bantam Books, 1985), p. 37. See also Shirley MacLaine, *Out on a Limb* (New York: Bantam Books, 1983).

46. MacLaine, *Dancing in the Light,* p. 111.

47. Daya Sarai Chocron, *Healing with Crystals and Gemstones* (York Beach, Maine: Samuel Weiser, 1983), p. 3. See also Stephan G. Ouseley, *Power of the Rays* (London: Fowler, 1981); Betty Wood, *Healing Power of Color* (New York: Destiny, 1984); and David Tansley, *Chakras—Rays and Radionics* (London: Saffron Walden, 1984).

48. Chocron, *Healing with Crystals* p. 4.

49. Charles von Reichenbach, *Vital Force: Physico-Physiological Researches on the Dynamics of Magnetism, Electricity, Heat, Light, Crystallization Chemism in their Relations to Vital Force* (New York: Redfield, Clinton-Hall, 1851), p. 81.

50. Chocron, *Healing with Crystals,* p. 34.

51. Korra Deaver, *Rock Crystal: The Magic Stone* (York Beach, Maine: Samuel Weiser, 1985), p. 36. Readers might also wish to consult Randall Baer and Vicki Baer, *Windows of Light* (New York: Harper and Row, 1984); Ra Bonewitz, *Cosmic Crystals* (Wellingborough, U.K.: Turnstone Press, 1983); William B. Crow, *Precious Stones: Their Occult Power and Hidden Significance* (York Beach, Maine: Samuel Weiser, 1968); Edgar Cayce, *Scientific Properties and Occult Aspects of 22 Gems, Stones and Metals* (Virginia Beach: ARE Press, 1974), Elizabeth Finch, *The Psychic Value of Gemstones* (Cottonwood, Ariz.: Esoteric Publications, 1979); and John Melville, *Crystal Gazing and Clairvoyance* (York Beach, Maine: Samuel Weiser, 1974).

52. Deaver, *Rock Crystal,* p. 17.

53. Ibid., p. 40.

54. An intriguing account of an American woman's self-proclaimed status as a shamaness and her psychopompic use of crystals is Lynn Andrews's *Crystal Woman* (New York: Warner Books, 1987).

55. Deaver, *Rock Crystal,* p. 2.

56. Ibid., p. 16.

57. Chocron, *Healing with Crystals,* p. 100.

58. Deaver, *Rock Crystal,* p. 46.

59. Katrina Raphael, *Crystal Healing: The Therapeutic Application of Crystals and Stones* (New York: Aurora Press, 1987), pp. 20–21. This volume complements Ms. Raphael's *Crystal Enlightenment: The Transforming Properties of Crystals and Healing Stones* (New York: Aurora Press, 1985).

60. Deaver, *Rock Crystal,* p. 17.

61. Ibid., p. 7.

62. *Prevention* magazine, for example, proselytizes for obedience to the God-given laws of nutrition and nonmedical healing. As with its companion volumes, *The Prevention Method For Better Health* (Emmaus, Penn.: Rodale Books, 1960) and *The Complete Book of Vitamins* (Emmaus, Penn.: Rodale Books, 1966), *Prevention* urges its readers to discipline their will in accordance with the divinely ordained laws of nature. However, Ronald Deutsch has pointed out that the founder of *Prevention,* Jerome Rodale, was occasionally prone to metaphysical jargon. Deutsch's fascinating *The New Nuts Among the Berries: How Nutrition Nonsense Captured America* (Palo Alto: Bull Publications, 1977) quotes Rodale recommending direct contact with plants because your hands can "drain their health-giving electrical charges into your body" (p. 10).

63. A helpful overview of the contemporary fusion of religion and healing among Afro-American traditions can be found in Albert J. Rabeteau's article, "Afro-American Traditions," in Ronald Numbers and Darrel Amundsen, eds., *Caring and Curing: Health and Medicine in the Western Religious Traditions* (New York: Macmillan, 1986). See also Jacquelyne J. Jackson's "Urban Black Americans," in Alan Hardwood, ed., *Ethnicity and Medical Care* (Cambridge, Mass.: Harvard University Press, 1981).

64. William McLoughlin, *Revivals, Awakenings and Reform* (Chicago: University of Chicago Press, 1978).

65. Ibid., p. 214.

66. Robert Ellwood, *Alternative Altars* (Chicago: University of Chicago Press, 1979), p. 33. Emphasis mine.

Chapter 6

1. See Larry Shiner, "The Concept of Secularization in Empirical Research," *Journal for the Scientific Study of Religion* 6 (1967): 207–220.

2. Robert Ellwood, *Alternative Altars* (Chicago: University of Chicago Press, 1979), p. 171.

3. *The Holistic Health Handbook* (Berkeley: And/Or Press, 1978), p. 13.

4. Ibid.

5. Dolores Krieger, *Therapeutic Touch* (Englewood Cliffs, N.J.: Prentice-Hall, Inc., 1979), p. 108.

6. Ambrose Worrall and Olga Worrall, *The Miracle Healers* (New York: Signet Books, 1968), p. 111. Emphasis mine.

7. Mircea Eliade, *Rites and Symbols of Initiation* (New York: Harper and Row, 1965), p. 3. The masculine gender is Eliade's.

8. Richard Katz's *Boiling Energy: Community Healing Among the Kalahari Kung* (Cambridge, Mass.: Harvard University Press, 1982) is an example of excellent scholarship concerning the role in which belief in a subtle energy (which the Kung call *num*) plays in both healing individuals and creating cultural cohesion.

9. Joy Lubove, "Dual Evolution," *The Chiropractor* 5 (1909): 74.

10. Krieger, *Therapeutic Touch*, p. 108.

11. Janet Quinn, "Therapeutic Touch: One Nurse's Evolution as a Healer," in Marianne Borelli and Patricia Heidt, eds., *Therapeutic Touch: A Book of Readings* (New York: Springer Pub. Co., 1981), p. 62.

12. See, for example, Patricia Heidt's "Scientific Research and Therapeutic Touch," Marianne Borelli's "Meditation and Therapeutic Touch," Janet Macrae's "Therapeutic Touch: A Way of Life," and Honore Fontes's "Self-Healing: Getting in Touch with Self to Promote Healing," all included in Borelli and Heidt, *Therapeutic Touch: A Book of Readings*.

13. See Arnold van Gennep, *The Rites of Passage* (London: Routledge and Kegan Paul, 1909); and Victor Turner, *The Ritual Process* (Ithaca: Cornell University Press, 1977).

14. Turner, *The Ritual Process*, p. 106.

15. Ibid., p. 139.

16. William Clebsch and Charles Jaekle, *Pastoral Care in Historical Perspective* (New York: Jason Aronson, 1975).

17. Karl Sabbagh, "The Psychopathology of Fringe Medicine," *Skeptical Inquirer* 10 (Winter 1985–86): 154–164.

18. William Nolen, *Healing: A Doctor in Search of a Miracle* (New York: Random House, 1974), p. 282.

19. See Ari Kiev, *Transcultural Psychiatry* (New York: The Free Press, 1972); E. Fuller Torrey, *The Mind Game* (New York: Bantam Books, 1973); and Jerome Frank, *Persuasion and Healing* (New York: Schocken Books, 1963).

20. Frank, *Persuasion and Healing*, p. 63.

21. Meredith McGuire, "Words of Power: Personal Empowerment and Healing," *Culture Medicine and Psychiatry* 7 (1983): 221–240.

22. Ibid., p. 230.

23. See, for example, the collection of essays in Zbigniew J. Lipowski, Don R. Lipsitt, and Peter C. Shybrow, eds., *Psychosomatic Medicine: Cur-*

rent Trends and Clinical Applications (New York: Oxford University Press, 1977).

24. See, for example, M. Friedman and R. Rosenman, "Type A Behavior Pattern: Its Association with Coronary Heart Disease," *Annals of Clinical Research* 3 (1971): 300–312; Michael Marmot, "Culture and Illness: Epidemiological Evidence," in Margaret J. Christie and Peter Mellett, eds., *Foundations of Psychosomatics* (New York: John Wiley and Sons, 1981); Victor Frankl, *Man's Search for Meaning* (Boston: Beacon Press, 1946); Robert Ader, *Psychoneuroimmunology* (New York: The Academic Press, 1981); and Jane Goldberg, *Psychotherapeutic Treatment of Cancer Patients* (New York: The Free Press, 1981).

25. See Lawrence Hinkle, "The Concept of 'Stress' in the Biological and Social Sciences," in Lipowski, Lipsitt, and Shybrow, *Psychosomatic Medicine*, pp. 14–26.

26. A great deal of this section is indebted to David Barnard's "Psychosomatic Medicine and the Problem of Meaning," *Bulletin of the Menninger Clinic* 49 (1985): 10–28.

27. Henry Guntrip, "Religion in Relation to Personal Integration," *The British Journal of Medical Psychology* 42 (1969): 323–333.

28. See Heinz Kohut, *The Search for the Self* (New York: International Universities Press, 1978); and Christopher Lasch, *The Culture of Narcissism* (New York: W. W. Norton, 1970).

29. Kohut, *The Search for the Self,* p. 459.

30. Otto and Knight, *Dimensions in Wholistic Healing* (Chicago: Nelson-Hall, 1979), p. 13.

31. D. W. Winnicott, *Playing and Reality* (London: Tavistock Publications, 1971), p. 14.

32. Marie Rizutto, *The Birth of the Living God* (Chicago: University of Chicago Press, 1979), p. 193.

33. Leon Eisenberg, "The Physician as Interpreter: Ascribing Meaning to the Illness Experience," *Comprehensive Psychiatry* 22 (1981): 239.

34. Jill Ireland, *Life Wish* (Boston: Little, Brown and Company, 1987).

35. Peter Homans, *Jung in Context* (Chicago: University of Chicago Press, 1979), p. 194.

36. Donald Capps, "Religion and Psychological Well-Being," in *The Sacred in a Secular Age* (Berkeley: University of California Press, 1985), p. 242.

37. William James, "The Will to Believe," in his *The Will to Believe* (New York: Dover Publications, 1956), p. 3.

Index

159

Tankers Full of Trouble

Tankers Full

The Perilous Journey

of Trouble

of Alaskan Crude

Eric Nalder

Grove Press
New York

Published simultaneously in Canada
Printed in the United States of America

FIRST EDITION

Library of Congress Cataloging-in-Publication Data

Nalder, Eric.
    Tankers full of trouble: the perilous journey of Alaskan crude /   Eric Nalder.
    ISBN 0-8021-1458-X
    1. Arco Anchorage (Oil tanker) 2. Petroleum—Transportation.
   3. Tankers—Accidents—Environmental aspects.   I. Title.
    VM455.N27   1994
    387.2′45—dc20   93-31198

Design by Laura Hough

Grove Press
841 Broadway
New York, NY 10003

10 9 8 7 6 5 4 3 2 1

To Jan Christiansen Nalder
My best friend

Acknowledgments

I was humbled by this project and am beholden to the people who made it possible. My wife, Jan Christiansen, could have been named a coauthor for all her work and advice. And I tip my watch cap to the tanker *Arco Anchorage,* while wishing it a following sea for the rest of its oceangoing life. I hope Captain Jack Carroll has a safe career and a great cook on every tour. And without Jerry Aspland, Arco fleet president, my task would have been impossible. Bryan Oettel was the best editor anyone could have hoped for. My agent Arnold Goodman inspired the whole thing and stayed with it when others might have paled. Grove Press, now part of Grove/Atlantic, was a generous publisher, and in that I am especially honored by the steady backing of Anton Mueller and Joan Bingham.

As for my search for the right language, I bow to my teachers: Kathy Triesch, Dave Boardman, Tom Brown, Joel Connelly, Tim Egan, and Bill Dietrich.

A special nod goes to four data collection services that generously supplied extra information: Arthur McKenzie's Tanker Advisory Center; the *Oil Spill Intelligence Report,* published by Cutter Information Corp.; Richard Golob's *Oil Pollution Bulletin;* and Lloyd's Maritime Information Services, Inc. (and special thanks to account executive Lorraine Parsons).

Acknowledgments

I applaud certain people who offered reams of material and ideas: James Atkinson, Charles Bookman, Fred Felleman, Bill Gossert, Charles Hamel, Virgil Keith, Dan Lawn, Norm Lemley, Arthur McKenzie, George Reinhard, Rene Roussel, Charles Thorne, Walter Parker, Tom Purtell, Mary Robey, Daniel Sheehan, and Ed Wenk.

Scores of other people explained to me the sea, the tanker trade, Alaska, and maritime politics, and the best among them were: Joe Angelo, James Card, William Chadwick, Dorothy Clifton, Charles Deschamps, Harry Dudley, Al Dujenksi, Steve Finley, Rich Fitzpatrick, William O. Gray, Kirk Greiner, Gene Henn, Hewitt Jackson, Roger Kohn, Larry Lockwood, Bill Masciarelli, Jack O'Dell, William Petersen, Robert Safarik, Steve Scalzo, John L. Sullivan, W. G. (Tom) Tomasovic, Thomas Tucker, John Waterhouse, Jim Watson, Ron Weightman, John Wiechert, and Tom Wyman. And thanks to James McFarlane for the artwork.

I appreciate the patience of the January 1992 crew of the *Arco Anchorage:* Svetko Lisica, Jean Holmes, Gregory Dean Davis, George Peloso, Scott Nehrenz, Ralph Schramm, Marvin Cropper, Mike Gussie, Pat Newman, Larry Bratnyk, Jimmy Doyle, James Vives, Robert Rich, Paul Hogan, William Harrison, Dennis Meehan, Daryl Akery, Neal Curtis, Ruben Garcia, and Thomas Hilken. I also appreciate the members of the May 1989 crew, especially Captain Robert Lawlor and chief engineer Paul Preziose.

I am grateful to the *Seattle Times* and to the *Seattle Times* library for their help and patience. And I thank my daughter Britt for just being there.

I aspire in this book to have been as diligent as others who have written about tankers before me, including Pat Coburn, Art Davidson, Noel Mostert, and Jonathan Wills, to name a few.

Contents

Contents

The Ship

S.S. *Arco Anchorage*

Deadweight tonnage: 120,357
Displacement weight, fully loaded: 160,160 (standard tons)
Tons of steel in the structure: 22,586
Length: 883 feet
Beam: 138 feet
Distance from keel to highest point: 160 feet
Depth of hull in water, fully loaded: 50 to 53 feet
Shaft horsepower: 26,000 h.p.
Standard cruising speed: 16 nautical miles per hour
Number of operating propellers: One
Diameter of propeller: 27 feet 6 inches
Weight of propeller: 47 tons
Number of rudders: One
Weight of rudder: 82 tons
Weight of one anchor: 29,800 pounds
Number of cargo tanks: 13
Maximum cargo capacity: 942,656 barrels* (39,591,552 gallons)
Cargo on January 1992 voyage: 820,700 barrels (34,469,400 gallons)
Oil cleanup capability: Limited amount of sorbent material on board
Year built: 1973

*1 barrel = 42 gallons

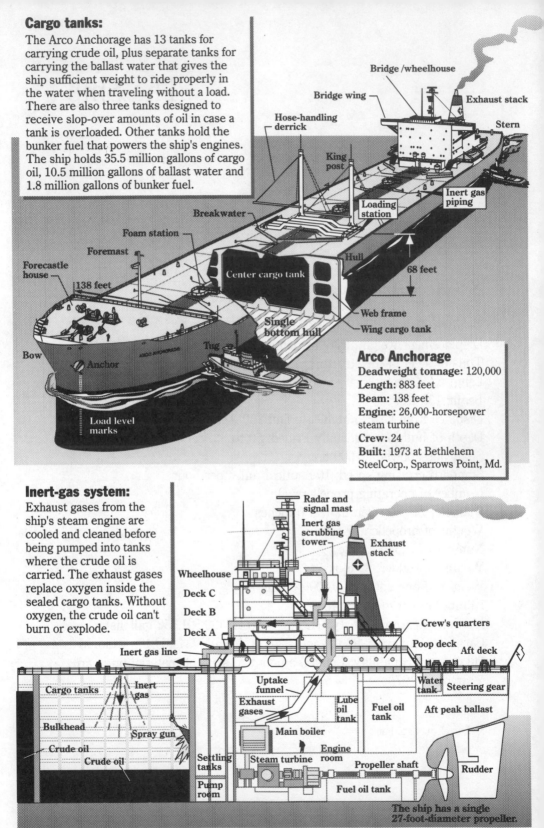

Cargo tanks:

The Arco Anchorage has 13 tanks for carrying crude oil, plus separate tanks for carrying the ballast water that gives the ship sufficient weight to ride properly in the water when traveling without a load. There are also three tanks designed to receive slop-over amounts of oil in case a tank is overloaded. Other tanks hold the bunker fuel that powers the ship's engines. The ship holds 35.5 million gallons of cargo oil, 10.5 million gallons of ballast water and 1.8 million gallons of bunker fuel.

Bridge /wheelhouse

Bridge wing

Exhaust stack

Stern

Hose-handling derrick

King post

Inert gas piping

Loading station

Breakwater

Foam station

Foremast

Forecastle house

138 feet

Center cargo tank

Hull

68 feet

Single bottom hull

Web frame

Wing cargo tank

Bow

Anchor

Tug

Load level marks

Arco Anchorage
Deadweight tonnage: 120,000
Length: 883 feet
Beam: 138 feet
Engine: 26,000-horsepower steam turbine
Crew: 24
Built: 1973 at Bethlehem SteelCorp., Sparrows Point, Md.

Inert-gas system:

Exhaust gases from the ship's steam engine are cooled and cleaned before being pumped into tanks where the crude oil is carried. The exhaust gases replace oxygen inside the sealed cargo tanks. Without oxygen, the crude oil can't burn or explode.

Radar and signal mast

Inert gas scrubbing tower

Exhaust stack

Wheelhouse

Deck C

Deck B

Deck A

Crew's quarters

Poop deck

Aft deck

Inert gas line

Cargo tanks

Inert gas

Bulkhead

Crude oil

Crude oil

Spray gun

Uptake funnel

Exhaust gases

Main boiler

Settling tanks

Pump room

Steam turbine

Engine room

Lube oil tank

Fuel oil tank

Water tank

Steering gear

Aft peak ballast

Propeller shaft

Fuel oil tank

Rudder

The ship has a single 27-foot-diameter propeller.

The Crew

Deck Officers

Captain: John A. (Jack) Carroll
Chief Mate: Svetko Lisica
Second mate: Jean M. Holmes
Third mate: Gregory Dean Davis
Radio officer: George J. Peloso

Deck Crew

Bosun: Scott Nehrenz
Able-bodied seaman (A/B): Ralph D. Schramm
A/B: Marvin S. Cropper
A/B: Mike Gussie
A/B: Patrick G. Newman
A/B: Lawrence (Larry) Bratnyk
Utility: James (Jimmy) E. Doyle
Pumpman: Dennis E. Meehan
Relief pumpman: Daryl Akery

Engine room officers

Chief Engineer: James Vives
First engineer: Robert F. Rich
Second engineer: Paul G. Hogan
Third engineer: William L. (Bill) Harrison

Engine room crew

Engineman: Neal T. Curtis
Engineman: Ruben J. Garcia
Engineman: Thomas C. Hilken

Galley Crew

Chief steward: Patrick T. Rogers
Cook/Baker: William J. (Willie) Herbert, Jr.
Messman: David A. Chun
Messman: Jon E. Niemisto

Preface

No machine has ever possessed the incredible mass, momentum, and physics of a modern oil tanker, and few other machines are capable of such environmental damage.

Like clockwork a crude-laden colossus sails half-hourly into an American port. Worldwide, there are billions of gallons of oil afloat on the oceans: water and oil—two incompatible fluids separated by a membrane of steel. Mathematicians say the odds-on likeliest sites for the next major American spill are the waters around the common tanker destinations: New York, Philadelphia, Houston, Long Beach, San Francisco Bay, or the Strait of Juan de Fuca. But don't count on it. Computers have never found a pattern to the tanker disaster, just a guarantee that another one will plague us before the year has passed. Randomly these ships blacken the beaches of the globe; one day it is the Strait of Malacca and another it is the Shetland Islands, or the coast of Spain, or the shores of Africa.

A world that guzzles thirty thousand gallons of oil a second makes no peace with any shoreline. Wherever salt water laps a continent, there is a sea lane used by one of the world's five thousand tankers. And there are more to come, for the number of oil ships entering U.S. ports sharply increases every year that the nation becomes more dependent on foreign sources. Wherever these huge vessels sail, there is a thin margin between the uneventful voyage and the

Preface

tragedy: a difference that may be in the strength of the steel, or the reliability of the technology, or the training and diligence of the crew.

I began my research into oil tankers in March 1989 when the *Exxon Valdez* went aground in Alaska's Prince William Sound, spilling an estimated eleven million gallons of oil. By the time I boarded the *Arco Anchorage* to take the January 1992 voyage described in this book, another eighty-four tankers had spilled sixty-five million gallons of oil—quite a record in just two years and ten months. But that record was overshadowed by the damage in the opening weeks of 1993 when tankers spilled eleven times more oil than the *Exxon Valdez*. The question is whether we have learned anything from this scourge, and if we have, why has it taken so long?

I knew little about oil ships when my editors at the *Seattle Times* gave me a rather broad assignment shortly after the *Exxon Valdez* grounding: to learn everything I could about them. I have always been fascinated by machines, especially the kind that are large and yet frail at the same time. As a reporter for the *Seattle Times,* I have explored the safety problems of nuclear weapons plants and space-shuttle rockets, and in every system of this type I have found that certain principles apply: Machines are never as safe as the builder would claim, they are never as well maintained as the owner would advertise, and the profit motive nearly always competes with the safety of the worker and the public.

I was not surprised to find this true in the tanker world, only surprised by the candor with which it is accepted and discussed. One former fleet manager told me the shipowners are like owls: "The more light you throw on them, the less they see."

To see the operation firsthand, I had to hitch a ride on a tanker. In April 1989 an Exxon public relations man listened impatiently when I asked whether I could ride on one of their ships, said no, and hung up the phone. Chevron considered my proposal for a day and gave the same answer. But Jerry Aspland, president of Arco's tanker subsidiary, invited me to take a ride during our first phone conversation.

My first voyage on the *Arco Anchorage* in May 1989, the one I used for the newspaper series, occurred in relatively calm weather. To write a book was another matter, though, so I needed more information and another trip at sea. I considered finding a different ship, maybe a bigger one from a foreign fleet, but I returned to the *Arco Anchorage* because it was a ship I had already explored. Having crawled around the beast once, I figured I could better understand its soul on a second visit. And I had no trouble deciding when I should make this reacquaintance because a crewman had given me good advice: "If you really want to see what happens on these ships, come back in the winter and puke your guts." So it was that, with Aspland's gracious invitation, I boarded the *Arco Anchorage* in January 1992.

No writer can take the pulse of a ship and come away with a meaningful diagnosis without a veteran guide to explain its quirks. In that I was lucky to draw a captain like Jack Carroll, a man both talkative and open, willing to share information even if it was embarrassing. My timing was good, too. The ship was overdue for an overhaul and facing an incredible winter storm. While the tanker seemed to suffer some, I at least did not puke, because I am blessed with some immunity to motion sickness, for which I am thankful. I did, however, hang on to my bunk for dear life a few times.

My apologies to avid mariners—there are places in this book where I use landlubber terms like "floor" instead of "deck" or "right side of the ship" instead of "starboard." My intention is to explain life on the high seas to an office worker who has never left the beach.

Into the story of my *Arco Anchorage* voyage I have woven a broader history of tanker misadventure worldwide. There is hope that new laws passed following the *Exxon Valdez* spill will slow the pace of spills, and there has been improvement in the United States. But spills increased in recent years in other parts of the world, and some say it is only a matter of time before another big one hits this country again.

To explore the reasons behind this trend, I asked some questions. Why did tanker owners:

- Reduce the steel in their ships while making the hulls bigger?
- Take decades to adopt a safety device that would cut back on explosions?
- Oppose a requirement for double hulls when statistics showed they would prevent spills?

And why did the Coast Guard:

· Cut back on inspectors when more were needed?
· Allow tugboats on tanker escort duty that were not designed for the task?
· Permit shipowners to reduce the size of crews when operator error and fatigue are the most common contributors to accidents?

I also wanted to know who was in charge, what the rules were, how they were enforced, and who should be held responsible for mistakes. I didn't expect to uncover the industry's flaws by riding a tanker in an Arco fleet known for its comparative diligence. I did so by reading scores of accident reports and government documents I obtained by asking for them or by filing requests under the federal Freedom of Information Act. In all, I perused more than one hundred thousand pages of documents and conducted hundreds of interviews. I crawled through the innards of a tanker during surgery in a shipyard, and I studied the schematics to understand their workings.

My voyage on the tanker is the center of this story because the first line of defense against oil spills is the crew that sails the ship. If you are awakened one day to the thick smell of crude oil in the air, the initial cause was probably human error. I wanted to understand the lives of the people who drive these ships, I wanted to see them bring an oil tanker through a Gulf of Alaska storm and guide it into a busy port.

As we chatted on the bridge, the captain asked me what kind of a book I was writing. I told him I intended to explore the history of the problems that have plagued this industry. I told him I would explore his ship, looking for signs of trouble and hope. I told him I'd be asking a lot of questions.

"I just hope you'll tell our story," he said, referring to his crew.

"It is your story," I said.

Seattle, Washington
March 12, 1993

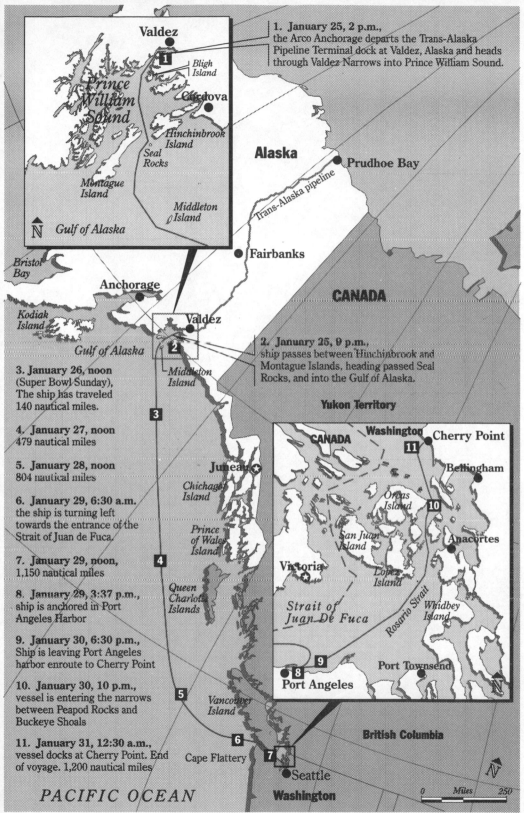

Valdez

1
Bligh Island

Cordova

Prince William Sound

Hinchinbrook Island

Seal Rocks

Montague Island

Middleton Island

N *Gulf of Alaska*

1. **January 25, 2 p.m.,** the Arco Anchorage departs the Trans-Alaska Pipeline Terminal dock at Valdez, Alaska and heads through Valdez Narrows into Prince William Sound.

Alaska

Prudhoe Bay

Trans-Alaska pipeline

Fairbanks

Bristol Bay

Anchorage

Kodiak Island

Valdez

2

Middleton Island

Gulf of Alaska

2. **January 25, 9 p.m.,** ship passes between Hinchinbrook and Montague Islands, heading passed Seal Rocks, and into the Gulf of Alaska.

Yukon Territory

3. **January 26, noon** (Super Bowl Sunday), The ship has traveled 140 nautical miles.

4. **January 27, noon** 479 nautical miles

5. **January 28, noon** 804 nautical miles

6. **January 29, 6:30 a.m.** the ship is turning left towards the entrance of the Strait of Juan de Fuca.

7. **January 29, noon,** 1,150 nautical miles

8. **January 29, 3:37 p.m.,** ship is anchored in Port Angeles Harbor

9. **January 30, 6:30 p.m.,** Ship is leaving Port Angeles harbor enroute to Cherry Point

10. **January 30, 10 p.m.,** vessel is entering the narrows between Peapod Rocks and Buckeye Shoals

11. **January 31, 12:30 a.m.,** vessel docks at Cherry Point. End of voyage. 1,200 nautical miles

Juneau

Chichagof Island

3

Prince of Wales Island

4

Queen Charlotte Islands

5

Vancouver Island

6

Cape Flattery

7

Seattle

Washington

CANADA

Washington **Cherry Point**

11

Bellingham

Orcas Island

10

San Juan Island

Anacortes

Victoria

Lopez Island

Whidbey Island

Strait of Juan De Fuca

Rosario Strait

9

8

Port Angeles

Port Townsend

N

British Columbia

PACIFIC OCEAN

0 Miles 250

JAMES MCFARLANE / SEATTLE TIMES

Tankers Full of Trouble

1

The Worst Winter

*(Hinchinbrook Island,
January 25, 9 P.M.)*

A fishing boat appears as a lighted dot ahead of us, bobbing like a scrap of driftwood on five-foot swells. The mood is gentle for these Alaskan waters, a soft ride compared to the January violence that churns the Gulf of Alaska a dozen miles south of here. The fisherman carries a load of cod toward home, past the sheltered wing of Hinchinbrook Island. A windbreak barely visible in the nine o'clock darkness, Hinchinbrook and another island called Montague enfold the southern end of Prince William Sound, sheltering the inside waters from the legendary southerly gales of the ocean. The furious noise of the gulf is completely muted, and the undulating waves are providing a nice nap to some sea otters relaxing in the channel. Nothing intrudes on the isolation of the place except the light on the fisherman's mast and two nearby beacons marking a couple of shallows.

Then the great prow of our oil ship appears, black and gloomy in the darkness, relentlessly plowing aside the rollers and making short work of the otters' lullaby. The gargantuan hull forces aside millions of gallons of water with every turn of the propeller. Anchors as big as fishing boats dangle like pirates' earrings from either side of the bow and the hull is as deep in the water as a five-story building.

At a relatively slow speed of eleven miles an hour, the nine-hundred-foot-long ship takes a minute to pass a spot on the water, with the momentum of eight Boeing 747s coming in for a landing. Even at this speed, if the tanker had to stop in an emergency, it would need a mile or two to do so.

The fisherman can't hear the tanker because the engine noise is muffled by three rows of cargo tanks containing thirty-five million gallons of Alaskan crude oil. But he is wisely out of the monster's path, a fact worth noting since a local halibut fisherman fell asleep at the wheel a few years back and awoke to the sound of his fifty-foot boat bouncing and spinning down the side of a tanker he'd collided with. He and his boat were lucky to survive.

Fully loaded, the broad ship sits so low in the water that nearly three-quarters of its 120,000-ton mass is submerged. Even so, it is a thirty-five-foot climb, straight up, from the water's surface to the deck where the anchor chain is hauled aboard, each link weighing nearly three hundred pounds. Near the top of the bull-nose bow, white letters announce that this is the steamship *Arco Anchorage*.

I am standing next to the windlass that hauls in the anchor, on a raised platform at the bow known as the foc's'le (forecastle) head, looking back more than seven hundred feet to a six-story building where the captain has control of the ship. I can't see him or anyone else in the darkened wheelhouse and, at this speed, the captain and the helmsman won't pass the stretch of water I am standing above for another forty-five seconds. Such is the dimension of this ship that from my perch on the bow I can see the water directly in front of me while, from his position on the bridge, the captain's view is blocked for several hundred feet by the mass of the hull. The skipper often posts a watchman here to look for objects in the water, but with the ship heading into a storm outside Hinchinbrook this spot will soon be swallowed by brine and the lookout has headed back in. When we enter the gulf, the seas will smash the bow and mercilessly sweep this spot clear of anything not grappled to steel.

Feeling the battle approaching, I walk back sixty-five feet to the rear of the foc's'le house and descend a dozen rungs of a steel ladder to the main deck. Standing there I am dwarfed by one hundred thousand square feet of gray paint and rust, and confused by a vast jumble of equipment. The two-acre deck between here and the wheelhouse is laced from front to rear and from side to side with two dozen pipes, the largest being nearly a foot and a half in diameter. The pipes have different purposes that a junior sailor must know. Some carry crude oil to and from the cargo tanks, others supply fuel oil to the engines, while the smallest ones are ready to deliver fire-fighting foam to the red nozzles that point out from five raised platforms evenly spaced down the deck. Huge red letters on the side of the foc's'le house say NO SMOKING, an uncompromising rule out here because the tanks contain enough explosives to demolish a small city.

The tanker is as wide as a ten-lane highway, but not as spacious, since the deck is cluttered with winches, cables, upright ventilation stacks, and miscellaneous equipment. As I walk toward the house, I must pick my way through this rusty maze, which reminds me of another rule sternly recited to me when I boarded the ship a week ago: "You must never run on deck." That seems obvious where a trot would end quickly against a taut cable or an upright ventilator pipe. The place does not have the look of recreation, but of business, and the business of this ship is underneath my feet, some thirteen cargo tanks containing sixteen million dollars' worth of crude oil.

The purpose of our twelve-hundred-nautical-mile journey from Valdez, Alaska, to Cherry Point, Washington, is to deliver this burden to an Arco refinery, which will then break it down into enough petroleum products to provide five million people living in western Washington and Oregon with a one-and-a-half-day supply of gasoline, diesel fuel, heating oil, jet fuel, butane, propane, coke, and lubricants. This oil, which was drilled from beneath the tundra of Alaska's North Slope, is so critical to the national economy, it accounts for four out of every five gallons of petroleum used by the people on the west coast of the United States.

Our task might be easier if we were not heading into one of the world's nastiest oceans, and if this were not the dead of winter at a latitude uncomfortably close to Arctic. The Atlantic-Richfield Company tosses the dice every time an Arco tanker leaves Alaska. If we lose the ship, we could send up the price at the pump. If we hit the rocks and spill our entire load, we could create a mess three times the size of the *Exxon Valdez* spill of 1989.

* * *

When I reach the front wall of the house—stark white, about sixty feet tall and nearly one hundred feet wide—I am looking at the only structure that rises high above the main deck. This is the ship's dividing line. Nearly everything in front of the house is cargo and nearly everything behind it is dedicated to the crew's comfort and the engines. The tanker is about 80 percent cargo and 20 percent everything else.

The bottom of the house looks like the deck in front of it—a jumble of pipes, railings, fire hoses, and other equipment collected against the baseboard like driftwood thrown against a seawall. Above that, the front facade is spartan and spotless, a white parapet marked only by two dozen round portholes, which is really a sparse number of openings for a five-story building. On top of the wall are the nine square windows of the wheelhouse centered over everything like a crown. The flying wings of the bridge jut out fifty feet from either side of the regal wheelhouse, creating two grand outdoor porches where the lookouts stand when they are not able to occupy the bow.

The wind is rising in pitch as I enter the side of the house and step into its neon-lit corridor, painted institutional green like a county hospital. I look back knowing this is my last stroll outdoors for some time. The sea will soon claim every inch of the main deck, not just the bow, and for the next few days and nights I will be imprisoned in the leviathan's drab interior. I wonder for a moment if there is an appropriate ritual to mark this loss of freedom. Underneath me hums the cavernous engine room, some eight stories high from the bottom of the ship to the top of the boiler pipes. Above me stands the apartment and office complex of the ship. The vibrating hallway with its ugly steel walls reminds one of how devoid these tankers are of ceremony. The largest ships in the world occupy a grimy crease in maritime history: they have never even generated a colorful jargon of their own, nor have the scribes honored their dangerous mission in literature. This is no glamorous cruise ship or romantic warship I am riding on tonight. This is a crude carrier heading into a sea of trouble.

I climb a switchback set of stairs five stories to the door of the wheelhouse, which is the command center of the entire vessel. On my way, I pass the galley, the crew quarters, the lounges, and the various offices, but I see no other crew members. I am often alone in this vast machine, for there are only twenty-four crew members, and they work in three shifts.

At the top of the stairs, more than sixty feet above sea level, with the wind now howling outside, the door to the wheelhouse is difficult to push open. As I crack it, it whistles with the sound of rushing air. Once inside, my eyes adjust to the darkness where the only light is the red glow from three radar screens mounted atop a couple of podiums in the middle of the room. Bright light isn't allowed in here, for it would obscure the night vision of the four men who are on duty: the captain, the third mate, the helmsman, and the lookout.

The word over the weather wire is that a sizable January storm is blowing outside Hinchinbrook Island. No sane mariner approaches Hinchinbrook this time of year without a feeling of awe and a buckling down of the nerves. By ritual, the mate is marking the word "departure" on the logbook, indifferently, noting for the record that this loaded oil tanker has begun its southbound voyage through the Gulf of Alaska. By reputation, the exit from Prince William Sound recalls a history of muggings.

The Gulf of Alaska is a brawling sea that claims the life of at least one fisherman a week. There was a time when seafarers thought the North Atlantic shipping route from New York to Rotterdam was the worst place in the Northern Hemisphere to sail a ship. But recent studies have shown that, by most measures, the Gulf of Alaska is more violence prone. Waves stand on end as tall as a hundred feet and, as if to prove that a ruthless god runs the place, temperatures drop to near one hundred degrees below zero while the winds roar at 150 miles per hour. Only madness, or its equivalent, oil, would make us toss our fate to these ballistic winds.

Captain Jack Carroll, the skipper of the *Arco Anchorage,* rests his right hand on the wooden railing that runs below the windows of the wheelhouse and stares outside with an expression of quiet anxiety, like a cop in a cruiser scanning a tough neighborhood.

At age thirty-five, Carroll looks unready to be in charge of a 120,000-ton oil ship. His cheeks, barely visible in the darkness, are covered by a five o'clock shadow but the face is still boyish. It's his first tour of duty as a captain, having been elevated from the position of chief mate just six months ago. Although this is his debut as a ship captain, he is no rookie to the sea or to this ship. He has walked the long decks of oil tankers since he graduated from the Kings Point Maritime Academy in 1978, and practiced the trade of chief mate aboard the *Anchorage*'s sister ship, the *Arco Fairbanks,* an identical 120,000-tonner.

Back home in Plano, Texas, today is his son's second birthday, but the captain must wait to see the party on a videotape his wife will mail to the ship. When he unwraps the tape a couple of port calls from now, and shoves it into the VCR in his suite, the lonesome skipper will wish he could join the festivities. Christmas and other milestones of family life come too often by instant replay, one of many reasons why divorce and instability claim the spirits of many sailors. Carroll quietly mentions his son's birthday to me and then drops the discussion altogether. This is not the gesture of a brittle man, but of a guy who would rather face the long night without thinking of impossible yearnings. Carroll does not hide his feelings in silence. He wears an elastic face that breaks into pantomime, sweeping the room with a wit as constant as a radar beacon. The jokes depend on timing and theatrics more than words. Tonight, for instance, he recreates a scene from his past when a brusque skipper caught him in the act of listening to an AM radio on the bridge, a sin serious enough to get a man fired. Carroll rolls his eyes back in his head to portray his own inattention to duty. He tells how the salt he had strewn under the door to make a warning noise—should the boss open it—failed to alert him because he wasn't listening. Then Carroll's imitation of the imperious captain snatching away his earphone, and of himself, the contrite mate, pleading for mercy—"Just trying to get the news, Cap"—soon has his audience in stitches.

Carroll's brown hair recedes slightly in front, and his unlined face displays an easy smile. Standing six feet, one inch, wearing a white-and-gray ski sweater and a red cotton turtleneck, he looks more like an executive on vacation than a ship captain about to enter the Gulf of Alaska in January. But if this is a vacation, we have made a wrong turn somewhere. The first of the large swells now thuds against the hull, and with a groan the tanker takes its first tentative roll, a pitch of things to come. Still miles from the open water, the ocean is telegraphing a warning.

The captain walks eight paces back to the lighted chart room behind the bridge, making no noise with the soft soles of his shoes. The shoes appear on the outside to be nothing but jogging footwear, athletic and casual like the captain himself. But inside they are reinforced with steel toes, a requirement for the industrial job.

Carroll pulls a map out of a flat drawer to get a picture of the battleground he is about to enter. In the brighter light, I see fatigue around his blue eyes. During the previous night in Valdez, as the ship loaded its cargo, Carroll caught seven hours of restless sleep. Since 7 A.M., he's been mostly on duty, wrestling the plights and predicaments that nip at a captain during cargo loading and departure from port. As we exit Hinchinbrook around 9 P.M., the young captain has sole responsibility for our safety and the protection of the ship. The harbor pilot who guided the tanker from the dock at Valdez departed on a little boat nearly five hours ago and the tug escorts are pulling away right now, no match for the weather outside Cape Hinchinbrook.

The captain and his crew have been absorbing storms like countless body blows over a period of months. In the decade and a half that Carroll has worked these waters, this is the worst winter he has ever seen. "This one is a horror."

Carroll studies the map he has spread on a drafting table in front of us, considering his options. The room is long and narrow and is lined with drab-colored imitation wood. We are surrounded by navigation machines, a gyrocompass, and writing tables. The other essentials are the logbook (a written diary of every trip), a fax machine that spits out weather maps, and a shelf of plastic binders that contain all the rules, procedures, and contingency plans for operating an oil tanker.

The captain reaches to the side and pulls a National Weather Service map off the fax machine. The smeared ink makes it hard to read, but it does not erase the news that a thug lurks just outside Hinchinbrook. In fact, one low-pressure system after another awaits us, circles on the map, scattered around the gulf like so many enemy mines. Carroll points at the shiny paper and says maybe we can skirt this one, and maybe we can get on the other side of that one, but it's probably wishful thinking. A ship is too slow to dodge bad weather, especially when everything out there is bad. There are services that guide ships, as best they can, around radar- and satellite-detected weather systems. Arco tried one service out a few years ago, but Carroll says the captains didn't like it. "It took away their prerogative." The *Arco Anchorage* will depend on the instincts of the captain tonight. No outside interference.

"There are three kinds of weather out here. Bad, real bad, and awful," says third mate Dean Davis, who comes into the chart room to mark the ship's position on the map. He shakes his head at the forecast. "This one looks awful."

More and more the ship shudders and rolls, nothing serious but it is a clear message of things to come. The crew has been telling me about these Gulf of Alaska storms, how the bow of the ship disappears in the waves, and how the seas rip apart the pipes. Lookout Ralph Schramm snaps the fur lining of his hood more tightly around his face and steps behind a barrier that serves as a windbreak on the bridge wing. Davis spreads his feet a little farther apart, bracing his sea legs for the oncoming battle.

Carroll can turn the tanker around if he thinks the weather is too dangerous for the ship. He considers it for a moment when we hear a radio report from another ship, the *BT Alaska,* which is approaching Hinchinbrook Island from the outside. The northbound traveler tells whoever is listening that he's being pounded by the tempest in the gulf.

"Bet you're glad to get inside Hinchinbrook," says another voice from some other ship in the night. "Sure am," comes the electronic reply.

But Carroll is not serious about stopping, not at this point anyway. He has a cargo to deliver. A ship like this costs thirty-five dollars a minute to operate, and it won't make any money sitting still.

Foremost in Carroll's mind is the pounding his hull is about to take. He studies the weather map, and the ocean chart, to find the path of least resistance. While he does so, his ear is tuned to the way his vessel is laboring. "You are just trying to feel the ship right now," he says. It is groaning.

Carroll must decide which direction to go once he exits Hinchinbrook and enters the gulf. His decision in this case is not influenced by obstacles on the surface but by the topography of the ocean bottom.

The depth of the ocean floor affects the behavior of the sea surface above it. The swells get bigger as the water gets shallower. If the captain turns left when we leave Prince William Sound, he'll take the ship over water less than forty fathoms deep (a fathom equals six feet). If he turns right, he'll go over a piece of ocean known as the "hundred-fathom curve" where, as the name implies, the water is much deeper.

The left turn is the shortest distance to Washington state, our destination, but it would be rougher tonight over such shallow water. The right turn takes us farther out in the ocean away from our course, but the water is likely to be smoother.

The captain says the odds-on favorite in winter conditions like this is the right-hand turn. Not only is it calmer out there, there is also more room to dodge the oncoming seas. But this course too has its dangers. Uppermost in Carroll's thinking is the hazard of potentially heavy swells rolling at him from the coast, forcing him even further off course. It happened to him once down south when near-hurricane-force winds and heavy seas blocked his turn into Washington state. "I've got my left turn signal going, but I can't turn left," he told the company dispatcher over the radio. Such an expensive delay tonight could tarnish the young captain's record.

Carroll isn't ready to make his decision yet. He will choose after he gets a chance to see the character of this storm firsthand. He returns to the wheelhouse window and stares outside. "Poke your nose out. Then you make your decision," he says. "Feel the ship."

The Gulf of Alaska's weather gets manufactured somewhere around Japan where cold air from Siberia meets warm air from the south, spinning, swirling, diving, and rising to form low-pressure cells. Like bubbles blown from a child's soap ring, the low-pressure systems then drift east across the ocean and collect in the Gulf of Alaska where they stick for a while against the mountain ranges. At the same time, cold air is trapped behind the mountains, forming high-pressure systems, another key ingredient in the recipe for terror.

Since air flows from high-pressure systems to low-pressure systems, the way water flows downhill, the air in these parts takes a pretty steep ride. You could say the wind here flows like Niagara Falls. Some Alaskan winters are cold and windy, and others are warmer and windy, but they are always windy.

The winter of 1988–89 produced wind gusts that exceeded one hundred miles an hour and temperatures dipped below minus 45 degrees Fahrenheit on a regular basis. With the windchill factor taken into account, one town recorded − 130 degrees. Over a dozen fishing vessels were lost and tankers arrived in port so caked with ice, the crewmen had to free the mooring winches from their encasement with baseball bats (carried on board for that purpose).

This winter is warmer—the temperatures are hovering above zero—but the winds are blowing ceaselessly. The reason for these strong and constant winds is a warm southern current called *El Niño* that has invaded the North Pacific a little farther than usual. The warmth pours more energy into the weather machine and out the other side come more low-pressure systems.

These constant winds blowing across the ocean have created monster waves. The key to wave making is not just the speed of the wind, but the length of time it blows. And the bigger the waves get, the more efficiently the wind will push and pull on them, the same way air lifts an airplane wing. It is a vicious cycle, and we are about to see the results: wall-to-wall, twenty-four-hour, seven-day-a-week horrendous rollers.

It's hard for a landlubber to imagine, looking at one of these great ships, why a captain of one would be the least bit concerned about waves. But as the soft rollers of Prince William Sound give way to the thundering oceans of the gulf, moving dunes of water crash over the prow with the power of the planet behind them. The long ship bends up and down from stem to stern, over and over again like an undulating lizard. The sound the steel makes, with all of its joints grinding, is like the sonorous complaint of a monster in death's jaws.

The bending is not subtle at all, but very visible, and somewhat alarming to the first-time visitor. It's called hogging and sagging: hogging when the hull bends upward in the middle like the arching spine of a hog and sagging when it bends downward like an old horse's back. A tanker will bend ten feet in either direction. From the bridge, I see a wave thunder over the foc's'le head; the nose of the ship lifts, and the long deck folds slightly upward, quivering and rippling on the way. Then the steel relaxes and the whole hull bends the other direction as the sea washes across the deck. The hull is designed to flex like that, to move like a tree branch in the wind; supple enough and yet strong enough to give and not to break. A friend of mine who sailed on Great Lakes ore ships—a second cousin to the tanker—remembers how veterans jokingly referred to the bending as the ship "waving good-bye."

Unfortunately, sometimes they actually are waving good-bye. There are limits to the design, and the history books are full of cases where tankers have snapped in half, cracked across the deck, or split down the side. The break can come as a result of a single blow, or months and years of bending.

One tanker, the *Stuyvesant,* cracked opened on two different occasions in the waters we are about to enter.

In January 1987 the southbound *Stuyvesant* was beaten senseless for three days and nights in winds and waves that grew fiercer and fiercer with each passing evening. At one point, the rolling seas buried the main deck under thirty feet of water, repeatedly turning the ship into an oil-carrying submarine. The skipper had seen this kind of weather before, but in the third night's darkness, at ten o'clock, the ship listed and oil started pouring out the bottom. A seventeen-foot crack released six hundred thousand gallons of crude oil into the ocean.

Seven months later, the patched-up *Stuyvesant* was once again bucking forty-five-foot waves and seventy-mile-per-hour winds while sailing south, fully loaded, in an October storm. For several hours, the heavy ocean waves chewed apart the eleven-hundred-foot-long ship. At 10 A.M., a big wave smashed a lifeboat away from the second deck. At 1:20 P.M., another one broke a huge winch to pieces. Fifteen minutes later, a wave that loomed as tall as the bridge—nearly ninety feet high—slammed into the ship. The great vessel shuddered and wrenched like a building hit by an earthquake. Immediately afterward, oil spilled into the Pacific Ocean; black, greasy stuff mixing with the angry rollers. It took another day before the waves had subsided enough so the crewmen could venture out onto the deck for a look. They found a crack in the side and broken machinery everywhere. Most disturbing, however, was the eighteen-foot-long fracture in one of the cargo tanks that released some 700,000 gallons of crude oil into the ocean.

The *Stuyvesant* story is not an isolated incident, and the crew was lucky the ship didn't sink in the lethally frigid northern waters of the gulf.

Tanker crewmen in other cases haven't been so lucky. Six months after the *Stuyvesant* incident, a Greek tanker broke in two and burned off Newfoundland, killing all twenty-four Polish seamen and five of their wives. Seven months after that, the Liberian tanker *Odyssey* broke in half some nine hundred miles from Newfoundland and caught fire with twenty-seven crewmen aboard. A Soviet rescue ship couldn't get close enough to help because of the intensity of the flames.

Even after the *Exxon Valdez* disaster riveted public attention to oil spills, the carnage far from shore continued without much notice. Organizations that keep track of tanker casualties say more oil and ore ships have cracked in recent years than ever before. Mariners seem to accept the toll as an occupational hazard. And since often the oil dissipates in the ocean far from land, shoresiders are able to overlook all but the most highly publicized cases.

Carroll is responsible for the lives of twenty-four people, a one-hundred-million-dollar ship, and a sixteen-million-dollar cargo as he crosses a thundering wilderness. And if the *Exxon Valdez* is any example, the cost of a major spill these days is more than three billion dollars. On our southbound journey, more than one hundred miles off the west coasts of Alaska and Canada, the ship will be pounded for three or four days. While enduring this, Carroll must avoid a freak wave like the one that tore apart the *Stuyvesant,* and point the ship into the trough of the rollers where the vessel won't take head-on impacts. He must keep in mind that this is a nineteen-year-old ship that has been at sea too long, and that it is months overdue for its two-year overhaul. By Carroll's own estimation, this is the poorest-maintained ship in the Arco fleet, and it has the roughest duty, since it makes the run between Valdez and Cherry Point once every eight or nine days on average. With this duty, the ship rarely leaves the mean northern seas to get a rest in southern waters. The *Arco Anchorage* is the gulf's punching bag.

"Jesus!" The sound of my own voice startles me. We have nosed into the first of the gulf's biggest rollers. As it slams into the bow, its broken waters shoot high into the sky like Old Faithful, forming a plume much wider and heavier than Yellowstone's famous geyser. "Here we go," says the mate, as the ship heaves into a roll. "God's country," says the guy at the helm. It is clear who is in charge out there.

These shipmates have been bracing themselves against storms like this for weeks. The fatigue is evident everywhere—eye sockets look darker, faces are scragglier, tempers are shorter, like a college dorm during final exams. I joined the ship only a week ago at the beginning of its northbound voyage from Washington state, but already my leg muscles are tired and my back aches from adjusting to this rolling world. I sleep fitfully in a bedroom that tilts as much as thirty degrees to a side. The only way to snooze is to jam something under the outer edge of the mattress, pushing it up at an angle so the body is wedged against the wall.

Third mate Dean Davis says the three kinds of weather out here require three different bed adjustments. "If it's bad, you put your life jacket under the mattress. Real bad, you put your life jacket and survival suit under the mattress. Awful—throw the mattress on the floor." The idea then is to turn the sleeping pad so it is rocking from head to foot rather than side to side.

A lot of mattresses have hit the deck this trip.

A few days ago, during our northbound trip, Carroll pulled out his logbook so he could recount what had happened during the first two months of his first tour of duty as a captain. "You'd think they would start me out on some nice summertime cruise, wouldn't you? But, nawwwwww, not for Jack Carroll." Instead, on one trip after another between Washington state and Alaska, the seas and the fates offered a menu of agony only a high-latitude tanker driver could understand. Here are the lowlights:

November 14: When Carroll took over the ship at the Cherry Point refinery north of Bellingham, Washington, there was, of course, no ceremony. Unlike a new Navy captain who gets piped aboard with whistles and ceremony, a tanker captain receives only a review of the paperwork and a brief meeting with the departing skipper who is usually in a hurry to get off. For weeks the seas had been placid for the previous captain, but that night as Carroll exited the Strait of Juan de Fuca into the big ocean, a major Pacific storm hit hard. The winds were blowing seventy miles an hour and the heavy seas forced Carroll to change directions several times, looking for the troughs in the waves. An unloaded tanker sits so high in the water, it acts like a sail, and the farther out the ship went, the tougher it became to navigate around the walls of water. The oncoming punches were so bad, the captain had to turn south to avoid them. Seaman Marvin Cropper said the ship at one point hit an incredible wall. "It stood this ship still for a moment. I mean, it just stood still." It wasn't until noon the next day that Carroll was able to resume the correct northbound course.

So it went for weeks as heavy weather pounded the ship on every voyage. One night Carroll had to turn on the main-deck spotlights just to figure out from which direction the crazy seas were coming. With the ship glowing like a football stadium, Carroll picked his way through the ocean at three nautical miles per hour. "At nighttime you are guessing. You can look at your radar and see where the seas are coming from, but other than that you are driving in the dark. You don't know how powerful those swells are."

Pausing as he read his logbook, Carroll wondered out loud how something as large as this ship could be tossed around like a cork or stopped dead in its tracks by water.

"The ocean is a very dangerous place. You gain a respect for the sea. A picture won't show you how really deep that swell is. A picture doesn't really tell the story."

December 14: Eight other tankers had been delayed by the storms when the *Arco Anchorage* pulled into Prince William Sound. They were stacked up at an anchorage called Knowles Head waiting for room to dock in Valdez. That night the winds gusted to one hundred miles per hour and some ships began to drag their anchors. "That's the most dangerous thing you can imagine." Carroll ordered his engines restarted, and called for the anchor to be pulled. The chief mate hung over the bow of the ship, guiding the anchor chain aboard with an icy wind tearing at his clothes, threatening to toss him off his perilous perch. The noise of the tumult made it nearly impossible for him to talk to the bridge over his two-way radio, so he tucked it deeper into his coat. "To know life at sea," said chief mate Svetko Lisica, "you have to be on the bow when you are soaked to the skin and the radio craps out on you."

Christmas Day: At one o'clock in the morning on this day of devotion, a little gizmo broke in the gyrocompass and, although the ship has a magnetic compass as well as a gyro, a tanker can't enter a port with a portion of its navigating equipment out of order. The Coast Guard ordered Carroll to anchor at Knowles Head, but Carroll told the Coast Guard he wasn't interested in parking again during a gale. After some negotiations the authorities allowed the ship to sail into Valdez with a tug escort, an expensive precaution usually required for loaded tankers going the other direction. Around midnight the ship was loaded with cargo, but it could not leave Valdez because the technician—who had been snowed in for a while in Anchorage—had not fixed the gyro. Each time he got it working, it broke again. By then, three other tankers were waiting to berth. Some fifty-two thousand gallons of hot oil flows out of the eight-hundred-mile-long pipeline every minute, and the stuff has only two places to go: to the ships or to a limited number of holding tanks at the Valdez facility. The authorities who regulate the oil terminal could not let the *Arco Anchorage* jam up the trans-Alaska pipeline.

The ship was given orders to sail with the gyro technician still on board fiddling with the equipment. He fixed the thing in the harbor and got off with the harbor pilot when the tanker reached the middle of Prince William Sound.

December 28: The tired crew was elated because their destination was Long Beach, California, a rare trip through calmer southern waters. "A little rest from the bangers," Carroll said. Five days later, the crew was enjoying sailing at top speed on softer oceans when an alarm sounded in the engine room. Some bearings had overheated, a dangerous condition that could destroy millions of dollars' worth of expensive machinery, or strand the ship or even set it on fire. The engineers made some adjustments and restarted the engines, but the main turbine was crippled and the ship had to limp into Long Beach at a speed of five nautical miles per hour again, as slowly as they had been forced to travel in the worst storms.

January 7: The next stop after Long Beach was a Chevron dock in San Francisco Bay. After unloading the last of the cargo there, past midnight, Carroll called for tugs and a harbor pilot to guide him out of the bay. Just then a crewman told him the radio officer was missing. The crew searched high and low for the man, while a tugboat and the harbor pilot waited, running up a huge bill for Arco. By federal law, the ship could not sail without a radio officer on board. Carroll was about to call headquarters when a van pulled up to the dock and out stepped, or shall we say, staggered, the radio officer. A merchant marine officer is prohibited by law from sailing while drunk, the definition of which is two and a half times stricter than the one commonly applied to motorists in the United States.

(The rule is a good one. Even a radio officer can get a tanker in trouble, such as the drunken sailor who hit an alarm in the eastern Mediterranean in December 1988, which signaled an emergency network that his American tanker had been seized by terrorists. By the time authorities discovered it was a hoax, the alert had gone up the chain of command to the White House.)

Carroll fired his radio officer at 3 A.M. With other tankers waiting to get in, the Coast Guard gave him permission to sail out and drop anchor in the middle of San Francisco Bay until a replacement arrived. At 7:30 A.M., retired radio officer George Peloso, sixty-six, got a telephone call at his Bridge City, Texas, home asking him to pack his gear and get to the airport immediately. A helicopter landed him on the main deck of the *Arco Anchorage* at around three o'clock that afternoon. Five minutes later, the crew pulled up the anchor and the good ship *Arco Anchorage* chugged out of San Francisco harbor.

January 20: One of the first things the captain complained about when I joined his northbound ship in Anacortes, Washington, was the niggling health problems plaguing his crew. A woman in the mess hall wrenched her arm when she slipped on a wet floor. An able-bodied seaman who had been with the company three weeks developed a disabling soreness in his wrist while using a vibrating needle-gun to clean rust off the main deck. Both crew members were classified as unfit for duty and sent home, statistics the bureaucrats at fleet headquarters always notice. Carroll was only half joking when he pondered the scorecard they are probably keeping, "Jack Carroll: Two unfit for duties." The clerks are probably clucking to themselves, "All this trouble on his first tour of duty."

Carroll reveals worry sometimes through a haze of humor, and in this case he was underlining the fact he has no job security. A senior captain might return to duty after running his ship aground, but a junior guy like Carroll could get demoted for the clumsiness of a mess hall worker.

"When a guy gets carpal tunnel, when a woman slips on a wet floor, out of nowhere, is it my fault?" the captain wonders out loud. "Naw. But tell that to the bean counters in Long Beach."

The trend continued after I arrived.

Bob Rich, the ship's first engineer, came down with a horrendous case of diarrhea as we sailed north through steadily worsening seas. I could see the illness draining his strength, his spirit, and his color. This time, though, Carroll had no inclination to joke, for he had lost an important player. Rich was the second in command down in the engine room, a distinguished graduate of the federal maritime academy at Kings Point, New York, a man trained to handle both the bridge and the engine room, something that is rare in this business. When things get rough, Carroll likes to know Rich is downstairs watching over the power plant. But now this valuable officer was confined to his bunk and his toilet. The captain said he would take the weather any day over the loss of his first engineer.

It didn't take long on our northbound voyage for me to see why Carroll worried about the loss of Rich. An old ship is like an aging airplane—the only way to keep it safe is to constantly renew its parts. To do so, you need the talents of expert tinkerers.

Nearing its third decade, the *Arco Anchorage* was a year away from the time when experts say a vessel should be retired. I could see the imprint of time when I toured the ship during a brief lull in the weather. A crewman painting the deck said his task was akin to "putting makeup on a dying cancer victim." Deck railings were broken and the mooring winches that helped docking were constantly breaking down. Behind the bridge, an acrid smell and a stinging in my eyes revealed that a leak had sprung in the exhaust-gas system. Down in the engine room, one of the two pumps that supply water to the boilers had failed. And the crew used a steam-driven pump normally reserved for fire fighting to replace a broken-down pump vital to the exhaust-gas system.

Yet the *Arco Anchorage* is a relatively sturdy ship in a fleet with a good reputation. When it was built in Maryland, it was state of the art and even ahead of its time. The business was brimming with optimism and shipyards all over the globe were churning out tankers. Now the industry is in the second decade of a long decline and, though this ship is not much older than average, tankers everywhere are going geriatric.

A new law requiring tankers to have double hulls—an outer one and an inner one, with a space in between—will eventually force tanker owners to build new ships to replace single-hulled vessels like this one. But it won't happen quickly because the law gives shipowners a generous amount of time to comply. The *Arco Anchorage* will not be forced off the seas until two years before the end of the millennium. Four out of ten single-hulled foreign tankers now visiting U.S. shores will continue coming here until the year 2005. Others won't go to the scrap yard until the year 2015.

Arco has scant financial incentive to build new ships. The *Arco Anchorage* and its sisters are sailing on a dying route. The trans-Alaska pipeline that was under construction during the early years of the *Arco Anchorage*'s life is now an old artery connected to Alaska oil fields that are drying up. If there is no oil to haul from Alaska, the country will be even more dependent on the overseas supply. But with the ship's thirty-five-dollar-a-minute operating cost several times higher than the cost of running a foreign ship with cheaper crews, the Arco fleet would find it tough competing in the international market for oil-hauling jobs. As long as the *Arco Anchorage* makes the run from Alaska to the Lower 48, it is protected from foreign competition by a law that says only a U.S.-registered vessel with an American crew can haul cargo between American ports.

As we sailed unloaded toward Prince William Sound, we were a couple of months away from the third anniversary of the *Exxon Valdez* oil spill. In the year that had just ended, we had witnessed the second-worst toll of oil spills in world history (the worst was 1979). The industry was in chaos. Nearly two decades of plummeting revenues had left many ships and companies in a shambles.

Knowing this, I felt empathy for the crew and its uncertain future. But when I mentioned this to Carroll, he said he ignores the stuff he can't fix and concentrates on the job ahead.

As he made that comment, we were making our northbound entrance into Prince William Sound, unloaded and thirsty for a load of oil. We still had another thirty-one hours to go before we would arrive back at Hinchinbrook, where Carroll would face the stormy decision of turning right or left in the gulf. The immediate job ahead of us was a journey into Valdez, where we had a date with the pipeline.

2

Pilots and Whales

*(Flashback: Prince William Sound,
January 24, 3 P.M.)*

As we sailed into Prince William Sound to fill our tanks with oil at the end of our northbound voyage from Washington yesterday, I was weary of the rolling seas and thirsty for signs of foliage and dirt. The heavy wind pushing at the side of the ship folded and unfolded the clouds so the low-lying sun glanced its light intermittently off the water, changing the hues from gray to gray-green to mystic blue. As the splendor of tall land appeared on all sides of us, the tanker seemed like an intruder in an innocent neighborhood.

Mother Nature saw no reason for lowlands in parts of Prince William Sound, no need to put anything between the sparkling water and the soaring mountains. Waves slap the sides of peaks without pausing at a beach. Where there is a shoreline, only a thin platoon of evergreen trees appears before everything is snow above them. The mountains aren't a picket line like the trees, though, but a battalion that marches peak after peak into the Alaskan frontier.

Glaciers flow out of the wilderness, so huge that, instead of plummeting down the sides of peaks, they surround the mountains, turning them into islands. Working patiently for millions of years, these ice rivers scoured out the waterways the tankers use, dredging some channels half as deep as the Grand Canyon and leaving others shallow and rocky. In the spring especially, they drop icebergs into the sound, some half the size of the *Arco Anchorage.*

Scattered around the sound, a body of water bigger than the state of Delaware, are islands where wildlife survives in abundance. During a spring voyage, I saw bears tumbling in play on a steep slope just shouting distance from the tanker deck. An eagle killed a salmon for dinner, swooping at free-fall speed and grabbing his prey with a practiced grip as we watched from the oil loading dock in Valdez Harbor.

Eagles aren't the only beasts who fish in Prince William Sound. Summer brings humpback whales to frolic and feed on small marine organisms. Like acrobats, they burst from the sea, rising high in the air before slapping their bodies hard onto the surface of the water. The killer whale resides here, too; a black-and-white ruler of the food chain who's built more like a monstrous dolphin than a whale.

There's poetic irony in the sight of a whale playing near a tanker. The maritime ancestors of these tanker crews obtained their oil not from a pipeline but from the harpooned corpses of these marine leviathans. The roster on the *Arco Anchorage* lists more than a few hometowns where sailors of another time were lured by the wages of whaling. The captain, Jack Carroll, was born in New York, the birthplace of Herman Melville, author of *Moby Dick.* The second mate, Jean Holmes, comes from an area in New Hampshire that probably spawned more than one crewman for Captain Ahab's ship. Bob Lawlor, the senior captain who commands the ship when Carroll isn't here, grew up breathing the same salty New England air that intoxicated the sailors aboard many a whaling vessel.

The petroleum carried in the belly of this ship is what supplanted the lamp oil extracted from the belly of the whale. Until Standard Oil's kerosene replaced Moby Dick's lamp oil (a process begun in the latter half of the nineteenth century), whales were dragged from the ocean by the thousands to be rendered into flammable goo. The whale oil was hauled in steel tanks on whaling boats. Later converted to kerosene ships, these were the predecessors of the modern tanker.

Of course, oil is found, like whales, in remote places where nature didn't make easy arrangements for ships. Like Ishmael on the *Pequod,* tanker crews wander far from home to get it. Prince William Sound is one of those places.

In the dimming light of a sub-Arctic afternoon, Captain Carroll prepared to pick up his harbor pilot, turning the ship to form a windbreak so the man could climb aboard without being blown into the water.

The purpose of a harbor pilot is to guide the ship safely through inland waters, keeping them away from the shoals. From here to the dock at Valdez, the pilot—a man Carroll has met only a few times— will give directions to the *Arco Anchorage* helmsman and call out the engine speeds to the mate. By law they must board and depart a ship at a certain point on the map. These hundred-thousand-dollar-a-year harbor guides are given room and board in a floating hotel, a boat to get to and from their clients, and a number of other perks financed by the fees assessed to the owner.

The qualifications of a pilot vary from state to state. Many are former ship captains, but it is possible under most state rules for merchant marine officers or tugboat captains to get a pilot's license without ever having commanded a large ship. Applicants for a pilot's license must travel the local waters a certain number of times and then sketch the harbor from memory in a test, accurately showing details like the depths of the water. In some states, including this one, pilots are required to take additional trips aboard a tanker with a senior pilot before they can guide an oil ship.

Our pilot's boat was a lighted dot on the water when it began motoring out to us from its station miles away. When the black-and-white boat with the word PILOT neatly painted on its hull pulled alongside, it was still toy-size against the mass of the oil ship. As it sidled up to the lee of the tanker, taking heavy seas over its bow, it performed a nautical dance, traveling with the ship at a speed around ten miles an hour. A man wearing a heavy coat above pressed slacks and polished hiking boots stepped confidently off the forward deck of the boat and onto a writhing rope ladder that had been suspended down the side of the tanker by *Arco Anchorage* crewmen. While the waters tossed below him, and the winds blew nearly sixty miles an hour, the pilot clambered some thirty-five feet up the side of the unloaded tanker. He was our first visitor in four days and he introduced himself, with a smile, as Richard Cochinos.

After his briefcase had been hauled up behind him in a box suspended by a rope, Cochinos greeted the crewmen who had helped him through the chained opening in the ship's railing. He brushed some moisture off his jacket, braced his six-foot, one-inch frame against the stiff wind and walked with a bossy gait toward the house. Cochinos sniffed a bit, his nose runny from the cold, and he looked relieved as he stepped into the doorway on the starboard (or right) side of the house. He climbed the stairs to the bridge and greeted the captain, the mate, and the helmsman in a quiet businesslike manner. Following tradition, he handed the captain a copy of the local newspaper, which the skipper then tossed onto a shelf. They exchanged information about the condition of the ship, not casual talk, but specific data required by regulations, things like the draft of the hull and the size of the load. The law says the captain must tell the pilot about any unusual handling conditions on the ship (there were none), but the information doesn't flow the other way. An attempt to require pilots to tell captains about the route they will travel, the speed they intend to go, and the docking methods they'll use was defeated two decades ago. I asked Cochinos about this and he said he doesn't have time for such chatter. "If he wants to argue about an order, we are going to have an accident while we are talking about it." I was amused to see, later, that Cochinos was quite a talkative guy.

In an unusual move, Arco recently invited pilots to train with its captains using a computer-simulated ship. Together, they would tackle fictional emergencies and build a sense of teamwork. Carroll and Cochinos have never trained together like that, but someday they probably will. The Arco captain remembered Cochinos from a previous voyage and liked his style. But Carroll kept one ear cocked to the action, peering out the window toward Bligh Reef, as the pilot began telling the helmsman which way to steer.

What makes the relationship between the pilot and captain a delicate one is not the legal codes, but tradition and the clumsy nature of having two people run the show. According to law, Carroll never relinquishes his control of the ship and he remains on the bridge all the way into Valdez. But when a pilot is on board, a ship really has two masters. The pilot gives directions and the captain stands by and watches, holding in reserve the ultimate authority over the vessel. I liken it to the relationship between a fare and a cabdriver. The customer doesn't ask the cabbie for details on the route because he assumes the driver knows where he is going. Ship captains are the same way with pilots.

Courts have ruled that a captain can countermand a pilot's order, and Carroll said he would not hesitate to do so. "If they are doing something you really don't like, you'd better take the ship away from them."

But practice says Carroll would probably avoid such a move. A captain who contradicts a pilot is risking an expensive layover. The pilot can throw up his hands and say, "All right, you've got it, she's all yours." By law, the tanker cannot then enter the harbor. Carroll would have to anchor and wait for a replacement sent by the same state-sponsored organization that provided the first one.

In each geographic area, pilots belong to associations, like medieval guilds, which hold the exclusive right to guide ships that enter and leave. In Prince William Sound, the franchise is held by the Southwest Alaska Pilots Association. The member pilots are independent contractors who pay a fee to keep the association going, and they have a lot of say over who gets to join.

The associations are policed—so to speak—by state boards appointed by the governor. In twenty-four maritime states, a total of eleven hundred pilots are governed by state boards made up mostly of appointees who have busy careers and no time to really play policeman. The boards are often dominated by the pilot associations and by the pilots who sit as members. I once watched a Washington state board member complain about pilots dictating his board's policy. "We normally do what you want us to do," he said to a pilot who was also a member of the board. Then the majority voted in favor of the measure put forward by the pilot.

Coast Guard statistics show that over a twenty-seven-year period, state pilotage boards have disciplined pilots in only 19 of the 390 cases where a potential wrongdoing was referred to them by the Coast Guard. The National Transportation Safety Board, a federal advisory agency that investigates accidents, has criticized this 5 percent conviction rate and called on Congress and the states to change the system, but to no avail. NTSB officials told me they were not surprised when a Florida commission, which had not disciplined a guide in five years, did nothing to discipline a pilot who guided a ship into a Tampa Bay bridge, causing thirty-five motorists and bus passengers to plunge to their deaths. Also not surprising was a case where a pilot sailed a gasoline tanker into another vessel in Upper Bay between New Jersey and New York; the same guy had been cleared by the New Jersey board for his involvement in seven prior accidents. And there was the case of a Louisiana pilot who caused or contributed to five accidents in a five-year period. He crowned his career by causing a collision between a huge bulk carrier ship and a barge near New Orleans. The maximum state fine for a pilot who does something wrong in Alaska is only five thousand dollars, and it is less in other states.

Posted on the wall of the *Arco Anchorage* wheelhouse is a list of three San Francisco pilots and one from the state of Washington who aren't allowed to work on Arco ships. They've screwed up in the past and have landed on a blacklist assembled by Jerry Aspland, the president of Arco Marine and Carroll's ultimate boss. Technically, ships must accept the pilot assigned to them and most vessel owners don't assemble blacklists, but Aspland once told me he was tired of pilot associations calling the shots so he has taken matters into his own hands. Two of his tankers, including this one, have been damaged in cases where a pilot was giving directions. The *Arco Anchorage* went aground in Port Angeles harbor in 1985, spilling 239,000 gallons of oil, when a pilot guided the ship into shallow water while the Arco captain said nothing to stop him. Aspland demoted the captain, but later allowed him to take command of another ship. Months afterward a San Francisco Bay pilot drove that second Arco tanker into the side of a bridge with the same captain at his side. Aspland said this sort of thing drives him crazy. "It scares me to death when people won't challenge the pilot. I think we can put all the equipment we want on board ships, and we can put on double bottoms . . . we can do this, we can do that.

Somehow we need to figure out why people do things they do when they are in positions of decision making."

Aspland isn't sure that the blacklist he posted on the bridge is legal, but he is waiting for the pilots to call his bluff.

As for Cochinos, he has a spotless record. Many pilots do, and they are exemplary mariners. To earn the six-figure salary he gets for six to ten months of work, Cochinos must hold two licenses: one from the federal government and one from the state. The federal license is required for piloting U.S.-flagged vessels. The state license is needed to guide foreign-flagged ships. The dual system is really part of the problem.

The states obtained jurisdiction over pilots in the earliest years of the republic. The federal government was supposed to come up with a better plan, but whenever it tried the well-connected pilot associations held their ground, with the help of local politicians, to keep regional control.

The federal government eventually got jurisdiction over pilots who guide U.S.-flagged ships, but not the foreign ones. When Cochinos guides an American ship he is using his federal license, and when he takes on a foreign vessel he is using his state license. (A local rule says both licenses are required to guide any ship in Prince William Sound, but that is not true elsewhere.) The courts have ruled that the federal government's authority is limited to U.S.-flagged vessels, and they cannot suspend or revoke a pilot's state license if he screws up guiding a foreign ship. Only the states can do that. Armed with this ruling, the pilots have vigorously and successfully opposed any attempt to put them under a single licensing system.

Cochinos gave me a pretty good lesson in ship handling before we got to the dock. He explained how he thinks three moves ahead before giving a command, and how he carefully times each turn. I had tried the wheel myself earlier in the day and could feel how the ship moves sluggishly against the resistance of the water and the momentum of its own enormous weight. At any speed, a tanker is a damn sight harder to handle than a big Buick. You turn the wheel and several seconds tick by before the ship responds. While you wait, you hope you've applied enough rudder to coax the ship in the direction you want it to go. You check one indicator to see that the bow is swinging in the right direction and another to see that the rudder is far enough over. Then you watch the compass to see if you achieved the course that was ordered. Several more seconds will pass before the compass clicks to the designated degree marker. Then, just as you reach the course you sought, the ship keeps swinging beyond it. With the skill of a soothsayer, you should have thought three moves ahead and turned the wheel the other direction to achieve a correction. The sailor at the helm tells me even a veteran struggles in tough conditions. "I've seen a current take this ship three to four degrees off, just like that. Sometimes you can bring it back on course. Sometimes the ass end wants to keep going. Sometimes you'll be fighting for half a degree."

Discipline and hard work were strong elements of Cochinos's upbringing. He got his start in restaurants, laboring long hours in the eateries his Greek immigrant dad operated in Vermont and upstate New York. His dad would tell him the only way to avoid a lifetime of hapless labor was to get a college education, but when he graduated from high school his dad's restaurant fortunes were in a slump. With no money for tuition, Cochinos followed a scholarship offer to the New York State Maritime College on Long Island Sound where he fell in love with ships. After graduating with a third mate's license and serving two years in the Navy, Cochinos worked on cargo vessels on the high seas for over a decade. But when he'd earned his license to be a ship captain, he decided he would rather get what he considers to be the Ph.D. of maritime work, the pilot's papers. You stay closer to home, he said, and when you are on the bridge you feel like "it's just you, the ship, and the weather."

He piloted vessels on the Saint Lawrence Seaway for nearly eleven years, but the tonnage was limited there by the width of the locks. In 1979, less than two years after tankers began calling on Valdez, he arrived in Alaska to take on the big ones.

Cochinos brought his family to the remotest corner of the United States because it is one of only two places in America that are visited by the world's biggest ships. The other is in the Gulf of Mexico near

Louisiana, where super tankers dock in deep water to unload, at the end of an eighteen-mile-long underwater pipeline, crude coming from the Persian Gulf.

Most American seaports can't accommodate super tankers because the water isn't deep enough. The continental United States is surrounded by a shallow shelf and many ports don't have more than forty feet of clearance, not enough to accommodate the *Arco Anchorage* with its fifty-two-foot loaded draft (twice as deep as most other cargo ships), and much less than the biggest tankers in the world, which draw eighty feet.

Prince William Sound, on the other hand, offers an average depth of nine hundred feet. Even against the shoreline, the docks at Valdez can accommodate ships four times the size of the *Arco Anchorage*.

The most common way to describe a tanker's size is deadweight tonnage, a measure of its burden when fully loaded. A deadweight ton equals 2,240 pounds, compared to the common ton, which is 2,000 pounds.

The biggest tanker in the world is a 564,000-deadweight-ton Norwegian-flagged freak that is over fifteen hundred feet long. Four college football games could be played simultaneously on its main deck along with two dozen basketball games in the gymnasium-sized cargo tanks underneath. A small midwestern town would fit inside the hull with room for a hundred-foot grain elevator. This behemoth, known as the *Jahre Viking*, occasionally visits the Louisiana port. Two 267,000-deadweight-ton Arco ships, the *Arco Spirit* and the *Arco Independence,* are among the largest super tankers that come here.

There is another waterway in America deep enough to accommodate the world's biggest tankers, the Puget Sound region of Washington state, the place we would be heading for soon. Evergreen State leaders realized back in the 1970s that their waters, carved deep by glaciers, could accommodate the most massive tankers in the world. With difficulty, they convinced federal officials to ban ships over 125,000-deadweight tons, the only place in the United States where such a rule is in force.

Barriers like the line in Washington state are reassuring, but in some ways they give a false sense of security. The 121,000-deadweight-ton *Torrey Canyon* would have qualified to visit Washington, and it produced the sixth-worst tanker disaster in world history, three times the magnitude of the spill caused by the *Exxon Valdez*. In America, the vast majority of tanker spills are caused by ships smaller than this one I was aboard. Worldwide, the story is similar. Although the top three global spills came from genuine super tankers (the *Castillo de Bellver, Amoco Cadiz,* and *Atlantic Empress*), the next seven on the list were around the size of the *Arco Anchorage*.

The cargo inside our tanks could destroy several hundred miles of beaches with one false turn of the wheel. Cochinos was there to make sure such a mishap didn't occur. He guided the *Arco Anchorage* unfalteringly through a slender passageway known as Valdez Narrows and, sailing between steep hillsides, brought the ship into a wide, oval, mountain-rimmed sanctuary known as Port Valdez. In the harbor, about twelve miles long and two and a half miles wide, the winds were blowing hard, and it was cold, snowing, and dark. It is a shame the sun goes down so quickly in winter up here, for it all too often turns out the lights on a magnificent scene.

Cochinos used plenty of caution, keeping the speed down, putting the ship through a wide J-shaped turn so it would end up at the dock facing the way it came. He said a pilot never puts more speed on the ship than he absolutely needs while docking.

"You can always add speed, but it's hard to take it off. You can't slow these big ships down very easily."

The stern swung out when Cochinos turned the bow in. He paid attention to both ends of the ship because they have a way of moving in opposite directions. I could see by watching the rudder indicator and the compass how we were being pushed by the currents, the tide, and the wind. To overcome these forces, and to control the ship's own momentum, Cochinos called for the mate to hit the engines. Tankers are so notoriously underpowered that piloting one has been described as the equivalent of driving a forty-foot cabin cruiser with a one-third-horsepower rowboat engine.

Carroll remarked that a good pilot parks a ship using the vessel's own engines, eschewing the tugboats until the last sideways shove to the dock. If you've got to call on the tugs too early, you've blown it. Cochinos knows all about that. We got as close to the dock as possible before he cut the engines.

Two growling tugs put their bumpered bows against the ship when we were a couple of city blocks from the dock. The tugs pressed the vessel inward, waiting for Cochinos's command to stop. Pushing on the bow was the nine-thousand-horsepower *Stalwart* while on the stern was the seven-thousand-horsepower *Pathfinder*—two tugs with over half the total power of the ship's own engines. With all that muscle under the hood, tugs must be careful to not press too hard in the wrong place and punch holes in tankers' sides. In fact, the *Arco Anchorage* still carries a patch on its side where an overly enthusiastic tug did so a few years back. To help prevent this kind of mishap, arrows on the side of the ship point to the place where the tugs are supposed to push.

A captain and a pilot are never very comfortable when a tug is pressing against a ship's hull. Just one and a half inches of steel is a pretty thin margin against a powerful tug and unmoving dock. Cochinos and Carroll walked out to the end of the bridge wing to get a better view of the approaching pier.

The tension rose the closer we got to the dock. Cochinos focused his attention alternately on the dock and on the churning tugs. The pilot ignored the cold as he and the skipper watched the procedure from the outdoor wing, some sixty feet above the approaching pier. The docking crew measured the shrinking distance between the ship's massive hull and the dock as crewmen on the ship's bridge and terminal workers on shore talked to each other over handheld radios. They repeated cryptic estimates of the closing distance. It was a slow-motion operation with enormous consequences. This monster has the momentum of a freight train even when it is crawling.

Everything went well until the radio Cochinos was using to direct the tugs quit on him. A crewman next to him was calling out the distance to the dock: "Five feet . . . four feet . . . three."

"Damn," Cochinos said as the bad-battery light on his radio flickered on. He twisted the dead battery off the bottom of his two-way and grabbed for a new one in his pocket just as the crewman said "two feet." He twisted the new power pack on just as the crewman said "one foot." He pushed the talk button and ordered the tugs to back off just as the ship touched rubber.

"Whew. Wow. That was close," he said. "You can never tell when the battery is going to go dead. It always goes dead at the worst possible time."

Despite the mini-emergency, Cochinos eased the *Arco Anchorage* into position the way a good maître d' slides your chair in at a restaurant.

3

Big Ships
and a Little Town

(Valdez, January 24, 9 P.M.)

T wo T-shaped docks protrude more than a thousand feet into the deep water at the Trans-Alaska Pipeline Terminal in Valdez, while two other docks sit closer to shore. Brightly lit in the clear night, the terminal looked like a lonely truck stop in a snowy wilderness. Two rows of rotund holding tanks squatted under the lights on a white mountainside and an array of switchback service roads snaked between them. My binoculars searched for signs of the main pipeline or the place where it ends its eight-hundred-mile journey from the frozen north, but most of the spigot for America's number one domestic oil supply is buried underground at this point. In the other direction, I could see the town's faint glow across the bathtub-shaped bay.

As the tugs eased us into berth 4, the near-freezing water was eighty feet deep below the hull of the *Arco Anchorage*. A crewman on the main deck made first contact with Alaska by tossing a "messenger" line to the dock. The thin rope, weighted at the end with a heavy ball, uncoiled in the air and landed on the pier where a dockworker retrieved it and attached it to a winch. The messenger line pulled over a much bigger polypropylene line, as thick as a man's arm and as heavy as a truck. Then the crew on the ship and the workers on the dock began the extremely dangerous work of tethering us to the pier with ten steel cables an inch and a half in diameter. Below me, a shipmate attentively listened to the cable as it went taut, knowing that a certain change in pitch meant the line was about to break. A heavy ship such as the *Arco Anchorage* can stretch a cable or rope like a violin string and break it in an instant. A line that snaps sounds like a cannon fired across the deck, and it rips apart flesh and equipment the way a knife cuts through bread. A coiled line can be a venomous trap as well. Three months from the day our ship docked at Valdez, a crewman on the deck of the tanker *Exxon New Orleans* was snared by an unrolling line that grabbed him and severed both legs.

Besides injuries, berthing accidents account for approximately 5 percent of the oil that tankers spill. The dribbles at the dock are generally small ones, but whenever chemicals hit the water near shore their impact on vulnerable marine life is more severe. A sign at the pipeline dock below me boasted OVER 10,000 VESSELS SAFELY LOADED SINCE AUGUST 1977. That all depends on how you define safe. Since the terminal began operation, there have been an average of thirty-three small spills a year.

It is a pretty good record, though, given the hazards of dockside operations. The cables and ropes must hold the ship snugly, for instance, or heavy seas and even the wake of passing vessels could jar the tanker loose and sever the pipes delivering the oil. The 807-foot-long tanker *Vic Bilh* was held by sixteen sturdy lines to a dock at Port Neches, Texas, but was pulled away when another ship passed within shouting distance. A smaller tanker, the *Jupiter,* was sucked away from a pipe at a Bay City, Michigan, dock by a ship passing sixty feet away. A spark from a broken electrical cable lit the gasoline that had spilled on the dock, and, like a scene from an action movie, the fire zipped from shore to the ship using the cargo hose as a fuse. Although most of the crew dove overboard just before the vessel erupted in a thunderous explosion, one man was killed.

When Captain Carroll declared that the ship was properly secured, the men on the dock maneuvered a high, arching gangway into place so crew and workers could walk between the ship and the shore. About half the ship's crew was working on deck at the time, and others were either asleep in their rooms or working elsewhere inside the ship. No one went ashore, which made sense since at this time of night there is nothing to do in Valdez. A representative of Alyeska, the consortium of oil companies that owns the terminal, boarded the ship to run down a checklist of safety items. He looked for cameras, cigarettes, and electrical devices: mechanisms that could emit a spark. Once the incendiaries were out of the way, though, he turned his attention to me. Who was I and what the hell was I doing here? I can understand him having concern about outsiders at an oil terminal critical to national security, but the way he eyed me I felt like a book of matches. With a special zeal he informed me that I could not go ashore unless I got permission from higher authorities and I could not take any pictures of him. I could see the pay phone beckoning me just one hundred feet away on the dock, but my jailer would allow no phone calls.

As I turned my attention back to the ship, the crew, heavily bundled against the cold, was to hook the ship to its mother lode of oil. A light snow was falling through the bright floodlights as I strolled along the main deck, watching the hookup and keeping one eye on the Alyeska official. Looming above us at the end of the dock was a tall contraption made of pipe that resembled the cocked forelegs of a praying mantis. The device, known as a hard arm, is the most prominent feature on any oil-loading dock.

Loading a tanker would be easy if the oil came aboard through a flexible rubber hose the way gasoline is pumped into a car. But because the flow of crude is very powerful, hundreds of gallons a second, the job requires rigid steel pipes that weigh tons. The four pipes of the hard arm soar straight up into the air and then down again. Each pipe has flexible joints at the elbows and ankles, so dockworkers can maneuver the heavy pipes into place, and once fastened to the ship, they are pliable enough to follow the vessel when it moves up and down with the tide.

A terminal worker on the edge of the dock directed the praying mantis toward the side of the ship by tapping buttons on a remote-control panel belted to his waist. Crewmen on the deck assisted the pipes into position with their hands, dangerous work because a hard arm moved too fast could crush a man. Everyone wore a hard hat.

With the pipes in the right place, the crew could hook the *Arco*

Anchorage to its oil supply. Each one of the four pipes was bolted to a corresponding twenty-inch manifold pipe located in the middle of the ship's deck. That done, the third mate signaled the chief mate by radio that they were ready for the next of many steps.

Chief mate Svetko Lisica, second in command to the captain and responsible for the loading operation, started preparing the ship for cargo long before we docked. First he got rid of ballast water, the fifteen million gallons of seawater the otherwise unloaded ship carries in its tanks to give it enough weight to keep the propeller underwater and to make it stable in the heavy seas. Clean ballast, having been carried in tanks reserved for ballast water only, was flushed directly into Prince William Sound through a grated hole in the bottom of the ship. The filthy ballast water, carried in cargo tanks, was pumped ashore after we docked. Pumped through the same four pipes that would bring on the cargo, this ballast would later be processed by terminal operators before being released into Valdez harbor. Dan Lawn, an environmental engineer who helped design and later inspect the terminal, says the terminal was originally designed to have sufficient equipment to thoroughly clean the ballast water, but there were cutbacks that diminished the capability. Critics say the water is now processed too quickly and returned to the bay nearly as toxic as it was when it came off the ship. Government investigators were called in recently to determine if ballast water was being dumped into the harbor before it was fully treated and if shipowners were pumping heavy metals from engine waste into the shoreside tanks to get rid of them. The investigators concluded that no laws were broken, but determined some allegations were true and fined tanker owners and terminal operators for sloppy practices. "Technically, they might say the letter of the law was not violated, but the spirit was surely bent," said Lawn.

It took five hours after the *Arco Anchorage* was bolted to the hard arm to deliver its dirty ballast water ashore. Then, shortly before 3 A.M., the crude oil cargo began coming on board with the sound of a bowling ball rolling down a gutter. It was the start of an operation that would last nine hours. In the beginning, the stream was moderate, but when the operators cranked open the faucet, oil poured through the pipes at a rate of more than eleven hundred gallons a second. A few seconds of inattention could spell disaster with oil under such high pressure. A small leak in a gasket would become a gusher very quickly, producing a spray with enough velocity to lacerate a man's skin. Adding to the danger of spills is the fact that the flow can only be stopped from shore; furthermore, it takes seven and a half seconds just to shut the valves.

While the oil came on the ship, the chief mate oversaw its distribution to thirteen cargo tanks from his command post inside a green, neon-lighted control room on the bottom floor of the ship's house. At age forty-five, Lisica has grown up with the sea, his father having been a Yugoslavian seaman before him. Although he is now a U.S. citizen and has worked for Arco for twelve years, Lisica's wife and three teenage daughters live in the homeland. Finding life in Long Beach, California, too crowded and dangerous, the family moved back to the Dalmatian coast only to be trapped when the civil war exploded soon after Lisica returned to America for his current tour of duty on board the *Arco Anchorage*. A short time ago, Lisica learned that a shell had hit the detached garage of his family's home. Although no one was hurt by the explosion, it is hard for Lisica to keep sailing, knowing that back home his loved ones are surrounded by danger. He scans the news bulletins that the radio operator posts in the mess hall, but he never gets enough detail. He calls home when he can, but that's no reassurance when he is half the world away, sailing in a cold, bitter sea. "They are determined to stay. That's my problem."

As he worked in the control room, Lisica was wearing the same thing he wore the day before, and the day before that: black shoes, brown pants, a greenish brown sweater, and a blue shirt. He allowed no interruptions as he manipulated the toggle switches to open and close valves in the piping system. When he finished moving a toggle switch, he placed a wooden spool over it so it could not be flipped accidentally. Occasionally he looked to the wall to check a device that looks a lot like a carpenter's level. He was making sure the ship stayed in trim as it loaded.

"If I load too much by the stern, the ship will lose speed. You don't want too much by the bow, either. Of course, you don't want to list the ship, either."

And, he added, "I also don't want to break it."

Loading or unloading a ship requires an intimate knowledge of its ability to take the stresses and strains of a shifting weight. Crewmen off-loading a 215,000-deadweight-ton tanker in Holland left too much oil and ballast in the front and rear while emptying the middle. The ship snapped in half; the heavy bow and tail sections pointed downward, raising the broken middle into the air. Not the kind of evening Lisica was anxious to have.

Lisica's round, Slavic face looked a little tired as he talked to crewmen out on the deck using his ever-present walkie-talkie. He would soon be able to catch some sleep, though. In an hour or so, the cargo mate, an Arco officer who lives in Valdez, would be relieving him of his loading duties. Not a member of the regular crew, he represents one of the many changes that have been imposed since the *Exxon Valdez* accident. Coast Guard investigators found that chief mates were being worked too hard, sometimes staying awake as many as thirty-six hours loading a ship and then standing watch on the bridge as the vessel was leaving port.

A federal law passed after the spill limited crewmen and officers on any American tanker from working more than fifteen hours in any twenty-four-hour period. Lisica is grateful for the relief. He said chief mates didn't complain in the days when they worked those hours, but that doesn't mean they were not fatigued. "They didn't know any better."

The captain also slept some during the cargo operation, but not until midnight, after he'd arranged for the first engineer to see a doctor in town. The sick engineer was the only one to venture outside the terminal. Carroll and the other crew members have not gone into town much since the days of the *Exxon Valdez* spill. When Valdez residents described tanker crewmen as drunks and misfits after the spill, they resented it. The *Arco Anchorage* was stuck at Knowles Head during the early stages of the *Exxon Valdez* disaster and the crew members heard the radio interviews as townsfolk told of wild parties involving tanker sailors and taxi drivers related how they delivered inebriated captains to the docks. Many of the anecdotes were true, spread over a period of years, but when concentrated into ten-second sound bites, the talk suggested the ships were run like brothels. "Those people in Valdez burned too many bridges," said the third mate Davis. "They told too many gray truths." Hard feelings die slowly on both sides of the fence. But while the crew might not have had much of a desire to visit Valdez, I very much wanted to see the town for the first time since the spill.

After the captain intervened, Alyeska terminal officials gave me permission to go to town, as long as I didn't stop along the way to examine the terminal itself. I awoke around 6 A.M. and on my way off the ship I learned there had been an emergency as I slept. A hydraulic line leading to one of the winches on the forward deck had broken, spilling oily fluid inside the foc's'le house. The captain and his officers were pretty upset about the mishap, worrying that the hydraulic fluid would spill into the water. But it was trapped and cleaned up. The only damage was a broken winch, lost sleep, and frayed nerves.

Clambering over the tall arching gangway on my way to the dock, I felt a little vertigo looking down the canyon between the ship and the pier. From the dock I looked back at the tanker, recalling how it had risen like a balloon during the night when the ballast was being pumped out and was now settling back down in the water under the load of its cargo. When loaded, an oil tanker looks like a sleek sword slicing through the water with the tall house at the back of the ship resembling the hilt. When empty, it looks more like an airplane hanger or a warehouse. Now, in the early morning hours, the hull of the ship was a steel wall blotting out the harbor and nearly half the mountain range behind it. While beauty eludes an oil ship, there is magnificence in its size.

The sun hadn't risen yet as I boarded a cab outside the terminal, but as we circled the harbor on our way into town the moon in a cloudless sky revealed a place surrounded by glistening white mountains. The town itself, a catch basin that averages 360 inches of snow each year, isn't likely to lift a visitor's spirits in winter. Everything is buried under a blanket of dirty snow, and the salt that is used to melt the road ice rusts anything made of metal. Some buildings have a Quonset-hut quality about them, which makes the hamlet look temporary, more like an encampment than an established town. Yet there are ordinary-looking houses as well, and somewhere under the snow there are sidewalks. It is a boom-and-bust place like so much of Alaska, with summer bringing tourists, fishermen, and hunters, and winter bringing long nights, card games, and gloom. Alaska is always in a rush of some sort, a gold rush or an oil rush.

Port Valdez was named in 1790 by a Spanish explorer. The oldest written record after that shows that in 1873 there were ninety-nine men in the Valdez area who owed money to someone "and for what it was never determined," said town historian Dorothy Clifton. The early debtors were probably miners, for Valdez was eventually overrun by indebted treasure hunters in the gold rush of 1898. Some prospectors found gold on the town side of the harbor and copper on the side where the oil terminal is now located, but plenty came up empty. "The town was full of promoters," said Clifton. "Everybody was making their buck. A lot of it wasn't on gold, it was on the gold miners."

Progress brought the area an army fort. Soon to follow were the fishermen, with their fish processing plants, seekers of a slippery kind of silver found in the sea. By then, more and more people were traveling to Valdez, by boat or by climbing over a glacier, but few stayed. In the 1940s, the army turned a trail into a steeply graded road across the mountains, the first motorcar access to the town. "The road wasn't a good road like you'd be used to," said Clifton. "It was a three-track road, if you know what I mean. There were two tracks under your car and one to the side so you could slide over if another car came the other way, which didn't happen too often."

When Clifton arrived in 1963 there were only four hundred inhabitants in Valdez. It was pretty quiet until the afternoon of March 27, 1964, when the earth moved. People in Alaska are accustomed to earthquakes, but this was among the largest ever recorded in North America, registering at least 8.4 on the Richter scale. Underwater landslides in Prince William Sound created enormous walls of water. Clifton said a monstrous wave "sashayed around inside Valdez Harbor like water sloshing in a bathtub." The breaker demolished the waterfront, killing thirty-one men who were unloading a supply ship. The earthquake also set off a 450-mile-an-hour wave that crossed the ocean and hit beaches more than 8,000 miles away. It killed eleven people in Crescent City, California, where a twenty-foot wave razed thirty city blocks. A total of 131 people died in all locations. Scientists who later surveyed the area found that the bottom of the sound had been raised in some places and whole shorelines had been moved. As for the town of Valdez, it was severely damaged. Government authorities worried about the stability of the gravel river delta where it sat, so the U.S. Corps of Engineers moved the whole community four miles away to its present site.

The next quake to hit town was a political and economic one. In 1968, when about five hundred people lived in town, Arco found oil under the frozen Arctic at Prudhoe Bay on the North Slope of Alaska some eight hundred miles away.

A growing environmental movement protested plans by a consortium of oil companies to drill for the stuff, while others debated how the oil would be transported. Numerous proposals were studied and discarded as impractical or silly, like ice-breaking tankers that would cross the top of Canada or oil-carrying submarines that would move under the ice. A pipeline across Canada would have eliminated the need for tankers altogether, but it was rejected because opponents said a valuable resource shouldn't cross foreign soil.

On a tie-breaking vote cast in the Senate by then–Vice President Spiro Agnew, an all-American, eight-hundred-mile-long pipeline between Prudhoe Bay and Valdez was approved in July 1973. The decision meant two things: Valdez would grow and the oil would be transported to the Lower 48 by ship across Prince William Sound and the Gulf of Alaska.

To ease environmental and safety concerns, President Nixon's secretary of the interior had earlier promised that ships carrying oil from Valdez would have double bottoms. But the Arco ships like the newly built *Arco Anchorage,* and most others, were nearly all constructed without them. There were a lot of broken promises to come.

Pipeline construction pushed the Valdez population to almost ten thousand people in the mid-1970s, making for a town full of strangers. Along with the population explosion came corruption and sloppy practices that helped push the pipeline's cost from nine hundred million dollars to over nine billion dollars.

By 1977, when the pipeline was almost ready for operation, no one had yet sailed a super tanker into Valdez Harbor. There were concerns about negotiating the three-quarter-mile-wide narrows between Valdez Harbor and Prince William Sound. To make sailing even more treacherous, there was Middle Rock, a pinnacle sticking up in the middle of these narrows. Adding to the navigation difficulties were extreme winds of up to one hundred miles per hour, and icebergs that clogged the waters just outside the narrows in spring and summer. Under public pressure, Arco sailed the *Arco Fairbanks,* sister ship to the *Arco Anchorage,* through the passageway as a test in April 1977 without incident, and movement of oil began shortly thereafter.

Early operations were cautious. The pilots boarded tankers at Hinchinbrook entrance, much farther out than Cochinos did yesterday. Sometimes, when sustained wind speeds exceeded forty nautical miles per hour, the tankers were not permitted to enter or leave the harbor at all. In times of extremely heavy ice, ships sailed only in daylight. But with the passing of time, safety practices corroded almost as quickly as the steel in the pipeline.

Although the endeavor was immensely profitable, the Alyeska Pipeline Service Company, the consortium of oil firms that operates the pipeline, scrapped a proposal to build extra oil storage tanks that might allow the terminal to shut down for longer periods during bad weather. James Woodle, Coast Guard captain of the port between 1979 and 1982, said his agency made adjustments in the weather criteria so the port wouldn't be closed as often. A requirement that tankers sail only in daylight during times of heavy ice went by the wayside, too. Then tanker captains were left alone to negotiate the ice floes in Prince William Sound when pilots found the weather too rough out at Hinchinbrook and had their boarding and off-boarding station moved back to a point just outside the Valdez Narrows.

In addition, a staff of Coast Guard traffic coordinators who guided the ships in and out of Valdez using radar and two-way radios was reduced in size. The staff's effectiveness was reduced even further when the radar system was downgraded in quality.

When Woodle retired from the Coast Guard and took a job with Alyeska in 1982, he discovered that consortium officials were telling the public one thing and doing another. Cleanup crews were cut back while the public was assured that the oil companies could handle any accident. Emergency drills were phony and on certain days of the week—like a Friday before a long weekend—there was nothing but a skeletal crew on staff. "They were there to make money. They cut corners," said Woodle.

Mike Cavett, the Coast Guard captain who replaced Woodle, said the Coast Guard operation was so slack, the post was nicknamed "Coast Guard Resort Valdez." Among the various offenses were Coast Guard enlisted personnel moonlighting as car mechanics for the townspeople and using drugs.

Meanwhile, Alyeska, like any major employer, enjoyed a cozy relationship with the town of Valdez. There were complainers, but most Alaskans were quite happy with a relationship that provided them with a tax-free life, with monthly stipends. When the *Exxon Valdez* spill occurred on a Friday before a long weekend—with too few Alyeska employees on duty to handle it—some people were stunned by the atrophied response system. Others knew they had paid the price for a pact with the devil.

"Like Faust, Alaskans came to an agreement with Mephistopheles and it didn't work out," wrote Alaskan writer and teacher Irving Warner in a letter to England's *Manchester Guardian*. "Many of us now want our state's soul back. We got our Helen of Troy, but she lied, cheated and is slowly corrupting our lands, waters and us."

But for the town of Valdez—which was itself never stained by oil—there was a brighter side to the spill. Like the gold rush and the oil rush before it, the spill rush brought in tons of money. The town was flooded with out-of-town visitors and the streets were crowded with job seekers. There were lines of people waiting to be hired to wipe oil off rocks for sixteen dollars an hour. Fishermen could lease a boat to the cleanup contractor for thousands of dollars a day. The spillionaires, as they were called, grew rich on the profits of smeared beaches. For a while, the nearly three-billion-dollar cleanup was the state's biggest industry. Some say Exxon sopped up more anger than oil with its dollar bills. That rush, too, came to an end, and in the end some were left to wonder if it wasn't another pact with the devil.

Before returning to the ship, my cabdriver took me on a tour of the town. The low winter sun had barely shaken itself clear of the powdered mountaintops and the village was still dozing. I was grateful for the all-night Safeway store where I paid for an armful of candy mints, camera film, and souvenirs. We passed the day care center where, back in the days of the spill, the proprietor had rented me his car. I recalled how the guy told me there were too many broken families in town, the result of a hard Alaskan life. We passed the restaurant where once old-timers had regaled me with frontier yarns, like the guy who played cat-and-mouse games from behind a tree with a very cantankerous moose. We passed the school where organizers had assembled cleanup crews, and the vacant lot where people had camped waiting for jobs. It was all familiar to me, except for the pace, which now seemed entirely too slow. The cabdriver explained that Valdez has quieted down a great deal since the days of the cleanup, and the result has been a business slump. For some, hard times had returned.

Back at the entrance to the terminal complex, I passed through a checkpoint where a guard examined me closely for signs of drunkenness. After *Exxon Valdez* captain Joseph Hazelwood was accused of drinking before the accident, a Breathalyzer machine was installed at this gate. This scrutiny has caught a few tanker crew members coming back drunk, including a captain, but no one is imbibing today. The precaution is good for public relations, but the fact is that not too many tanker accidents have been caused by drunkenness.

The guy who drove me from the gate to the ship, past the rows of holding tanks glistening in the snow, was under orders not to talk to any writers. It's an old Alyeska rule that creates bizarre "conversations." I asked him whether the pipeline snakes down the hill and he said, "No, it does not do that." I said, "Well, what does it do?" and he replied, "I cannot answer that." I said, "Well, does it just come straight in out of the mountains?" and he said, "Something like that."

The pipeline consortium has a well-earned reputation for paranoia. They have fired whistle-blowers, but probably the most damaging case to their image began when Charles Hamel, a one-time tanker operator and entrepreneur from Alexandria, Virginia, began leaking information about Alyeska's operations to the Environmental Protection Agency, congressional committees, and the media. Alyeska hired a Florida-based security agency, the Wackenhut Corporation, to investigate him. Wackenhut conducted a black-bag operation that included the use of women, undercover agents, electronic surveillance gear, and a phony environmental organization to lure him into revealing his sources inside of Alyeska. They watched his home, picked through his trash, and obtained his banking and telephone records. Alyeska and its police-state contractor didn't stop there, either. They targeted other critics as well, including the chairman of the House Interior Committee, George Miller, a Democrat from California, who was responsible for Alyeska oversight.

When the Alyeska escort dropped me at the ship, he told me to board without talking to dockworkers. The stringent security had both amused and irritated me enough to think about climbing a ladder to talk with one of the hard-arm operators, just to set off the alarms. In the past the hard-arm operators have told me some pretty wild stories about sotted crew members knee-walking their way onto the ships. But I wanted to get back to the *Arco Anchorage* so I wouldn't miss any of the action that surrounds the final stages of loading. I chatted for a moment with one of the dockworkers, who responded with some easygoing banter, then I walked up the gangway, noticing on my way how much lower the ship was sitting in the water.

On board, the crew was topping off the tanks. They wore breathing masks on their faces, another recent change brought about by reports that petroleum fumes may cause cancer.

Topping off is a delicate operation that requires crew members to stand near tank tops measuring the rising oil so no tank is overfilled. Overfill the ship, and oil will spray into the air out of a mast riser near the front of the ship's main deck. Underfill it and you'll waste money. Three seamen and the third mate radioed their measurements to the control room while they shuffled their feet to keep warm. As the loading operation came to an end, the mate went down to the dock and checked a line on the side of the hull to assure that the ship was sitting low enough in the water to be fully loaded, but not too low so that it would violate the load-line laws. Each inch of immersion represents about thirty-six thousand dollars' worth of oil at today's prices, so accurately filling the ship is important. Then there are variables a landlubber would never think of: When looking at the load line, the mate takes into account that a tanker sits lower in the less salty water of the stream-fed bay than it does out in the ocean, among many other things.

All the time we were topping off, Tech Leepansen, an independent petroleum inspector, also known as a gauger, was on board. An auditor of sorts, he frequently used a sophisticated dipstick to determine exactly how much oil was on the ship so that neither the buyer nor the seller felt cheated. Although Arco is a member of the Alyeska consortium that owns the pipeline, the company is a buyer like anyone else when one of its ships pulls up to the dock.

The oil is still hot after it makes its eight-hundred-mile pipeline trip over three mountain ranges and eight hundred rivers and streams. But by the time it gets to the ship after sitting in holding tanks, it ranges in temperature between 60 and 120 degrees. The warm oil contains water; if there is too much, it becomes a loss to the buyer. Leepansen's dipstick beeped with a different sound when the end of it passed through the oil and reached the water that settled at the bottom of the tank. He determined to his satisfaction that our load did not contain too much water.

Hamel, the target of the Wackenhut investigation, says Alyeska spiked some of the oil he purchased from the pipeline ten years ago. The consortium added water to his oil to punish him for operating a tanker at prices that were undercutting the major shipowners. "I got an extra jolt of it. The worst voyage was with seven hundred thousand dollars' worth of water. I'll tell you, it hurts right here—uuuuuh," he told me, pointing to his groin. Alyeska denied the claim.

When Leepansen finished his gauging work, he met with chief mate Lisica and they began what is a traditional argument over the actual amount of the load. They huddled in the chief mate's office in front of a computer that contained all the data. Lisica closed the door when I tried to listen. Nobody blindly trusts anybody in the oil business.

Captain Carroll was by then on the bridge with a new pilot, Timothy Christy, getting ready to leave the dock. With bitter winds whipping around them, crewmen on the bow jury-rigged a system of ropes and cables to replace the winch that broke last night and began the painfully slow task of pulling in the lines. Over the radio, the captain learned that, because the gusts were blowing over fifty miles an hour in the Valdez Narrows, he would have four escort boats to follow him out, just in case he lost power or steering. Normally there are two, but with such high wind conditions the Coast Guard can require more. One boat had on board a modest amount of booming equipment and a man whose only job it was to sit there ready to direct a cleanup operation in case of another spill.

Months after our voyage, a Prince William Sound tug would save a disabled tanker from hitting Middle Rock. But as we sailed toward Middle Rock, Carroll knew that his escort service was not what it could be. Escort tugs should be able to throw a line to a tanker in all sorts of conditions and take it under control. But there are two kinds of tugboats: the ordinary kind that are designed to push ships or pull barges, and tractor tugs specially designed to wrestle with wayward tankers.

Escort services in Europe and Japan rely upon tractor tugs, equipped with a vertical fanlike propeller underneath the belly. The tractors have an uncanny ability to maintain traction while pulling or pushing on a ship in conditions when a regular tug would be overwhelmed. During the 1970s, the Coast Guard sent Captain James Atkinson around the world to learn about tug escorts. After witnessing the effectiveness of tractor tugs, he tried to get Alyeska and the Coast Guard interested in using them in Valdez. Despite a demonstration he set up in Valdez Harbor in 1977 that clearly demonstrated the bumbling inabilities of conventional tugs, no one was interested in tractor tugs because they were substantially more expensive than the conventional ones. The drive system alone is priced at one million dollars.

Atkinson retired shortly afterward and the tugs in Prince William Sound remained the same.

Finally, a decade and a half later, there may be a change in the works. After the tug company Foss Maritime bought some tractor tugs and put them to work in Washington waters, Arco and British Petroleum announced in 1992 that they would allow only Foss tractors to escort tankers in that state. The Coast Guard's regional office recommended that the agency require other tanker companies to do the same, but the Washington, D.C., headquarters backed down and left the choice up to the discretion of the tanker captain. Although tractor tugs would cost pipeline owners only a few days' profits, things haven't changed yet in Alaska. But some hope the move in Washington state will pressure the Valdez port and others to do the same.

Some people have faith in the present system, though. As we left the dock and headed for Valdez Narrows, our pilot Christy told me he believes the many reforms instituted since the *Exxon Valdez* accident are enough to guarantee safety. After passing through Valdez Narrows under a speed limit of six nautical miles per hour, the *Arco Anchorage* had to obey an additional new speed limit of ten nautical miles per hour all the way to Hinchinbrook. In the old days, ships could hit top speed as soon as they left the narrows. Also, Christy would be getting off the ship at a new, slightly more distant location near Bligh Reef so that, among other things, captains will no longer sail through iceberg territory without a pilot the way Hazelwood did on the *Exxon Valdez*. We were also being guided by new Coast Guard radar equipment and the escort tugs followed us all the way out to a point near Hinchinbrook.

"We have done so many things for safety up here that the chances of an accident are really remote," said Christy. "A BP study says it is a 1-in-64,000 chance."

The evening before the *Exxon Valdez* accident, Alyeska officials declined an invitation from Valdez townspeople to send a speaker to a meeting regarding tanker risks. But Riki Ott, a fisherwoman from the nearby town of Cordova who also holds a doctorate in water pollution, told the group by speaker phone they had plenty to fear from the oil ships. When Hazelwood boarded the tanker that fateful evening, not even Ott could have predicted what he and his crew would do. After the pilot left the ship, Hazelwood stayed in his cabin, something no tanker captain would normally do while sailing in inland waters. An overconfident and weary third mate and a helmsman with a reputation for poor steering were left to guide the tanker around an unusually enormous flow of icebergs known as "growlers." For reasons no one can figure out, the ship's steering was placed on automatic pilot, another no-no in inland waters. The vessel sailed out of the tanker lanes, out of sight of the sometimes blinded Coast Guard radar, and onto Bligh Reef.

Won't happen again, said Christy.

Probably not, but I thought about the observations of a member of the Alaska Oil Spill Commission, a citizens' group that investigated the accident and made recommendations for change. Ed Wenk, Jr., an emeritus professor of engineering and public affairs at the University of Washington, knows a great deal about the strength of ships. He was a structural designer at the Boston Navy shipyard in 1941 and conducted the maiden tests on the hull strength of the world's first nuclear submarine. He was a science adviser to three presidents—John Kennedy, Lyndon Johnson, and Richard Nixon—and a researcher in Congress. He was in Europe with Vice President Hubert Humphrey when the *Torrey Canyon* went aground, rushing to the scene in time to catch a scent of the noxious oil. For the past twenty-five years he has earned a reputation as both an irritating gadfly and an incisive commentator with his calls for safety reform.

Wenk believes that almost all systems have "operating instructions," and the most important one in the tanker industry is that safety costs money. That implies that safety is too expensive. "As long as that is one of the operating instructions, nothing will change.

"They want to ship oil in the largest ships, with the thinnest hulls, with the smallest crews, to save money. They use their political power to make their case, to block safety."

When an airplane goes down, the voter and the congressman can identify with that since they fly in airplanes. But most don't ride on ships, so the impact of a ship disaster is usually not as powerful.

"The only thing that will beat the system is when you have a major accident. A major accident, like the *Exxon Valdez,* has a fantastic virtue. An accident agitates the system so much that now you see things with your eyes shut that you couldn't have seen with your eyes open."

Wenk says of the changes now being adopted by the tanker industry in the wake of the *Exxon Valdez* disaster that most have been "on the books" as recommendations for twenty-five years. Since the attitude that allowed people to ignore them for so long hasn't changed, he predicts the industry will return to old practices once the Valdez spill fades from memory.

"What we are not doing is going back and asking ourselves, why were these recommendations of five years ago, ten years ago, twenty years ago, ignored. And we need to make sure that the lessons of the past become the operating instructions of the future. Otherwise, we'll just keep repeating the errors."

The ship nosed through Valdez Narrows like a slow freight train chugging through a narrow canyon. As the space between steep white slopes tapered in front of us, the wind tunnel tore at our flags and ripped white froth from the chop of the waves. Middle Rock passed several hundred yards away on our right, not a stone's throw for a guy like me but perhaps within range of a bionic arm. As we exited the narrows and lumbered into the middle waters of Prince William Sound, the magical basin showed us one more sleight of hand. The fierce windstorm that had buffeted us in the narrows suddenly and completely vanished. I don't know where all that air went, but we were now sailing in total calm. In the space of a few miles we had changed weather as quickly as a magician switches cards.

The pilot boat arrived and in a continuing calm I walked with our harbor guide across the main deck to see him off. It was 4:20 P.M., but, given the short working hours of the winter sun, dusk had already arrived. He was grateful for the lack of gusts as he crossed the railing under a darkening sky and lowered himself to his boat. The ladder was shorter now with the loaded boat sitting low in the water. Many pilots rue the idea that the public will pressure regulators to force them to meet and depart ships out at Hinchinbrook rather than here. Maybe a pilot will break his leg climbing a ship ladder in these waters, but you could die playing rope-ladder games on the edge of the Gulf of Alaska, Christy told me.

As I said good-bye to our Alaskan pilot, I knew I would not see another stranger until we reached Washington state. Up on the bridge, Carroll was relieved to regain full control of his ship, and he seemed anxious to reenter the ocean where he could pick a fight with nature without so many rules to follow. I've never met a ship captain who liked people telling him what to do. In the darkness, Carroll complained about the ten-nautical-mile-an-hour speed limit that forced him to crawl so slowly across the last stretches of Prince William Sound.

"It used to take five hours from Valdez to Hinchinbrook, now it takes seven."

4

The Captain

*(Outside Hinchinbrook Island,
January 25, 9:15 P.M.)*

"**F**eel that?" the captain asks, as though I could overlook a gut
punch from the Pacific Ocean. It's serious business out here, a
full-force gale. The low-pressure system we saw on the weather map
as we approached Hinchinbrook was no joke. Now that we are out in
the Gulf of Alaska, the winds are blowing over seventy miles an hour,
coming at our face from the southeast. The tanker feels like a rowboat
and the fury of this frontal assault makes the gusts in Valdez Narrows
seem downright gentle. This is Mother Nature on angel dust, Sonny
Liston versus Twiggy.

Captain Carroll is not asking whether I feel the obvious sensations
of the ocean at our throats. He is inquiring whether I sense the subtle
sounds of the ship writhing in pain. He is "feeling the ship" to get a
sense of the storm. The volume of the grinding and groaning will tell
him whether he should turn left on a shortcut over the shallower water
or right for a softer ride in the deep.

Once again the ship is jolted, and a white wall of water rises high
in the air above the bow. The winches on top of the foc's'le house,
visible a moment ago, disappear under a wave as though they were
flotsam on a beach. The main deck is closed to all on board for there
is no muscle in a man's body strong enough to grip a railing against
such a fierce ocean. Outside on the bridge wing, the lookout is standing

in a horizontal rain. Stinging remnants of the wave that hit the bow now blow past his face. Everywhere there's a steel joint in the ship, the metal is complaining. I'm excited and a little leery. I haven't gotten seasick on this trip yet, but this tempest has the look of a true test.

The mate, though, has an expression on his face that says, "You ain't seen nothing yet." Sure this is a storm, but we aren't talking hurricane yet. Tanker sailors are accustomed to frothy waves soaking the deck machines. With the belly of the tanker more than fifty feet underwater, there is only seventeen feet of clearance between the mean waterline and the first railing of the main deck—not enough of an obstacle to stop one of these thirty-foot rollers. The veterans, however, don't get excited until they see a solid wall of green water crossing the bow. That is when the pipes break and the ship takes a solid nosedive.

Sometimes a tanker will soar too high off the top of a wave and slam down so hard it will bash the steel asunder. On one Arco ship the extra propeller bolted to the main deck broke loose and the forty-seven-ton object, as big around as a three-story building, wandered down the deck tearing pipes loose. "I've seen the gangway wrapped up around the port king post. Tank tops torn off, and oil out in the open," says the captain. "I've seen the sea break crude wash pipelines in half."

Tonight, the massive main deck looks like a coastal seawall facing a blistering tempest. Waves slap against the steel breakwaters that are arranged like fences in front of the equipment. They strip enough energy from the waves that they flatten to fast-moving streams by the time they reach the house. It will get worse, I'm told. Said one veteran crewman: "You know you are in trouble when the waves start breaking over the bridge."

"Then we just hope and hang on," said another.

Carroll notes the direction of the wind and says that if we were to turn left, and head on a true course to the Lower 48 over the shallower water, we'd hit the storm right on the nose and bang into the heaviest seas.

"So I'm going to go that way," he says, pointing right.

He gives the order, and the helmsman steers the ship on a heading that would put us in Hawaii if we stayed on it. We'll turn back to the main highway south, the captain explains, when we pass Middleton Island, an inhospitable outcropping of rock surrounded by vast reefs some fifty miles south of Hinchinbrook. The route he's chosen will take us over the hundred-fathom curve of deep water where the seas should be less angry. "Stay in the canyon, it's good for the ship."

The ship takes a hard roll and Carroll notices a blip on the radar screen. Another tanker, the *Prince William Sound,* has chosen to go left on a beeline to the states. He'll check in a few days to see who fares better. I pencil a reminder in my notebook.

The captain's decision to turn right is the kind of move that could add years of life to the ship and hours to the trip. It could also be a bad one if he loses the pinball game that sailors play against the violence-prone low-pressure systems drifting around the gulf. A lot of bad wagers have been made by desperate mariners out here.

But the captain's decision tells a lot about his style. Some masters drive a ship hard, pushing it head-on into heavy seas at a schedule-keeping speed. Others slow down and turn into the trough. By turning right, Carroll underlines the fact that he is a cautious guy who spares the equipment. Maybe it is a unique glimpse into his future. Maybe it portends that Carroll will retire in comfortable anonymity rather than going out in a blaze of worldwide notoriety like Joseph Hazelwood.

A study the Coast Guard was reluctant to release (until my newspaper threatened legal action) shows that tankers are too often driven in heavy seas as though this were a demolition derby. It isn't pluck that inspires these lead-footed captains so much as the fear of the shipowners, who worry that money will be lost if their tankers arrive too late in port. An unnamed ship with a reputation for cracking was required by the owners to maintain an average speed of over fourteen nautical miles per hour for several months. The bureaucrats who kept track of the ship's schedule included the time spent in port when they figured the speed. To keep that pace, the harried master had to sail the vessel at sixteen knots, which is nearly top speed for the *Arco Anchorage,* regardless of weather, fog, or traffic. When the captain complained, the front office told him to do whatever was necessary to keep up. The anonymous skipper said he'd heard of captains being fired for not meeting the schedule, but never for driving a ship too hard.

Carroll says that such demands are no longer part of the Arco operation. "That's not even talked about. If you slow down a ship for a good reason, nothing is ever said." Jerry Aspland, the fleet president, says he worries more about captains who sail too fast than he does about missing a schedule. He thinks sailing a ship too hard is a matter of personality, not necessity. Skippers in their seventh to twentieth year are the worst speedsters, and Aspland is not sure why. He hopes Carroll remains cautious even as he gains experience.

"I would hope people would say, I take care of the ship," says Carroll. "I don't bang 'em."

Carroll never dreamed of being a ship captain when he was a child. Some of his first views of the world were from a bar stool in New York City. His grandfather was an Irish barkeeper in Queens who played minor league baseball on the side. The old guy would set up shots, talk sports, and collect wagers while his grandson sat back and took in the wonders of this world. Carroll's dad ran his own company making name tags until heart problems forced him to go into sales. Carroll is dedicated to his dad, and proud of him, noting how the older man would drive two hours a day just to make sure his son could play sports after school.

Maybe it was Grandpa's influence, but Carroll grew up as an athlete not as a scholar. The skipper still looks ready to play as he paces the bridge of his tanker in his steel-toed running shoes. The grace hasn't left his lanky body in its fourth decade of life. That's how it was when he was a kid. Young Jack seemed like a natural athlete even as a toddler in Queens. He kept it up in the Long Island suburb of Farmington, some forty miles from New York City, when his family moved there as he was entering grade school. He eventually lettered in soccer, basketball, and baseball at St. Anthony's all-male Catholic high school in neighboring Smithtown.

The ball always felt easier in Carroll's hands than the schoolbook. But the ship captain figures he got the best lessons in self-discipline not from any coach, but from a man of the cloth. A teacher at St. Anthony's paid him $1.50 an hour to do chores after class and to garden during the summer. Carroll remembers resenting the old padre at first, but his parents urged him to stick with the job.

"He was a demanding guy, tough, tough, very tough. He would keep people there. He would preach at 'em, yell at 'em. Boy, when I first got to know him, I was afraid of him."

Later, when Carroll was an altar boy he got to know the clergyman better and to like him a little more. When the priest died, Carroll learned that, all along, the strict cleric had been helping his family pay his high school tuition. It wasn't just the family finances the priest was supplementing, though, but, in good Catholic tradition, the health of the youngster's soul.

"He kept me out of trouble while I was growing up. I never got into the drug scene. A little beer, maybe, but not much."

Although he was never a great all-around student, Carroll did well on tests. With a high Scholastic Aptitude Test score he caught the attention of the registrar at the prestigious U.S. Merchant Marine Academy in Kings Point, New York. Carroll had applied for a congressional appointment to the school not because he yearned for a life at sea, but because the tuition and boarding were free. It was also easier to get admitted there than at the other service academies like Annapolis. The day Carroll got word he was accepted to Kings Point, he was also named athlete of the year at his high school. As it turned out, admission to the merchant marine equivalent of Harvard turned out to be more important.

The uniformed underclassmen and women at Kings Point are required to march around and salute like Navy plebes, but the setting for all this militarism is nothing short of spectacular: an eighty-acre beachfront property with a dazzling view of the Manhattan skyline. Multimillionaire Henry Chrysler built the Long Island estate in the 1920s so he could watch his Chrysler Building go up in the city across from him. The federal government formed the academy in 1938 and purchased the Chrysler estate for a song during World War II—just one hundred thousand dollars. The demands of the war—in which 140 academy graduates lost their lives—forced the government to compress the academy curriculum from four years to two. By the time Carroll arrived in 1974, however, it was once again a four-year institution with an enrollment of around one thousand. The school is run by the nation's most obscure uniformed corps, the U.S. Maritime Service, an arm of the Department of Transportation whose only job is to train future deck and engine room commanders. It is not a service with a bright future. With each passing year, as the nation's merchant marine fleet shrinks, the academy enrollment declines.

Carroll brought muscle and grace to the ball fields of Kings Point, but he struggled in the classroom. He needed a 2.0 grade average (out of a possible 4.0) to stay in school, and managed a 2.4 with a lot of work. In the end, he got his bachelor of science degree in engineering, his third mate's license, and an ensign's commission in the Navy reserve. And in the years that followed he did better than most academy graduates, by attaining the rank of captain.

He never gets an easy start at anything, however. His first day on a ship was no more auspicious than his debut as a ship captain. Like other academy cadets, young Carroll had to serve an internship on a couple of cargo vessels during his sophomore and junior years. His first on-the-job classroom was a container ship docked at Staten Island. Shortly after he stepped on board, the chief mate told him to follow a crewman to a container so he could sweep it out. "I'm twenty feet behind this guy. He goes around the corner and I hear a shout." The crewman had fallen one hundred feet into a cargo hold. When Carroll got to him, he was dead. Carroll helped the mate put the battered body into a plastic bag and move it to a cooler. At a later court hearing Carroll learned that the victim was a young man with a wife and two children. The cause of his death "was a little grease on the deck."

"It was, like, welcome to the sea."

During another internship on an Arco ship, the seventy-one-thousand-ton *Arco Sag River,* Carroll peered into a tank and was overcome by fumes, a common tanker mistake that can be fatal. Despite the chilling experience, he liked the work on tankers and mastered the job quickly. He impressed the Arco officers and when he graduated from Kings Point in 1978 the company gave him a job as a third mate on the now-defunct *Arco Prestige.*

"I was fired my first day on the job," says Carroll, pausing for a moment as another wave crosses the *Arco Anchorage* deck. "It was Blackie Bristow who did it." Bristow was a legendary Arco captain, a terror in the fleet. Carroll remembers how he reported for duty that first day with a short haircut, a scrubbed face, and a sea bag full of schoolbooks. Bristow was unimpressed. "I know who the fuck you are," he said. "You are the new green third mate. Don't unpack your bags until I tell you to because you may get fired before you are done with your first watch."

The ship was sailing out of Houston into waters famous for heavy traffic when Bristow turned it over to Carroll and went downstairs. Carroll white-knuckled it past a multitude of dots on the radar screen. "My arms were sweaty and I was exhausted." When the watch ended at midnight, an academy buddy, then working in the engine room, invited Carroll to his quarters to celebrate their first night of watch standing. The friend brought out a bottle and glasses were passed around. The alcohol policy wasn't very strict in those days, but Bristow was on the prowl. "Blackie walked the ship at night, trying to catch people." Bristow charged through the door, saw the bottle, and said, 'Get up to my office. You are fired.'"

The dismissal turned out to be a bluff. He kept Carroll "fired" until they arrived in Delaware, then he rehired him. "Blackie fired people and then hired them back, just to be a gruffy old guy."

Carroll had a few more run-ins with Bristow until one day he confronted him and stood his ground. From then on, the tough captain treated him with respect. Bristow gave him an unusually glowing performance report, which helped Carroll rise fast in the company. By 1985 he was chief mate on the *Sag River,* the same ship he'd fainted on as a lowly cadet nine years earlier. Six years after making chief mate, he was a captain.

Carroll may have benefited from Bristow, but he didn't adopt the old captain's style. Instead, Carroll's mentor is Arco Captain John Piotrowski, a man who is the exact opposite of the Bristow model. As Carroll experiments with the job of master, he regularly thinks back to the way Piotrowski would do things. The veteran skipper, who now commands the *Arco Prudhoe Bay,* is widely admired in the fleet for his evenhanded style and fairness. He commands by example rather than terror. Carroll says the main lesson Piotrowski taught him was that leadership begins with a self-examination. "Just be yourself," the senior captain told Carroll before he took over this assignment. "Carry yourself, and you'll have no trouble as a captain."

Carroll said cooperation is the most important lesson he learned from the men and women he sailed with. "You can sit here and you can make a happy ship, or you can make a sad ship."

My landlubber legs respond clumsily to the rolling motion of the ship as we hit more thirty-foot seas. I'm surprised at how far over a fully loaded tanker can heel and I'm grateful for a railing to grab on to.

As Carroll guides the *Arco Anchorage* into the gulf tonight, his wife Ann is recovering from their son's birthday party while watching over their daughter as well. In her spare time, she is selling their three-bedroom, twenty-three-hundred-square-foot house in Plano, Texas, so they can move into a thirty-eight-hundred-square-foot replacement they have purchased on thirteen acres in nearby Argyle. There's room enough there for the two kids, the horses they own, and the black Labrador retriever named Tanker. Carroll can't wait to drive through the gate of his new estate in his gas-guzzling Cadillac.

Carroll says an Arco officer's most important benefit is the one day of vacation he earns for every day he sails. Even so, the best relationship he can hope for is a part-time one, a couple of months at home and then two at sea. The ninety-two thousand dollars a year he earns make the time pass more easily, but it doesn't buy harmony. "You've got to have an understanding wife, or this could be a horrible job."

Carroll first encountered Ann when he was a sophomore at the academy. True to his ways, it was not a promising beginning. His family had moved from Long Island to Plano, a booming suburb north of Dallas, seeking a better life. Carroll was home on vacation when Ann, who played basketball with Carroll's sister on the local high school team, telephoned their home one night asking for a ride home because her car had broken down. Carroll said his sister wasn't home and hung up the phone abruptly, leaving Ann stranded. When Ann asked her friend afterward who the hell that was, she replied: "It was my brother Jack. He hates Texas." It would be years before the couple began dating. By the time they got married, in 1982, Carroll was working for Arco.

A sailor's marriage is not *Ozzie and Harriet* by any means. Carroll is at sea so often the couple celebrates their November 6 anniversary only once every other year. With adjustments, they do well. Ann makes a modest living—or at least breaks even—teaching horses to run and jump the obstacle courses of equestrian competition. She studied horse training at a college in Missouri. Standing five feet, seven inches tall, with a cheery face and an easy sense of humor, the captain's wife is as athletic as he is. When Carroll comes home, she challenges her cocky husband to a game of one-on-one basketball. She says if he didn't foul her so much, she could beat him.

When Carroll is gone, he and his wife have faced more than one crisis. The worst was the day Ann's father died suddenly and unexpectedly, leaving the entire family in shock. Billy Bruce Arledge had been a Navy pilot, an oil-well wildcatter, a dairy farmer and rancher. He brought home fancy cars in good times and debt in bad times, like when the Oklahoma oil fields began to trickle rather than gush. He shared with his daughter a love of horses. It was a powerful bond. Ann's dad put her on the back of a small Shetland pony before she was old enough to walk. When they moved to Plano, where there wasn't room for horses, he made adjustments so she would have a pony by the time she was in her early teens. Ann was numb at the news of his death, cold and unable to talk. As the fifty-fifty luck of a sailor's wife would have it, Carroll was out on the tanker. She had never telephoned her husband on the ship before, because a call like that costs at least forty dollars just for the first few words. Carroll knew something was wrong when the radio officer came to get him. It was a stormy night in 1990, just like this one, and Carroll's tanker was leaving Hinchinbrook with a full load of oil. The first words out of Ann's mouth were, "My father is dead," and then she could talk no more. Her brother had to get on the line to explain the rest. Although the captain let Carroll call home every night for free, he was filled with sorrow and worry for the remainder of the ship's tumultuous twelve-hundred-mile trip to Port Angeles. The pilot boat took him to shore, but he couldn't catch a flight home until the next day. Carroll landed in Texas just as the undertaker's limousine was stopping at the beer-and-wine store on the way home from the burial. Carroll made it to the party that Billy Bruce had always wanted for his wake. He was relieved to finally hold his wife in his arms.

Carroll is an attentive dad when he's home, but parenting has been another long-distance challenge. Their first child, Kristin, was born with rare chromosomal damage that caused everything from hearing to heart problems. Two days after she was born, doctors told the new parents their daughter might not live. One of the biggest scares came when, as an infant, the child stopped breathing and had to be revived on the kitchen floor by her mom. Today she is a sweet and lively five-year-old who needs extra medical attention and help in school; as any parent of a handicapped child knows, the special needs tug on the soul.

As for the boy, they named him Billy Bruce after Ann's father, and he inherited spunk from both sides of the family. He has no health problems, which is a good thing for Ann, but he is a high-speed toddler with a mind of his own.

Though he is dedicated to his job, Carroll says the best days of his life are the first ones after he arrives home and the worst are the last when he leaves. "People are out here to make money, earn vacation, and go home."

The *Exxon Valdez* accident gave some people a cut-and-paste image of tanker captains—irresponsible rascals who, like Joseph Hazelwood, dip in and out of alcohol treatment while commanding an oil ship. But unlike Hazelwood, Carroll has not mixed alcohol with ship work since his run-in with Bristow. Even so, he must prove he is not Hazelwood every time he prepares to sail from the dock. As now prescribed by law, a mate watches him blow into a handheld breath analyzer device to check for alcohol in his system; a humiliating precaution, but one he must live with it. Carroll won't drink any alcohol until he boards the plane for his flight home on vacation, and even then he'll palm his identity so the public doesn't get aroused. When fellow passengers ask, he will tell them he is a marine insurance salesman, not a tanker captain. He doesn't want anyone telling the folks at home that there was another Hazelwood on the plane, sipping martinis.

The annals of marine history are filled with descriptions of ship captains who made horrendous mistakes, but less recorded are the routine times when they protected our shores. Skippers like Carroll didn't build the modern oil tanker with the thinnest possible hull, they just have to drive them.

If the experts are right that human error causes 80 percent of tanker accidents, then Carroll is probably more important to this ship than a double hull. Before we fling our arrows at these guys, we should examine them more carefully. Maybe Carroll could be called a front-line environmentalist for the way he's handled his tanker in this storm. Maybe his caution is the difference between a clean beach and an oiled one.

There is no cookie-cutter way to describe the typical tanker commander. The two skippers who alternately drive the *Arco Anchorage* certainly come out of a different mold. Robert Lawlor, more than a decade older than Carroll, stands at parade rest most of the time he is on the bridge; his feet spread apart so he resembles a sturdy, five-foot, eight-inch-tall A-frame. The eyes are disapproving and piercing, as though they are searching for something in a mist. Although he has a keen sense of humor, Lawlor's manner is dismissive and he expects the audience around him to listen intently when he speaks. He believes in the symbols of power and order, even going so far as to say he would fire a crewman for sitting in the captain's chair. His demand for formality carries over into the officer's mess hall where there is a rigid seating arrangement. Lawlor is the strong father figure, a patriarch.

By contrast, Carroll is much more convivial with those around him. And although he's reputed to have a fierce temper, it comes and goes as quickly as a Texas rainstorm. He's also more apt to engage in self-criticism than the battened-down Lawlor. A crewman can sit in the captain's chair if he likes, and a little rearranging of the seating at dinner never disturbed Carroll.

However, Carroll might be tougher by some measures than Lawlor. For one thing, he is unhappy with the condition of the ship as

Lawlor has left it. He told me the other day he will turn it around even if it takes an overdue black mark on some officer's performance evaluation. It would be a mistake to assume that Carroll's good humor and his desire to make a "happy ship" mean he would coddle a slacker. Fleet president Jerry Aspland says some older captains talk tough but give out glowing annual appraisals to people who don't deserve them. Carroll hasn't filled out the paperwork yet, but I think some people are in for a surprise.

Trust, of course, is the fullest measure of a ship captain, whether it is public trust or the confidence of the crew. The *Arco Anchorage* crew praised both Carroll and Lawlor. They said they'd steam into a typhoon with either man, and expect fairness from both in case of discipline.

Outside in the gulf, the one-sided pummeling continues. The ocean delivers its punches and the ship tries to duck the worst ones. Jack Carroll must catch some sleep, but he is taking no chances with the thin hull of the *Arco Anchorage*. As he hands over the bridge to third mate Dean Davis, he gives him instructions to maintain a slow speed and to call him if conditions get worse. Although the skipper's veteran legs have adjusted to the pitching ship, he prudently grips both handrails as he pads down a flight of stairs to the three-room suite he calls home. His door is the closest to the stairway, a design statement about the importance of a master near the helm.

His office, lounge, and bedroom look out at the bow through portholes that are sealed shut tonight by latched hatches. "Years ago, I'd walk by this office and look in. This room to me used to have a real mystique."

The office is businesslike—a metal desk, copy machine, computer, file cabinets, small conference table, and rack of three-ring binders containing the company rules and federal regulations a skipper needs at his fingertips. Taking me into his adjacent lounge, Carroll apologizes for the discount store decorations—a cartoonish picture of an owl, a poster of Arco ships, and a reprinted painting of Venice. He'd have something classier, he says, but the adornments are Lawlor's. The refrigerator contents are his, of course: smoked salmon and halibut,

Brie, and a special brand of tostada chips he brought from Texas. Completing the lounge's decor are a stereo, TV, VCR, bookcase, couch, and table. In the bedroom, there's a mattress on the floor and another on the bed. He's ready for any kind of weather.

Carroll clicks a tape into his Sony Walkman. As a young man, he loved disco music and even wore the black garb and cloggy high-heeled shoes made famous by actor John Travolta. Nowadays, he favors jazz and Motown music. The jazz and a warm shower settle him down for sleep. It's around midnight and upstairs second mate Jean Holmes has assumed control of the ship from Davis. The gulf is pounding the hull harder as she begins her 12-to-4 A.M. watch.

5

Death by Design

(Near Middleton Island,
Latitude 59° North, Longitude 147° West,
January 26, 1 A.M.)

Leaving Carroll in his quarters, I ease down another flight of stairs to my private room. Tossing my shoes into the closet, but not bothering to undress, I shove the survival suit under my mattress and wedge myself against the wall. *Huuuuumph. Grrrrrrrr. Huuuuumph. Grrrrrrr.* I lie there captive to the ship's constant murmuring and the ocean's endless flailing. For a while I try to separate the metallic sounds, to hear maybe an individual joint or a plate grinding itself into filings. But the noise seems to be one voice grieving the fate of tankers.

I need some sleep, but I'm reluctant to drift off, for I would not want to miss the worst storm of the trip. Then again, maybe it isn't the worst storm. I remember how the weather service map was covered with swirls, each one the fingerprint of another felonious storm waiting to pounce on us in the dark. Tomorrow could be a doozy, or nothing at all, depending on which side of the swirl we end up on. Sleep would be easier if the ship rocked evenly, but that isn't the way of this storm. One moment the ship is still, and the next it is shuddering and rolling. Never a pattern, just an anarchy of . . .

Bam! My tape recorder hits the floor, followed by a stack of papers and a book. Then my camera case careens off the bedroom wall and something else slams into the bathroom wall. It's funny how I hear the sounds first, and then realize the ship has taken a thirty-degree roll.

I leap out of bed, too thrilled by the brute force of this storm to stay cooped up in my room. In another room I hear something else crashing and breaking but I ignore the damage and scramble upstairs to the bridge, determined to see the assailant in action. The rolling stairwell is a little trickier this time. Second mate Jean Holmes chuckles when I arrive, saying, without words, "Oh, it's you again?" I've been anticipating this storm like an amusement ride, and now I seem like an excited puppy.

It is 1 A.M. and the ocean is throwing roundhouse punches. Green water crosses the deck and the ship rocks at a steeper angle than ever. The grinding noise in the hull and the howling wind combine to create a chorus of doom. Holmes picked up the bridge phone long before I arrived and rang the captain in his quarters. Not yet in a deep sleep, Carroll ordered her to slow the ship and hurried upstairs to join her. He changes course and for another hour and a half he watches the ocean play rock-and-roll games with his command. Focusing on the sea, he alters our course repeatedly and slows the speed even more. Speechless in concentration, he peers into the darkness, watching the way the ocean plays across the deck, looking for an advantage, for some way to get this sucker under control. Like searching for a pattern on a shattered windshield, he hunts for the trough in the wave, a better place to be, because the ship rolls without hitting a wave head-on. Every time he locates the seam, though, the ocean changes its mind. What is the rhythm of this cussed storm, anyway? Slowing the ship even more, Carroll finally finds what he is looking for. He gets the tanker into uneasy harmony with the raging beat of the rollers. By now it's 2:30 A.M. and Carroll's had only an hour's sleep since his wake up in Valdez twenty hours earlier. He doesn't feel secure leaving the bridge in these conditions, so he grabs a set of ear covers and lies down in a bunk reserved for him at the back of the bridge. Before doing so, he tells Holmes to call him and to reduce the propeller speed by five RPMs if things don't get better soon. He reclines there half asleep, never quite dozing, while the ocean drums at his ship.

We are climbing the uphill side of a big low-pressure system, rough terrain for any size of ship, but maybe worse for a long bend-y one like this than for a short one. Suddenly I feel alone with the other members of the crew—a long ways from home. I can see how the captain and the second mate must trust their skills for this battle with the gulf. No one else will help them this far from land.

All the while there is this assumption that the people who designed the hull two decades ago made it sturdy enough for such savage seas. The ship's birth certificate is on the wall at the back of the bridge, but it provides only bare details:

Port of Registry: Philadelphia, Pennsylvania

Builder: Bethlehem Steel, Sparrows Point, Md.

Contract date: June 10, 1969

Keel laid: March 1, 1972

Delivery date: June 5, 1973

If the certificate tells us little about the strength of this ship, the history of oil tanker construction tells us a lot. Unfortunately, it's not the kind of tale that bodes confidence.

The naval architects and engineers at the Bethlehem Steel shipyard in Sparrows Point said they considered nights like this when they blueprinted the *Arco Anchorage* in 1969. The architects and engineers divide their duties on a ship the same way it is done on a skyscraper— one produces the concept and the other figures out the details. But a building never experiences the kind of continual stresses that confront a ship. A structural engineer must consider how a skyscraper will support its own weight against the pull of gravity and resist the lateral forces of wind and earth tremors. Designing a ship, a naval engineer must contemplate a lifetime of "earthquakes" in a medium that is alien to man's logic. As we push farther into the gulf, rollers twist the hull from one direction and pound it from another. The groaning structure tells its own story, how it must resist one stress and at the same time give in to another. Job in the Bible didn't face the rigors of a ship in an ocean gale.

It would be comforting to know that tanker designers overbuilt these ships to withstand the worst blows an ocean could deliver. But the price of construction worried the shipyards and the owners more than the mischief of nature. Steel is the highest-priced item on a tanker, and a ton of steel in the structure is one less ton of cargo it can carry; the owners don't hanker to buy or carry more steel than necessary. The architect and the engineer must find a happy medium between strength and cost. Sometimes the meeting point isn't so happy.

Starting shortly after the end of the Second World War, tanker builders engaged in a giant experiment. They produced the largest machines ever known to man, while slowly cutting back on the thickness of steel that went into them. It was a gamble in which lives were lost and oil was spilled.

You could enter this story almost anywhere during the postwar era, but a good place to start might be December 10, 1960, the day that second mate Jean Holmes was born in Newmarket, New Hampshire. Holmes is taking a long drag off a cigarette over near the bridge window right now, a quiet tomboy with nearly a decade of sea time under her belt. But this thirty-one-year-old graduate of Maine Maritime Academy is still learning the officer's trade, adding to her knowledge of the craft with each trip. When she was born, tankers were undergoing some mighty changes of their own.

Back then, tankers the size of the *Arco Anchorage* were as unknown as a woman in charge of a ship. But in the industrial seaport city of Quincy, Massachusetts, not far from Jean's birthplace, Bethlehem Steel engineers and architects were laying plans for a 114,000-deadweight-ton tanker they expected to be the largest in the world. Ordered by a Greek entrepreneur, the *Manhattan* would have carved a place in history had it not been for the fact that other ships were under construction in other countries that would soon be larger. When Holmes entered kindergarten, ships over 200,000 deadweight tons had emerged from Japanese shipyards. When she was in third grade, there was a 300,000-tonner under construction. Before she was old enough to hold a driver's license, a half-million-tonner, the largest ship in the world, had slid out of the dry dock. The term "super tanker" was being redefined annually.

Ships had never grown so fast. The first oil ships, launched in response to mid-nineteenth-century Pennsylvania oil discoveries, were sailing vessels adapted to carry oil in containers. The first deep-sea tanker to carry oil loose inside its riveted steel hull was the 3,500-deadweight-ton *Gluckauf* launched in England in 1886. Riveted ships—too leaky—were replaced by welded hulls and the framing was improved to make it possible to build bigger tankers. But between World War I and World War II, the average tanker grew in size from only 12,000 deadweight tons to 16,600 deadweight tons.

The explosion in size after World War II was sparked by avarice. Oil in the postwar boom was profitable beyond belief, and a ship that could carry ten times more oil with no increase in crew size and only a modest hike in horsepower could make its owner fabulously wealthy. A 1948 article in a technical journal predicted that a 50,000-ton tanker would cut the cost of shipping a gallon of oil by 60 percent over a 12,000-tonner.

Naval architect Tom Robinson thought the 25,000-tonners built right after the war were super tankers. But the young designer, who worked on the *Arco Anchorage,* had to adjust his thinking as 50,000-, 60,000-, and 70,000-tonners came out of the yards. It seemed the only limit on the size of the tanker was the construction capacity of the world's shipyards.

There were prudent exceptions to the rule that ships should be built with the least amount of steel possible. The *Manhattan,* for instance, was designed using the old-fashioned principle that a bigger structure needs similarly bigger parts. The ship's bones were so abundantly thick, it had nearly twice the steel used on the slightly larger *Arco Anchorage.* But investors were loath to spend their up-front cash on something as robust as the *Manhattan* when some of the newer breed of ships were paying for themselves.

On the bridge of the *Arco Anchorage,* Holmes wanders back to the chart room to mark our position on the map. I follow her, adjusting my eyes to the light, noting that like me she is wearing the same clothing she had on yesterday, a rugby shirt and jeans. While she plots the course, I rummage through some papers, stopping at a set of blueprints that show the skeletal structure of the *Arco Anchorage.* The plans show a pretty hefty ship, even if it is less muscular than the *Manhattan.* The cloak of steel this tanker wears around the hull is about one and three-eighths inches thick. As time went on, and fashions changed, more modern ships were dressed in seven-eighths-inch-thick armor. And the bones got thinner, too.

With the trend going so fast toward giant ships, owners needed someone to establish new standards for the way they were built. That meant adjusting the "scantling" rules. (The term describes the size of materials used in construction of a vessel.) For that, they turned to an institution unique to the maritime world—the classification society.

The first classification society regulated the qualifications of ship masters in the mid-nineteenth century. Over time, they got out of the personnel-qualification business and concentrated on ship designs, a service that was more in demand. In most maritime countries of the world, there are classification societies that inspect ships, write rules for maintenance and repair, review blueprints, and monitor vessel construction. In most countries owners are not required to "class" a ship, but a vessel not "in class" is usually uninsurable and difficult to market.

Trouble is, classification societies have proliferated to a point where there are forty-two of them today, and less than ten are what anyone could call responsible. Examples of the better ones are the American Bureau of Shipping in the United States, Det Norkse Veritas in Norway, Lloyd's Register of Shipping in the United Kingdom, Germanischer Lloyd in Germany, Nippon Kaiji Kyokai in Japan, and Registro Italiano Navale in Italy.

Standards decline with outfits like Bureau Veritas of France, the Korean Register of Shipping, the China Classification Society, Polski Rejestr Statkow of Poland, and the Yugoslavian Registar Brodova.

Below them are obscure societies described by Rear Admiral Gene Henn, chief of the Coast Guard's safety and environmental protection office, as "Tinkertoy" organizations willing to "put a stamp on a ham sandwich." He says the worst ones consist of "two men and a dog in a room with a television set—and the dog has the highest IQ."

The flaw in these so-called watchdog societies, even the best ones, is that they are too easily manipulated by the ship-owning customers they serve. Although they are nonprofit, they compete fiercely for customers around the world. If a shipowner doesn't like the way the

Norwegians enforce the standards, he can always take his business to the French (provided the laws of the country his ship is registered in would allow him to do so).

So the shipowners and shipyards had little trouble getting these competing societies to set the standards they wanted for the scantest steel scantlings. Starting in the late 1960s, the societies began juggling the requirements; they established "reasonable" guidelines that reduced the steel requirements for these oversized ships. A. Dudley Haff, once the top naval architect for Bethlehem Steel, recalls how insiders at the American Bureau of Shipping resisted the push for lighter steel. "Our representative on the technical committee raised hell about it." But the Japanese and British were already doing it.

"No one was going to class a ship with ABS if they had to have heavier scantlings than they would if they did it with Lloyd's." ABS fell in line, as did the others.

The designers and owners were not malicious but what they were doing was dangerous. Like an athlete who ignores medical warnings and builds his body with steroids, these ships grew to have inherent and self-destructive weaknesses. In storms not much stronger than the one we face tonight, tankers and their second cousins, the ore and bulk carriers, split and spilled oil, or in some cases actually sank. One study showed that during a five-year period between 1969 and 1973, the greatest single cause of massive oil spills from tankers was structural failure. Sailors died by the dozens.

Yet designers kept looking for better ways to bloat their ships while slimming the metal surrounding them. During the late 1970s and the 1980s, classification societies allowed designers to shave even more steel off their creations, to produce what became known as "reduced scantling" ships. By the late 1980s, after two decades, the amount of steel on an average tanker had been reduced by 18 percent. By then, the industry was aware of the hazard. A 1989 Coast Guard report noted that, "Even the vessel owners have complained that it is impossible to build a vessel to last under the current rules." Haff says the Americans acted as responsibly as they could, designing ships as robustly as possible under tough competitive conditions. His own shipyard even went so far as to jimmy the statistics so the owner believed he was paying for the least amount of steel while the designer knew there was an extra margin.

One engineer told me he was shocked that the insurance companies who paid for the cracked and sunken ships never stepped in to stop the trend. But the insurers in the maritime world are influenced by ship-owners nearly as much as the classification societies. The leading maritime insurance groups were created as shipowner-controlled co-ops, known as hull clubs or P & I clubs (for Protection and Indemnity). Since rates were not based on track records, but on competition, the insurers sat on the sidelines paying little attention to tanker quality. Not until the companies began to suffer crippling losses in the early 1990s did they move to address the situation. "Their problem is they have three hundred years of tradition behind them unmarred by prog-ress," says the Coast Guard's Henn.

Further misleading regulators and insurers were the poorly trained, poorly funded, and, in some cases, biased accident investiga-tors, who seemed to look for every reason other than steel to explain disasters. Maybe the broken ship was overloaded, they said, or the captain was driving it too hard. Maybe the owner allowed corrosion to eat the girders and shell, or maybe it was improperly repaired during its last shipyard visit. Maybe the last inspection wasn't good enough. All are defensible conclusions, but none are more legitimate than the obvious one: If the designer had put a sufficient margin of strength into a ship, corrosion, overloading, rough seas, and poor seamanship would not so easily have cracked it.

When Coast Guard officers investigated the 1971 sinking of the tanker *Texaco Oklahoma,* they should have sounded a clear and early warning. The skipper of the American tanker, on a loaded voyage from Port Arthur, Texas, to Boston, slowed down the way Carroll did to-night in the face of a similar sixty-five-mile-an-hour gale and heavy seas. The crewmen heard a loud crack as the 660-foot-long ship rolled in heavy swells off the North Carolina coast. Racing to the deck, they saw the front half of the ship broken completely away and drifting toward them. Tankers had two houses in those days, one at the rear of the ship where crewmen and engineers lived and the other in the middle where deck officers slept. The ship split just aft of the middle house, so the captain and twelve other men were trapped up front while thirty-one other crewmen were stranded in the rear. The two halves of the ship scraped past each other and the last sign of life aboard the front section was a flashlight signal from the wheelhouse. The seas toyed with the broken rear section for a full day and night, ripping away the remaining lifeboats until it began to sink in the wee morning hours. Only eleven men, exhausted and nauseated by the fuel they'd swallowed, managed to get aboard a life raft. They were rescued that afternoon by a passing Liberian tanker. Two others were found clutching life rings hours later. In all, thirty-one men died and more than eight million gallons of oil spilled or went down with the ship.

A Coast Guard investigation concluded that the vessel split where the most powerful bending stresses would be expected. But the agency noted that some tanks had not been examined for cracks at the last dry-docking and said it was likely the thirteen-year-old ship was the victim of corrosion.

The National Transportation Safety Board disagreed, saying the problem wasn't so much that the ship had deteriorated, but that it had been poorly built and too heavily loaded. The NTSB, an independent advisory agency, said the Coast Guard and the American Bureau of Shipping were not doing enough to assure that ships of this size were strong enough to survive the ocean's stresses.

In response, the Coast Guard stepped up inspections and began collecting data on ship accidents for analysis of ship structures. But it would be another two decades before anyone would look closely at the data and do something about it.

Meanwhile, the reduction in steel scantlings accelerated, as did the number of cracked and foundering ships. Pick any time period, and the record books contain gruesome stories of tankers and ore ships cracking or breaking up in heavy seas.

George Reinhard, a consultant from Port Washington, New York, says that because it is in their nature, tanker and ore shipowners chose to abide the death and destruction rather than spend money. With thirty-seven years experience as a ship manager himself, Reinhard saw the reckless behavior firsthand. During the 1970s, he began openly criticizing the industry and in 1978 he wrote a scathing letter to a retiring Coast Guard admiral predicting more disasters unless tanker owners stopped their policy of "build now, pray later." Two years later, he took a liking to a clean-cut British merchant marine officer who was testifying in a ship accident case in which Reinhard was serving as the arbitrator. "During a luncheon break there was the usual small talk, and the twenty-six-year-old man told me he was anxious to get back to Britain because he was committed to one more trip at sea before taking up a shore post with his owners, Bibby [Tankers, Ltd.]. He was so happy about coming ashore because he was just married."

As a wedding present, the company let the young man take his wife with him on his last voyage aboard the 170,000-ton *Derbyshire*. In July 1980, the four-year-old oil-and-ore ship sank in a Pacific typhoon south of Japan. It took with it forty-three people, including the young man Reinhard had befriended and his new spouse. The sudden loss caught the attention of the British government, but not enough to stop the death toll. During the next seven years, while designers looked for more ways to reduce steel, more than three dozen other oil and ore ships sank in storms because of structural failures.

Despite cries for reform, and criticism of classification societies, too little has changed. In the year prior to my voyage on the *Arco Anchorage*, twenty tankers were lost or damaged. This year it was reported that the annual toll of broken ships had increased yet again. Three months after my voyage, the *Katina P,* a 70,000-deadweight-ton tanker, split apart in heavy seas off the coast of Mozambique, spilling one million gallons of oil onto the African beaches. Although racked by civil war, the Mozambique government hired experts to survey the damage, and when the tanker company refused to turn over some records, the captain was arrested, a rare instance of law enforcement in the shipping business.

How could all this go on for so long?

Greed was not the only factor. Improved technology encouraged the trend toward larger ships, and then the drive toward steel reduction. For instance, the military developed a special class of steel alloy for submarines during World War II, which was superior in strength to previous steels. Tanker designers embraced the new "high-tensile-strength" steel after the war, figuring they could use less of the alloys since they were rated tougher than the old-fashioned "mild" steel. Problem is, while high-strength steel was more resistant to stretching and breaking when pulled than mild steel, it was no better at resisting cracks caused by fatigue when it was bent back and forth. Metal fatigue is a major problem on tankers.

High-tensile steel also proved more difficult to weld, and there were weak spots wherever high-tensile steel butted up against mild steel. Nevertheless, ship designers put in the new metal wherever they expected high stresses on a ship, and cut back on plate thickness because of the new alloys' sturdy reputation.

Better tank coatings were also developed to reduce the rust that withered the steel inside the tanks. That, too, encouraged further rounds of steel reduction, but the new coatings worked only if they were properly maintained.

Finally, the computer gave engineers another tool to make larger and proportionately lighter ships. A sixty-seven-thousand-ton tanker built by Esso in the early 1960s was the first ship designed with the aid of a computer. As time went on, designers used the computer to find ways to build larger structures and to scan every nook and cranny of a ship's blueprint looking for metal to eliminate. In the guts of this ship tonight, there are thousands of steel parts that are welded together. During the design stage, if an engineer can slice an ounce from one joint and then punch a computer button to apply that same reduction to hundreds of others, you can see the result.

Ship designers were excited when they discovered that the computer could calculate the forces that plague a ship with an accuracy and sophistication never attained by an engineer with a slide rule. But the computer programs and machines used in the tanker-building boom were not up to the task. As tankers grew exponentially, so too did the forces that would twist and bend them. While engineers needed a mathematical model that would closely approximate all the dynamic stresses a thousand-foot-long tanker experiences at sea, what they got were programs that didn't take into account the increasing nuances— the rolling, pitching, and yawing that occur all at once on a ship that large. Of course, a computer is only as good as the assumptions we humans feed into it.

Looking out the window tonight, I could say we should reinforce the right side of the ship because the seas are coming at us diagonally from the right. I would be wrong, of course, because the forces in a fluid world change direction constantly. Scientists would never make that mistake, but more subtle errors arose because the early computer models could not duplicate the capricious ways of the ocean. While they could imitate the basic pummeling, they missed subtle but vicious ways a ship is tortured by storms.

Man has studied the ocean for centuries but not unlocked all its secrets. Instrumented buoys, scientists, and sailors have calculated the size of waves, but researchers recommend taking the scientific readings with a grain of salt and the stories of seafarers with a whole bottle. Yet this same wave data is what designers use to decide where to reinforce a hull. They must also consider how waves heft long tankers at either end, leaving the middle to bend like a slat laid across two sawhorses. They must calculate how the cargo sloshes against a bulkhead, how the ship reacts with its own motion, and how the ocean throws an endless variety of gut punches.

And then there is the problem of fatigue. Even with ships built to withstand a typhoon, designers must look farther into the future to gird against the longterm effects of steel bending back and forth. In the past, they have miscalculated or ignored this danger.

To understand the effects of all this, and to uncover their mistakes, tanker designers and regulators needed to consult the ship casualty data they had been gathering since the days of the *Texaco Oklahoma*. But the Coast Guard didn't step up to the task until 1987, and when officers went looking they found many of their records were incomplete. The agency had no formal procedure for filing structural failure reports, and even when one was filed it was often less than helpful. Structural failures are difficult to investigate, anyway, since they are gradual events that occur in remote corners of a ship's hull. Also, they are seldom witnessed, and when a ship goes down the best evidence is gone altogether.

However, after studying casualties involving American-flagged tankers during a three-year period in the mid-1980s, Coast Guard investigators were able to describe which tankers they thought were most likely to crack: tankers sailing in the Gulf of Alaska, longer than seven hundred feet and less than twenty-one years old. The fact that the younger ones were included is significant, since they were built with lighter scantlings and high-tensile steel.

Of course, there were other contributing problems. When inspectors found poor welds in a class of tankers built at Seatrain Shipbuilding in New York (including the *Stuyvesant,* which cracked twice in the Gulf of Alaska), they determined that trainees from a special program had been doing the work. And another factor was poor maintenance; not the niggling troubles Carroll is having on this ship but serious cases of neglect.

The economic woes that hit the tanker business contributed to poor upkeep.

A decade and a half of declining charter rates and an oversupply of ships following the Arab oil embargo of 1973 led to financial hardship for owners and a deterioration of the ships. Norwegian ship manager Erik Kruse assessed the state of the industry at an October 1988 tanker conference in New York: "There was only one thing to do in order to survive. Cut costs, to meet the competition, and hang on for dear life." Ships were automated, crews were reduced and disillusioned mariners left the industry. With no incentive to build, owners were running tankers well past their expected life span, all the while chopping maintenance to the bone.

"We operated on rates somewhere between lay-up and operational breakeven. As for interests and down payments, it was pointless to even think of them. We all suffered. Owners, shipyards, banks, equipment manufacturers, brokers, insurers, and many more. Prestigious companies became merely names for the history books, individuals went broke, bankers bled—it was just one huge gloomy picture."

In the bargain, the recession also halted the development of jumbo tankers. A writer during the heady days of 1973 predicted the construction of a million-tonner, but it never happened. What was to become the biggest ship ever built began life as the *Oppama.* It slid out of a

Japanese shipyard in September 1975 at 418,000 deadweight tons, only to face bad economic times that forced its owners to put it into mothballs. The tanker resurfaced in the late 1970s under the ownership of Hong Kong tanker magnate C. Y. Tung, who spent thirty-five million dollars to have it expanded to 565,000 deadweight tons; renamed *Seawise Giant,* it leapfrogged past two other ships to become the largest machine ever built.

Tung's gamble didn't pay off. The expanded *Seawise Giant,* with its seven-acre deck, completed only two more cargo-hauling trips before it was retired again in a bad economy. By then, there were useless tankers parked in Norwegian fjords, and new oil discoveries in Alaska, the North Sea, and Mexico had made smaller ships like the *Arco Anchorage* the vessel of choice.

The obsolete *Seawise Giant* served ignominiously as a floating storage tank in the Gulf of Mexico and the Strait of Hormuz before Iraqi warplanes bombed it into a blackened hulk in May 1988. Three years later, after a tug towed it across three oceans, it resurfaced once again as a tanker. Fitted out with twenty miles of new pipe and sixteen acres of fresh paint, the newly named *Jahre Viking,* flying a Norwegian flag, is hauling oil from the Persian Gulf to Asia. As big as ever, the ship will always be a humbled symbol of man's folly.

In the wake of all this turmoil, ship designers and regulators are finally taking another look at tanker design. When the *Exxon Valdez* accident focused new attention on the frailties of these big ships, classification societies like the American Bureau of Shipping began reviewing the steel requirements. Now the Coast Guard is requiring tankers sailing the Gulf of Alaska, like this one, to undergo more thorough hull inspections. Some of the more frail ones sailing the gulf were reinforced with extra steel, and the worst were retired to other oceans or to the scrap yard.

After conducting a major review of ship construction standards, American Bureau of Shipping Senior Vice President Donald Liu says his classification society will require a new approach in which the computer will be part of the solution, not part of the problem. More sophisticated computer models using the latest technology will give ship designers a better model of the ocean and of the stresses applied to a ship. Using them, engineers will pay better attention to the details of the design, and the computer will be asked the question—Just how strong is that joint?—rather than simply looking for ways to lighten it.

"We say, the second time around, let's do it right," said Y. N. Chen, a former college professor who is studying ocean stresses for Liu and the ABS.

I hope he is right, but there are reasons to be skeptical. Even as Liu's organization issues new guidelines, the faultfinders on the bookkeeping side are questioning whether ABS-classed vessels will be too heavy with steel. Reacting to that concern, Liu says the new guidelines will add little weight to the ships. Steel will be redistributed to vulnerable areas of the structure, not added to the whole ship. For critics who care about safety, however, Liu's words raise another question. Will the classification society, in its effort to stay competitive, simply shift the problem from one part of the ship to another? Some say tankers should be 30 percent beefier over the entire structure, but Liu's plan would add less than 1 percent to the weight. He says there is no reason to worry about strength, since the solution is not in adding more steel but in placing it where it is most needed. "To beef them all up blindly, it doesn't take a genius to do that."

Whatever new rules classification societies set, the new U.S. legislation requiring double hulls will inspire new construction. However, the legislation says nothing about how much steel these new ships should contain. With charter rates depressed, tanker owners are still tempted to conserve on steel. Some experts worry that the next generation will be as lightly built as the last, and that the classification societies will allow it.

As another roller crosses the bow of the *Arco Anchorage* tonight, I feel better that this twenty-year-old trooper is what they call a "full-scantling" tanker. Even if it isn't the *Manhattan,* it was built long before the engineers took their heftiest whacks at the steel in the body of the hull. When inspectors crawl inside this baby at the shipyard later this year, they will find hundreds of hairline cracks in the steel structure. But unlike the mess they have found in some of the newer tankers that ply the Alaskan trade, there will be no major holes that could spill oil or rip apart the ship.

Holmes says it looks like the worst part of this gale is over. The low-pressure system has wandered a bit east and we have slipped a little south of its fist. It's still rough, however. It takes time for the ocean to smooth itself, so we are doomed to another night of rolling. But as I wander sleepy-eyed back to my quarters I expect to awaken to a different world. The ship rocks me into oblivion in my bunk, and down in the hull a load of crude oil sloshes around in thirteen cargo tanks built of steel.

6

White-Line Fever

(Gulf of Alaska,
60 nautical miles south of Middleton Island,
240 miles west of Chichagof Island,
January 26, 9 A.M.)

The steel leviathan shrugs off another roller in a calming morning ocean. The seas still wash the main deck, but the wind and waves are half what they were last night. When my gaze drifts beyond the ship the only reference points are the curve of the earth and the lights of the heavens. The blue expanse leaves one feeling a bit lost, but rest assured, I am told, we are pointed in the right direction.

Far from land like this, the weather is our landscape and the sea is our terrain. A storm is a mountain to be climbed and a fog bank is a forest to be reckoned with. This morning, when I awoke, we were sailing on a plain of rolling hillocks after easing ourselves down the back slope of last night's tempest. The next obstacle on the map is another low-pressure system converging on our course.

Outside, on the left wing of the bridge, able-bodied seaman Ralph Schramm is standing watch in a state of limbo, his lookout duties made irrelevant by the fact there is nothing to avoid out here. The ship's twin radars have been scanning the horizon for twenty-four miles in every direction and they haven't seen another vessel for an hour. The nearest coastline is more than two hundred miles away. The third mate Dean Davis is out of sight in the chart room penciling our position on a map. No one is standing at the wheel because a computer is steering the ship.

Early this morning, after the ship slipped south of the low-pressure wind machine, the mate flipped a switch near the steering wheel that set the autopilot to a southbound compass course. The autopilot—a computerized helmsman known to all sailors as "Iron Mike"—then took control of the ship, turning the rudder whenever the wind and waves diverted us from our course. The seaman who had been steering us through the ocean's upheaval was relieved of his duties so he could do other work. They say a good seaman does a smoother job of steering than the computer inside the green box, but Iron Mike is plenty good out here on the open ocean.

We are a robot ship traveling a straight line. The autopilot will keep us on this vector forever, regardless of what lies ahead, until someone changes its instructions. A Japanese tanker was sailing the Strait of Juan de Fuca on autopilot when the second mate fell asleep and the computer drove the ship straight onto the beach. Sometimes a small boat will disappear on the high seas without a trace. Speculation inevitably runs to the possibility that a big ship, with Iron Mike at the wheel, ran the smaller vessel down. Fortunately, Arco has a rule requiring someone on the bridge at all times. The bridge includes the chart room which leaves Dean Davis technically on the bridge.

Standing alone in the wheelhouse, I experience for a moment the solitude of the officer's watch, plus the satisfaction of a well-trimmed vessel under "my" command. The sea is such a clean place, and holding a cup of tea with a great ship under my feet, I feel . . . well . . . satisfied.

The mate walks back into the wheelhouse and gives a distracted glance to a radar screen located on the right side of the thirty-foot-long room. Arranged in a straight row to the right of the steering wheel are three round radar screens, each one with its own set of dials and each one mounted on its own podium.

The right and left screens are hooked to independent antennas rotating slowly on the roof one hundred feet above the water. Each antenna can be adjusted to scan the horizon as far out as 120 miles or as close as three-quarters of a mile. With help from the mate, I adjust the antenna range, and when I zoom it in close, I call up details as small as the tops of waves. When I zoom it out, the wave interference disappears but, voilà, a single blip appears. We have found a ship sailing twenty-five miles from us. Each time the radar beacon sweeps the screen—like the second hand on a clock—the blip reappears at a slightly different position. Our fellow wanderer is too far away to cause concern, but his sudden appearance gives the mate a chance to demonstrate what the radar screen in the middle will do.

The middle screen gets information from both the radar antennas and decodes it using a computer. The computer can tell us how fast the "target" ship is traveling, what direction it is heading in, and when it might cross our path. To demonstrate, the mate "captures" the other ship's dot with an electronic cursor and hits a button to call up the information. The computer tells us the other ship is heading north at around fifteen nautical miles per hour. We can't get its name or description unless we contact it by radio, but, at that speed, it is probably a container ship. No need to chat since the computer says we are on a course that will not bring us near the other ship.

If the vessel was getting too close, anyway, the computer would have sounded an alarm. The mate shows me how he sets the "collision avoidance system" (CAS) warning fence to a twenty-four-mile radius on the open ocean. If anything gets closer than twenty-four miles, a buzzer goes off. By some estimates, CAS eliminates nearly half a deck officer's headaches by simply watching out for other vessels. But the mate warns me, "It is only an aid, definitely not something you want to stake your life on."

Iron Mike and his cohort, CAS, are devices newer than the ship itself. Even the radar was unheard of on merchant ships four decades ago. When it was introduced, it was so unreliable, some captains turned it off. The early versions of the collision avoidance system were also troublesome, sounding a false alarm at the appearance of a taller-than-normal wave. But the radar, Iron Mike, and the CAS are better now and nearly as trusted as the compass. That trust is translating into a loss of jobs.

The *Arco Anchorage* is only a partially automated ship, but machines like Iron Mike and CAS have made it possible for Arco to cut back on seamen. In Japan and Germany there are experiments with computer-controlled loading systems, automated winches, and tank-cleaning robots. Ships with engine rooms bigger than this one run at night with no human being in attendance. The bridge, which was once dominated by the wooden steering wheel and the magnetic compass, now looks like a video parlor. And in the future all the information coming from the radar, the CAS, and the navigation machines will be fed into one device that will give us a constantly changing picture of our position and everything around us.

Then there's the human cost. A person like Schramm may be more interesting to me than a machine built by Sperry, but from an accountant's point of view Schramm is a thirty-thousand-dollar-a-year salary, who needs medical insurance and a retirement plan.

Because crew salaries are a major portion of any ship's budget, there is a worldwide competition to design ships that run with fewer people. The Europeans started the trend in response to a labor shortage during the 1960s. The Japanese surged ahead in the 1980s, experimenting with ships crewed by only sixteen people. By 1987 they were trying out eleven-person crews, nearly all officers, on vessels larger than the *Arco Anchorage*.

The reduction in American crews has been almost as dramatic, but not as deep. Thirty years ago the average U.S.-flagged ship sailed with forty-five crew members. Today they have twenty-two. Not all crew reductions were the result of automation: a toilet on the bridge eliminated the need for an extra watch stander; better coatings reduced the number of deckhands needed to chip paint.

So does the industry need a guy like Schramm? The answer is not a simple one, and the debate troubles nearly everyone on this ship, especially the able-bodied seamen. Owners are anxious to dump salaries, and the unlicensed sailors like Schramm are usually the first to go.

Out on the bridge wing, Schramm's steel-rimmed spectacles are reflecting the morning light and a gloved hand is resting on the rail. His thin, pale face is surrounded by the fur trim on the hood of his heavy brown coat. It's cold and breezy today, in the low twenties, but Schramm is amply defended by heavy winter clothing. Luckily, he's not facing the kind of deep-freeze weather that at times reaches thirty degrees below zero and limits a sailor's outside work to short bursts.

Schramm is an introverted guy who ponders life quietly while it passes by. He doesn't talk loudly or engage in the vulgar banter down in the galley, but instead enjoys the contemplative times on the job. He says the steady movement of the ship through the water anesthetizes him. "Some people find it soothing. Like a truck driver with white-line fever."

When I ask about his life, he scrolls through a rolling checklist of way points. In four and a half decades, he's been the son of a prominent NASA rocket engineer, an Army helicopter mechanic in Vietnam, a community college student in California (liberal arts) and Washington (oceanography), and an able-bodied seaman on Arco tankers (for six years). He's been married twice and had an equal number of divorces, for reasons he is still trying to figure out. He has lived in Ohio and Alabama and is now staying in a bedroom-community that's a ferry ride across Puget Sound from Seattle. One of the benefits of merchant marine work is that you can live just about anywhere you want. Arco will fly a crew member back and forth from any address he or she calls home, as long as it is within the United States. Other crew members hail from an island in Florida, a high desert in California, a farm in New Jersey, and towns in New Hampshire and Missouri, just to mention a few. Schramm is thinking of moving to a hot, dry place in eastern Washington, where he can look at sagebrush rather than the sea during his days off.

For sailors, vacation time is the goal. They talk longingly of "the beach" and they refer to the ship as "the bitch." Long respites cost the company plenty of money, since every ship must have two crews. But furloughs are as important to the crew as pay, and will be considered as such every time the officer's and seamen's unions negotiate a contract with Arco. A few decades ago seamen spent eleven months at sea and got only a month of vacation at home. But now the contract says a seaman like Schramm will sail seventy-five days and get fifty days off, less than the one-to-one ratio an officer gets, but not bad. Schramm says time off is part of the appeal that keeps him and others coming back. The other is the lifestyle. "The thing I like about going to sea is that I've got somebody else taking care of me so many months of the year. No grocery bills, no rent, et cetera. That's why we get so many ex-Navy people out here."

Schramm doesn't mull the fate of the merchant marine as much as he thinks over and over again about the way he would live his life differently, how maybe he might have preserved a failed marriage.

"I've got a lot of time to think about things out here. I've got to live with myself, you know. Up on the bridge, all I do is pace back and forth and think. I find myself thinking the same thing over and over again.

"The hours are long. Living quarters are limited. Time is synchronized. It gets lonely and boring sometimes."

I find as I ride this tanker, talking to people like Schramm, that the merchant sailor is a bit dwarfed by the dimensions out here. We are surrounded by an ocean so large that the ship is like a scrap of debris. If we lost radio and radar contact with land, it would take a search plane days to find us despite the tanker's size. And on a ship where I need binoculars to recognize a crewman walking halfway up the deck, one is further miniaturized. We are a ranch in the wilderness patrolled by walkie-talkie cowboys.

The truth is that, just like the Western cowboy, the country no longer needs the American merchant seaman. At one time in the 1950s there were thirty-five hundred merchant ships flying the Stars and Stripes. Today, there are less than five hundred. The number of American citizens earning salaries at sea has dropped from one hundred thousand to twenty-seven thousand during the same period of time. An entire industry that was once a proud arm of a seafaring nation now employs about as many people as the New York City Police Department.

It was only four decades ago that American ships dominated the trade; now only one of every fifteen tankers flies the Stars and Stripes. Liberia has the largest fleet. Owners, which include Americans trading in foreign waters, prefer foreign flags because the taxes are lower and they can hire crew members from any country they wish. A typical U.S.-flagged tanker shells out three million dollars a year for its American crew while it is possible to hire Russians these days for two hundred thousand dollars. And benefits are so minimal that a ship pilot once told me of a foreign vessel he guided into an Alaskan port that had crewmen from Bangladesh wearing newspapers packed around their legs to protect them from the cold. At least on Arco ships the company gives crew members a twenty-eight-dollar-a-month allowance for winter gear.

Arco uses American crews because of an old American law, the Jones Act, that requires anyone hauling cargo between U.S. ports to use a U.S.-flagged and U.S.-crewed ship. The *Arco Anchorage* crew consists of twenty-four people, including the captain, three mates, one radio officer, one chief engineer, three assistant engineers, one bosun, one pumpman, five able-bodied seaman like Schramm, three enginemen, one lower-ranked utilityman, and, in the galley, one chief steward, one cook-baker, and two lower-ranked galleymen—a relatively bigger complement than some modern tankers that are more automated.

Nearly everybody I talked to said it's a sufficient crew, although a bit thin when the ship is loading, docking, and unloading. Nobody said a smaller crew would be a safe idea on this ship.

However, a Coast Guard certificate on the bridge of the *Arco Anchorage* would permit the ship to sail with a complement of eighteen officers and crew members, not counting the kitchen gang. That's at least two fewer crew members than even fleet president Jerry Aspland would be comfortable with. Although Aspland admits his company requested the reduced manning level in the first place—and got it—he says the current crew size is "probably about where we need it to be," with the possible exception of the radio officer, who is considered expendable because of advancements in communication equipment.

One surprising argument made in favor of smaller crews is that having fewer people will reduce the number of mishaps. Proponents of this idea say that, if human error causes 80 percent of accidents, then the solution is to get rid of people. As crazy as this argument sounds, a National Research Council board completed a study of crew size in 1990 and suggested the industry take a closer look at the notion. While the council admitted to finding insufficient data to make conclusions, their report went on to say that the American shipping industry was dying because it was unable to compete with foreign ships that had smaller crews earning lower wages. It lamented the inability of American shipowners to experiment with reduced manpower and called on Congress to change the laws. Half the members of the twelve-person research council board were associated with shipping line management while only three had connections to unions.

There may be some wisdom in these arguments, but the logic has its limits. A smaller crew invariably means more work for each member and more fatigue. When the *Exxon Valdez* went aground, the third mate who was threading an obstacle course of icebergs had gotten less than six hours of sleep in the previous twenty-four hours and was described as dead tired. But if he was fatigued, then the blundering captain of the Greek tanker *World Prodigy* must have been comatose when he hit a reef spilling nearly three hundred thousand gallons of diesel oil into the waters of Rhode Island Sound and Narragansett Bay three months later. He had been on duty for thirty-three hours without any significant rest.

I can see on this ship how the weather and the hours wear people down. Just look at the schedule. Each work day is divided into shifts called watches and by tradition, everyone on the tanker, except the captain, the chief engineer, and the mess hall worker, is assigned to 2 four-hour watches, each one separated by eight-hour gaps. The chief mate has the four-to-eight watch, which means he goes to the bridge from 4 A.M. until 8 A.M. and from 4 P.M. until 8 P.M. The second mate has the twelve-to-four, with each watch starting at midnight and noon. The third mate starts his watches at 8 P.M. and 8 A.M. The officers also work four hours of mandatory overtime, every day, seven days a week.

What is left over is reserved, supposedly, for sleeping, eating, and relaxing. But officers often have extra paperwork to handle and crew members may have to work more hours cleaning tanks or helping in a difficult port call. Sleep is a rare commodity, usually accomplished in four-hour naps between split shifts. When the seas are tossing, it is difficult to get any shut-eye. I experience that myself. I lie on my mattress wedged against the wall, dozing off, feeling like maybe the rocking ship will soothe me into a slumber. Then, all of a sudden, the vessel lurches and groans loudly and I wake again. I ask crew members whether the fatigue I feel is a result of inexperience, but they tell me everyone has the same problem. Bosun Scott Nehrenz says people get cranky after four or five days of rough seas. "You get up on the helm and you are asleep at the wheel," adds seaman Pat Newman.

Guys like Newman say a shorthanded crew can't adequately fight fires or handle other emergencies. He also points to the illness that has confined the first engineer in his bunk. He asks what happens to an eleven-person crew if there is a flu epidemic or someone goes overboard? Two decades ago—when crews were larger—a seventy-thousand-ton Chevron tanker was bucking heavy waves near our current location in the Gulf of Alaska when some barrels broke loose on the rear deck. Four crew members went back to lash the containers in place and a tremendous wave washed three of them away, including the captain and chief mate. The ship returned to port, but the outcome might not have been the same had there been only seven crew members left.

No doubt robots can handle many jobs on the open sea as long as there are no storms and rocks to contend with. But how many seamen does it take to run a safe ship on an unpredictable ocean when they constantly have to rely on machines that are a computer chip away from disaster? It is a hotly contested issue between management and unions, with regulators like the Coast Guard caught in between. The Coast Guard tends to approve the size of rosters on a ship-by-ship basis, since vessels are not built to standard designs like airplanes. Sometimes Coast Guard officers make manning decisions with only a cursory examination of a particular ship. When Exxon was petitioning the Coast Guard to reduce crews on some 75,000-deadweight-ton tankers operating along the West Coast, the company ordered chief engineers to make sure, during the test period, that overtime was "essentially nonexistent" on the paperwork. Since the Coast Guard did not examine the ships closely, there was no way of telling whether the newly reduced crews were being overworked or whether their hours were simply being kept off the books. Shortly afterwards, two of the Exxon ships lost power and were set adrift near the coastline of Washington state because of minor problems that grew into big ones. In one case, a ship lost all power and electricity when an inexpensive part smaller than a pencil eraser failed. A crewman from the other vessel told me a key portion of its newly automated system had been shut off because it kept sounding false alarms.

Crewmen and officers who showed me around the *Arco Anchor-*

age say crew cutbacks have resulted in poor maintenance, and it doesn't take a trained eye to spot the rust and broken railings. In the days of larger crews, the ship had low-level helpers who took care of these kinds of things.

Some crew members look bitterly on what is happening, fully expecting to lose their jobs someday. Others are adapting, learning to do more with less. Able-bodied seaman Pat Newman and third mate Dean Davis exemplify the opposite sides of this battle.

Newman is a hard-core union man who sees his world crumbling around him as he reaches midlife. The merchant marine is being ruined by "actively arrogant assholes," the "triple As", as he calls them. "It doesn't have to be a horseshit job, some people just want to make it that way."

Tall as a thundercloud, with deep lines carved in his stubbly face, Newman is an unlicensed seaman, the merchant marine equivalent of an enlisted man. A Southerner who delights in his own colorful language, he has theories about everything. He believes that the invention of the TV and the automobile spelled the end of the "neighborly lifestyle" in this country. And, of course, the triple As are bringing an end to the good life at sea.

"I knew it was a dying profession when I got out once in 1984. Business kind of cratered. They'd laid up my third ship in a row. Just shot it out from under me."

Shortly before that happened, Newman's ship was in a Mississippi dry dock when then–Secretary of Transportation Elizabeth Dole visited the shipyard to make a speech. "There was quite a buildup. People thought, she's going to say something, do something for the industry.

"You know what her speech was about? It was about the third taillight on the automobile. That went over like a screen door in a submarine."

After the demise of his third ship, Newman hit the beach in disgust, figuring he'd never go to sea again. "I sold dirt. I sold insurance, I got a real estate license. I worked property management. Anything to make a buck."

The only reason he went back to sea was that things were even worse for him on land. "Economy changed. Wife got laid off when her job went south. I needed a steady paycheck. Things are fucked everywhere."

He found it easy to get another tanker job because of the high turnover rate among able-bodied seamen—around 25 percent, according to Newman. With the crew reductions and lack of pay raises, "nobody wants the job anymore."

Unions could do something, but if there is anything that Newman and other crew members argue about on this ship, it is the union issue. When he was younger, Newman sailed on ships crewed by members of a national union, and, by his own description, he was happier. But Arco has company unions, one for the officers and one for the unlicensed seamen, that are independent, according to management. Newman, however, says they are nothing more than "the personnel arm of the company." As proof of their complicity, he points to the fact that because of a drastic pay cut in 1985 he makes the same money today (something over thirty thousand dollars a year) that he made six years ago. A strong union, Newman says, wouldn't allow that. He would like to rejoin the national union, but the organization has plenty of detractors. Some of the other seamen think the national unions are corrupt, and internal divisions have split one of the organizations in two. The crewmen also object to the way national unions turn sailors into gypsies. National union members are assigned for short periods of time to one ship after another, all based on a hiring-hall list. Sometimes a sailor must travel from hall to hall and wait months for a job to open up. With Arco, at least, these sailors are guaranteed a job.

But right now the Arco seamen are without a contract and the protracted negotiations between the company union and Arco are making everyone nervous. The company wants to impose a twelve-hour working day, seven days a week, in exchange for higher pay and benefits. The seamen—who usually volunteer to work twelve-hour days for the extra pay—would nevertheless like to retain their right to work an eight-hour day when they feel like it. The company promises better benefits and longer vacations in exchange for the twelve-hour requirement, but the crew members are skeptical. "Right now, I have an option to sleep more," said one. "When you tell somebody you have to work twelve hours a day, every day, in port, or out of port, your body says screw it."

With all this going on, paranoia is pretty high. When I first joined the ship, a crew member saw me reading union memos posted on the mess hall bulletin board and taking notes. Newman told me the rumor spread afterward that I was a management spy. Only after I showed my reporter's union card, and explained my intentions, did they accept me.

As much as he distrusts shipowners and company unions, Newman also feels the people on the beach don't care about sailors. He notes how they make a big fuss about oil spills, but care little when a ship blows up and a crewman gets killed. He is right to some degree. A United Nations study found that during a fifteen-year period more than twelve hundred people lost their lives in tanker accidents. That's an average of eighty-one a year, or more than one a week. As horrible as that sounds, the UN statistics are probably low. The National Research Council tried to tally crew deaths and injuries but found that industry records are unreliable. Deaths were often not tallied unless they were accompanied by an oil spill or a major equipment loss. One expert told me that one tanker seaman dies, on average, every three days.

"Does anyone give a shit?" asked Newman.

Dean Davis is just the opposite of Newman. He loves his job and to give him a task is like handing a hungry puppy a fresh bowl of food. The light on the forward mast was broken in the storm last night and Davis is nearly salivating at the opportunity to climb up a wet ladder to fix it. The twenty-nine-year-old third mate performs one job and is already thinking of the next one. That is how he came up through the ranks from sailor to officer, "through the hawsepipe," as a seaman would say, referring to the steel tunnel that guides an anchor chain up to the deck.

He started his career as a lowly messman, waiting tables in the galley and making beds rather than coming out of an academy the way many officers do. He was fresh out of high school, broke and without a job, when an Arco captain who was dating his mother suggested he take a chance on tankers. "Being as I had five dollars at the time, I said sure. The first trip out, I loved it. The camaraderie. Everything." The old captain married his mom and became Davis's mentor, but he died before he could see Davis become an officer.

Davis worked his way up to able-bodied seaman and then took a course during his vacation time that enabled him to pass the third mate's exam.

Like Newman, Davis is a member of a union, but his officers' union took a predictably different tack in negotiations with the company. They accepted the twelve-hour-a-day, seven-day-a-week work schedule in exchange for pay raises. Davis fully embraced the idea. Prior to the new contract, the captain doled out overtime hours to officers as though it was a privilege, and the ones who got it made more money. The chief mate and the first engineer got the most hours, sometimes more than one hundred a week, and as a result they were richer and got less sleep. "The blood pressure hits sky high. Eyeballs about to fall out of his head," commented one officer. The second and third mate got the least overtime hours, and their paychecks were much smaller. "They were the captain's little budget-saving people," said Carroll.

Then, in 1990, the U.S. Congress threw a curveball into the system. Concerned about fatigue following the *Exxon Valdez* spill, Congress passed a law prohibiting any tanker crew member or officer from working longer than fifteen hours in any twenty-four-hour period, or thirty-six hours in any seventy-two-hour period. The practical effect is a twelve-hour daily limit.

To adapt to this problem, Arco negotiated a new contract with the officers' union that requires every mate and engineer to work no less than twelve hours a day, seven days a week. And they will also not work longer than twelve hours a day. An eighty-four-hour work week might sound onerous to landlubbers, but it had an appeal to guys like Davis. While overtime pay was eliminated, the officers got a hefty base pay raise. Chief mates don't work as long as they used to and third mates make more money. Some officers told me they would rather have the choice of when to work overtime and when to take a full night off but Davis loves it, and not just because of the money. The reorganization of the work schedule also allowed him to grab a wrench and do maintenance work he had not been allowed to do before. To understand why takes a further explanation of the division of labor, and how the twelve-hour rule changed it.

In the old days, on most ships of the world, the deck crew and the engine room crew were as divided as former East and West Germany. The deck officers drove the ship, the engine room crew fixed things, and rarely did they mix. In the mess hall, they sat at separate tables, and I am told that on some ships they didn't even talk to each other. Deck officers referred to engine room officers as snipes because they work in dark places like the marsh bird of the same name. The engineers called deck officers coneheads because they didn't have the brains to work on machines. "The snipes used to think the coneheads only break things," said Davis. "The coneheads used to think the snipes were just jealous and wanted to be on deck."

But when deck officers were required to work a twelve-hour day, every day of the week, the captain had to find more for them to do besides standing watch on the bridge. The most logical thing was to have them perform maintenance. Since the law still technically forbids deck officers from working in the engine room, they get their hands dirty on the main deck, fixing pipelines, gauges, and winches. But Davis—ever in search of more challenges—has been wandering recently into the once-forbidden territory of the engine room.

The third mate has struck an unlikely friendship with third assistant engineer Bill Harrison. Davis is a muscular weight lifter and an aggressive snow skier when he is home in Oregon. The dark hair is sculpted so it dangles down the back of his neck and the clothing is sporty and colorful. He is unmarried, although he has a steady girl-friend.

Harrison is rounder of body and has a mussy head of red hair with a mustache to match. He wears a small hoop earring in one ear—a pirate touch—and is almost always garbed in a frumpy blue coverall. He is a decade older than Davis, married, and has two grown stepchildren.

But they talk the same crescent-wrench language, which gives them a bond. Davis drives a Corvette, and when Harrison is home in Buena Park, California, he tinkers with a restored 1978 Pontiac Firebird.

Today at lunch, Harrison invites Davis to help him change a huge valve down in the engine room, a task that requires the heavy piece of equipment to be jimmied around with a complex set of blocks and tackles. The third mate accepts with a huge smile on his face. "Damn right. I'll be there."

This collaboration means more to the future of the merchant marine than would seem at first glance. While Davis is getting on-the-job experience, the academy at Kings Point, under a program introduced in 1989, is churning out two dozen graduates annually with dual training in the deck and engine room, what the school calls the "officers of the future." Arco fleet president Jerry Aspland told Davis at a meeting one day that he was looking for officers with both skills.

The academy and Aspland have their eye on the Japanese fleets, where the lines between deck officers and engine room workers have been all but eliminated. The all-officer crews on these scantily manned ships are expected to do everything. If U.S. ships are to survive against that kind of competition, American officers must fall into line. Davis may be riding the top of a wave into the future.

But some maritime experts worry that fatigue won't be the only problem on ships as thinly crewed as the Japanese tankers. The intellectual vacuum could also be dangerous. Ships that sail for weeks at a time between the Persian Gulf and Japan, or Valdez and Panama, might become floating dead zones where an officer never sees another human being except during a change of watch.

"I think the question is bigger than just saying I can cut the cost by umpteen million dollars by going to twelve crew members," said Virgil Keith, a Maryland ship safety consultant. "What if those twelve go goofy on you out there?"

And George Peloso, the sixty-six-year-old radio officer on the *Arco Anchorage,* worries about the effect on young people who hanker to go to sea. With no low-level training jobs, where are they going to get experience?

"How are we going to encourage young people to take up this career?"

7

A House Away from Home

(Gulf of Alaska,
100 nautical miles south of Middleton Island,
January 26, 1 P.M.)

Today is Super Bowl Sunday and the crew had hoped to see the championship game on TV. They were wishing for a little breakdown in Valdez, nothing serious, just enough to keep us close to land where we would get good reception. But we are far out in the ocean at kickoff time and the only way to follow the game is by Armed Forces Radio. Washington Redskins quarterback Mark Rypien is backpedaling to pass when the play-by-play announcer's voice—already scratchy and intermittent—fades into an inaudible mess for good. As we sail into an oceanic black hole, the faithful are reduced to reading typewritten quarter-by-quarter summaries ripped from the radio officer's telex machine, a fan's equivalent of a bad blind date. An engineman and a seaman mutter cryptic words of disgust as they wander out of the crew lounge.

The remoteness of the Gulf of Alaska explains why videos are the main source of entertainment on a ship like this. A sizable collection of canned entertainment stands ready at all hours in a hallway closet, videos ranging from Hollywood's best down to raunchy violence, but nothing X-rated since company policy outlaws that stuff.

The lounges, located on the galley deck, are divided along rigid class lines, one for the unlicensed seamen and the other for the officers. Like in the military, these shipmates watch movies, socialize, eat, and sleep as though it is healthy to be separated by the happenstance of education and rank. Newman has lived with it for years, but he still despises the system. "They put their pants on the same way we do, they pick their nose the same way we do, but they think they are so goddamn special.

"When you get new guys out of college making twice what the senior unlicensed make, you create a lot of resentment," he says.

The unlicensed crew lounge reminds me of hangouts I inhabited in college and the Army. The walls are off-white, the carpet is brown, the clock is institutional, and the mismatched furniture is ratty. Although the place is ventilated, the air retains a tobacco stench. Smoking is allowed inside the house but not on outdoor decks where the cargo tanks are located. There are usually a couple of guys scrunched down into well-worn chairs watching the boob tube. On one occasion I saw a pair sitting at a table talking, but I never saw a dart thrown at the board on the wall. The movie *Dances with Wolves* is quite popular with this crowd, but it alternates with a couple of violent karate-type flicks.

The officers' lounge is tidier, by contrast, but less used. The only time I saw officers in there was when the chief mate and the radio officer were enjoying a quiet, but truncated, chess game.

Life on an oil tanker eddies around three activities—eating, sleeping, and working. When it comes to sleeping, the lower-ranked crew members occupy the lower floors of the house and the higher-ranked get the upper decks. Of course, the quality increases the higher you go, as does the view. On the low-rent first deck there are twenty side-by-side bedrooms for unlicensed crew members (some of which are now used for storage). The floor would be roomier if the engine room didn't jut up into the middle of it, and if there weren't also two big food storage rooms, the cargo control room, several tool rooms, and the crew laundry. The sailors' private sixteen-by-nine-foot bedrooms are not much bigger than a four-man jail cell, especially when closet lockers and other furniture are counted in. But it is a vast improvement over the days when forty-man crews were crammed into shared rooms.

Some rooms are cluttered and others are neat, but there is enough space in one for a guy to paint a seascape on an artist's easel or have an elaborate stereo system. Schramm says a sailor has only three places to go for relaxation—the galley, lounge, and stateroom—"and only one is truly private." Schramm spends most of his free time in his room where he closes the door and drifts back to the shore aboard a magic carpet of compact disc music that consists of New Age music, country and western, and a little bit of rock. "That's a way to escape any conflict on a ship." His round porthole looks out the side of the house at a main deck cluttered with equipment. The officers get the panoramas.

The main attraction on Schramm's deck is the exercise room, which is shared by the officers and unlicensed crew members alike. It is a hurled-together gym of weight machines and barbells occupying a space designed for storage. The stationary bike and the treadmill are the only aerobic workouts a person can get on a ship where running is prohibited. At one time, the *Arco Anchorage* had a basketball hoop on the rear deck where I'm told a lot of misplayed shots went overboard. The company removed the hoop, however, when a crew member playing a pickup game suffered a sprained ankle (and became another unfit for duty). Other oil tankers—including two owned by Arco— have swimming pools in the rear deck. A pool wouldn't get much use up here in the Gulf of Alaska, but on ships sailing for weeks at a time without a port call—like the jumbos on the Persian Gulf run—it is a welcome distraction. The folks on this ship will have to make do with warm showers. "Life on the sea does not go by what you like," jokes chief mate Svetko Lisica. "It's what you can get."

Up a flight of stairs from the first deck is the poop deck, which contains the galley, the crew and officers' mess hall, the crew and officers' lounge, and living quarters for the pumpman, bosun, chief steward, cook, and messmen. These guys are unlicensed, too, but— except for the messmen—they are the merchant marine equivalent of noncommissioned officers, a position that affords them slightly better views and accommodations.

Next up is "A" deck, which houses the chief engineer's three-room suite, the first assistant engineer's two-room suite, the ship's hospital, the officers' laundry, and bedrooms for the third assistant engineer and a guest. The engineers occupy this floor so they have quick access to the engine room.

Above them is "B" deck and the domain of the deck officers. With slightly less square footage than lower decks, it holds the chief mate's two-room suite and bedrooms for the second mate, third mate, guest (me), pilot, and a cadet from a merchant marine academy (whenever there is one; it was empty this time around). One reason the floor is smaller is the addition of porches high enough to be out of reach of waves during a storm, an important feature when tossing waters claim the main deck and confine the spirit. The eighty-by-eighty-eight-foot house, some sixty feet tall from the main deck to the top of the bridge, feels pretty dreary when the winter Alaskan sun disappears after 4:30 P.M.

My room is outfitted the same as the third mate's, including a steel door so powerfully sprung I must be careful not to let it slam lest I wake the neighbors. The sixteen-by-ten-foot bedroom has a separate closet and a private bathroom with a toilet, a sink, and a welcome morning refuge—a three-foot-square walk-in shower. The bedroom is faded like an old motel room, with a metal desk, a well-worn lounge chair (with loose springs), and reddish-brown carpets and curtains. A chest with five drawers holds a lot of winter clothing and the slightly lumpy bed has two additional drawers underneath. These containers, and an ample walk-in closet that dwarfs my two coats, provide more than enough storage space for the average sailor. They don't need many changes of clothing, since a ship is not a fashion show.

Everywhere you look on the ship you can see how these shipmates protect themselves from the hurling motion of the ship. Whether it is a toothbrush carefully placed in a holder, a medicine cabinet sealed by a metal latch, a mouthwash bottle wrapped in soft cloth, or clothing stored in locking drawers, these people must think differently about stowing their gear when a mile of unruly water lurks underneath their feet. Even sitting on the toilet a sailor needs a hefty handrail within reach. The veterans tell me they memorize the location of important items in their room, and they keep it neat, for you will die when the lights go out and the ship breaks apart if you can't find your survival gear and a flashlight.

Then there are the luxuries. Every day a messman cleans the officers' rooms, and there is no limit to the hot water you can use in a shower since the engine room boilers produce plenty. As if to underline that point, the messman has equipped my bathroom with five different bars of soap—Lava, Zest, Dial, Irish Spring, and Dove.

Up another flight of stairs is the high-rent district, or "C" deck, where the captain's three-room suite has the best view through three portholes facing forward. Next to Carroll's office is a room called the slop chest, which is the ship's equivalent of a 7-Eleven store. By tradition, the captain is allowed to make a profit off the items he sells. The bare metal racks display toothbrushes, cigarettes, shaving cream, razor blades, aftershave lotion, deodorant, and T-shirts decorated with a drawing of the *Arco Anchorage*. Carroll says he makes only a few bucks a month because he sets the price to be more popular than profitable. He hopes the senior captain, Robert Lawlor, raises prices when he returns. "They'll all be mad at him, and they'll appreciate me," Carroll says with a snicker.

When I ask Carroll why the pecking order on a tanker is so rigid, he says it is not for the benefit of his ego but for the discipline that keeps a ship running safely. He is the top of the heap, of course, more powerful than most bosses in any workplace on shore. Hundreds of miles from assistance, he is the banker, doctor, and guidance counselor for all on board. As the sheriff, he has the power to confine an unruly crew member to his quarters on a diet that is the equivalent of bread and water. Just in case of trouble, he keeps a straitjacket and a .357 Magnum pistol with fifty rounds of ammunition in a cabinet in his office. While the gun is mostly symbolic, the captain does keep cash and medicinal drugs, including opiates, that he must protect. His real weapon, though, is the power to fire any crew member, an absolute unquestioned authority to hand out pink slips. Some of his underlings have similar power over the folks below them. Although the company has an appeals board, it usually upholds the skipper. On this tour, the captain has already fired the drunken radio officer and it is general knowledge he wouldn't hesitate to do it again. As if to prove the point, there is another crew member on board right now who was fired by Carroll back when the skipper was a chief mate. In the maritime world, the willingness to ax a seaman is an officer's badge of honor and crew members are well aware of it. At the same time, it is a matter of pride among some seamen that they do not act like favorites or sycophants.

Below the captain, nine officers run the deck and engine departments and below them are a couple of noncommissioned officers, the bosun and the steward, who run the deck and the kitchen.

At the bottom of the pecking order is Jimmy Doyle, twenty-six, a "utility" who splits his duties between the engine room and the deck. He wipes up grease, throws out garbage, and runs errands, standing alone as the only remnant of a disappearing rank known as the ordinary seaman. With the "ordinaries" gone—chopped out for budgetary reasons—Doyle's position is the only entry-level job left on a tanker, outside of the galley, where someone with no experience can get on-the-job training.

Doyle is the wiry son of an engineman who served on Arco ships for twenty years. Sipping coffee in the mess hall, he has a friendly smile that belies his tough-Irish-kid-from-the-city look—dark hair and dark eyes, black jeans and a black T-shirt, a little scar on the cheek. Raised in Philadelphia, he tried for seven years to get a job on Arco ships before he landed one last year. Being on the bottom of the pecking order, he is still pretty shaky and unsure on the job. One night the skipper told him to wax the floors and make them look good. Early the next morning I heard Jimmy banging around in the hallway with a big electric buffer. After sunrise, the captain was out in the hallway, inspecting the dull floors, coated with something that resembled butter or grease. When the captain smelled the wax on the buffer pad he shook his head knowingly. Jimmy didn't remember that these floors are a self-waxing type that must be finished with a special liquid, not with a buffer. Later, we were up on the bridge, when Doyle came up looking all excited. "Captain, I think I know what happened about the floors. I buffed 'em. I shouldn't have buffed 'em."

"You're right, Jimmy," said the captain, keeping a straight face.

Doyle walked away kind of proud of his discovery. "Doggone. I did all that for nothing." Carroll chuckled.

Back down in the mess hall afterwards, I eat some pie with Doyle and wander into the kitchen just before dinnertime, snatching a peanut butter cookie from a drawer on my way. The formal meal hours are strictly enforced on the ship, but for people who can't make it to sit-down meals the mess halls offer plenty of opportunity for round-the-clock grazing. We can select from among high-octane Oreo cookies, Fig Newtons, chocolate-and-marshmallow munchies, crackers, bread, jam, peanut butter, and several brands of ice cream. Nothing fancy about it, but the coffeepot is always warm.

The class system is well enforced at mealtime. The kitchen stands like a Berlin wall between the officers' dining room and the crew mess hall. Time was when the officers' dining room on a merchant ship was fitted out with stiff white linens and the dinners were formal, complete with uniforms and other trappings. On this ship, the officers dine at round tables covered by a white cloth, but it is a limp one. The clothing is casual (sometimes stained with grease). Over on the unlicensed side, the crew eats at two long tables sans tablecloth, of course.

I have been given permission to eat wherever I want so I split my time between the two mess halls. Tonight I grab a chair across from the captain and next to the chief mate. Lisica has a wry sense of humor that is unsettling at times. I ask him how many languages he speaks and he says "none." I ask him how the weather is outside and he says "Salty." If the chief mate can be called reserved, then Carroll is chatty. He grabs my tape recorder and does a parody of a reporter interviewing a tanker captain. "Why you drive this boat onto the rocks, guy? You hate otters?"

Carroll looks over the menu critically. Good food makes a happy ship and he is an expert, since his favorite leisure-time reading is cookbooks and gourmet magazines. Although he admits his favorite food is an Oreo cookie dipped in chocolate, the captain has gourmet credentials. While he delegates menu planning to the steward, he freely expresses his opinions about the food and has ultimate authority over the offerings. The ship has a budget, but the captain has discretion over the details of what he buys. The dinner tonight includes choices of prime rib, baked potato with the works, roast duckling with orange sauce, steamed rice, vegetarian Italian casserole topped with mozzarella cheese, carrots, broccoli, snow peas, dinner rolls, and iced tea with lemon wedge. Dessert is pie, or your choice of cookies (including Oreos) and ice cream. The captain nods his approval.

Messman Jon Niemisto takes our order and walks to and from the kitchen with our food. It is low-level work for a middle-aged man like Niemisto, but he is grateful for the employment. His previous job, helping run a restaurant, was dependent upon his wife's family, who owned the business. When the marriage fell apart so did the paycheck. He was scratching around for work when a chance conversation with a friend led him to Arco. He had never worked aboard a merchant ship before, but like many others he found the wages attractive: A cook can earn forty-five thousand dollars a year and a waiter/bed-maker like Niemisto gets thirty thousand dollars. Given the circumstances, Niemisto doesn't mind mopping floors, making orange juice, setting out food, and cleaning four rooms a day. Someday, he says, he might try for a higher-paying job as a seaman.

He might need to, since the kitchen crew is a target for manning reductions. At one time ships employed more waiters and bedroom servants, and as recently as the mid-1960s hotel services were the costliest operational expense on a merchant ship. Today that isn't true, and accountants envision a day when prepackaged food is served in a cafeteria line, or in a vending machine. For now, though, the galley crew can clatter around busily in its thirty-by-twenty-foot kitchen packed with industrial-sized food processors and ovens. The man in charge is chief steward Patrick Rogers, who stoops a little to fit his puffy chef's hat and his six-foot, eight-inch frame under the seven-foot ceiling. With a slightly gray mustache and thinning hair, Rogers is casual enough to have hailed from Southern California, obscene enough to have spent four years in the Navy, loyal enough to have put in ten years with Arco, and sufficiently organized to keep his meal plans on a computer. He is an unlicensed crew member by definition, but like a noncommissioned officer in the military he has his own squad to oversee—one cook-baker and two messmen.

The galley comes to life around 5:30 A.M. regardless of weather or circumstances. "The main factor is that fucking clock over there," said cook-baker Willie Herbert. "I have to be ready by 7:30 A.M. or it's my ass." The kitchen crew gets midday breaks and someone wipes the last rag across the last counter around 7:15 P.M.

Making a casserole or controlling a hot and sloppy frying pan during a thirty-degree roll is a culinary adventure to behold. The seas are kicking up now, and I watch Herbert bracing himself. As he rotates his body between a hot oven and a pan full of meat, holding a huge knife in one hand and a tray in the other, I ask how he dodges injury. "When we take a big roll in the galley, we just stand by the side and let her go. There's nothing you can do."

If TV dinners replace fresh-cooked meals someday, most ships will lose some character. Galley crews are famous for being mixing bowls of odd individuals. Herbert is twenty-seven years old, ex-Navy, at sea since he was eighteen, and one of the tanker's true oddballs. Holding court in the galley, he sees himself as a twisted source of entertainment. A self-described walking library of pornography, he also claims to give directions, from memory, to the sauna parlors of any city he's visited. But even more important are the magazines: Herbert's world revolves around them and it was through one that he says he met his wife. He saw an ad for a "mail-order bride" from the Philippines and after corresponding briefly they married two and a half years ago. They have two children, but it hasn't changed his style. When he talks, Herbert cocks his crewcut head and his hand to one side, a gesture that gives him a slightly demented look. "I could screw anything," he says to another messman as they sip coffee after dinner. He then lists various objects, animate and inanimate, that would fill the bill.

Seaman Larry Bratnyk stands up from the other table and gives the cook-baker a disgusted look. "Why don't you go back to the Navy?" he says. Bratnyk is an elder in the Mormon church, a quiet guy who wears scratched round glasses tightly over his heavyset face. "The Navy is his religion," Bratnyk explains afterward. "I know from past experience that people in the Navy like to drink, lie, and tell jokes. If you can throw them a curve once in a while, they have to think twice about what they say." I'm not sure Willie got the point.

Then there is David Chun, a quiet, intense, twenty-five-year-old messman who enjoys needling Herbert, picking at his words and making him back up what he says. Originally from Honolulu, he worked in a restaurant in Ashland, Oregon, before coming to sea, attracted by high wages and long vacations. His favorite pastime seems to be poking holes in the stories people tell, and there are more than enough stories to challenge on a ship like this one. At home, Chun is an avid member of the Society of Creative Anachronism, a group that dresses in Middle Age costumes and playacts the ceremonies of the era. When Chun enters his time machine, he is an archer.

Ships are breeding grounds for claustrophobia, and a crew will chafe if it doesn't find a way to live together. The Navy understands that, carefully choosing members of a submarine crew. Common courtesies keep harmony on a tanker. Bratnyk knows there is an unwritten rule against talking religion or politics, despite his strong feelings regarding church. With people sleeping at all hours, there is no running, slamming the door, or shouting. One night I discovered to my chagrin that I had violated a rule by leaving my bedroom porthole uncovered. A seaman informed me that the light pollution troubles the officers on the bridge.

Nobody is immune, though, to the constant pounding of the sea. Tempers get short, and if the lack of talk about politics keeps down the debate, the same cannot be said for union matters. The other day, Newman was pulling out all stops, laying out the reasons why he hates the company union. Suddenly, the bosun's face reddened and he jumped up from his chair, hurling a verbal barrage at Newman. "Every time I come in here you are talking the same crap," he said, stomping out of the room. Newman was embarrassed, but laughed it off. Rogers, the steward, said that in the old days a bosun might have slugged a seaman who offended him. In more blatant cases, gangs of sailors would corner a repeat offender and treat him to a "blanket party," a beating where the victim is wrapped in a blanket so he can't see his assailants. Nowadays, crew members either walk away from an argument, or risk being fired.

Engineman Ruben Garcia says sea duty is a little like a marriage. When you see some guys seventy-five days a tour, it can magnify small problems and make the big ones intolerable.

If you are a racial minority—like Garcia, messman Chun, and able-bodied seaman Marvin Cropper—there is a special investment in harmony. Racism is not tolerated the way the class system is, but there are subtle reminders. Arco officials say they have an aggressive affirmative action program, and I have no reason to doubt them. But it wasn't until recently that higher positions were filled by people other than whites.

History shows that, while the American merchant marine has employed people of other races for quite some time, the jobs were often menial. Even until recently the Navy made racial ghettos out of some servantlike jobs. On some foreign ships, racial divisions are strictly enforced and the bosses don't speak the same language as the crew.

The only African-American on this cruise is Cropper, a friendly bear of a man with a mustache and glasses. Called "Starvin' Marvin" because of his appetite, he's one of the most popular guys on the ship. He is the second generation to work for Arco; his dad, Booker Cropper, was employed at a company refinery in Philadelphia for thirty-six years before retiring in 1982.

His folks live on a small farm in New Jersey where Cropper spends much of his vacation time. He was married once but it was an unhappy union with a nurse that lasted just two years and turned him into a "gun-shy dog" when it comes to matrimony. His forty-four years of life have been salted with fifteen years on Arco ships and six in the Navy, including time spent in Vietnam. As one of the most experienced crew members, he bristles with hair-raising sea stories, like the time a Navy destroyer took a record-breaking fifty-two-degree roll, dipping its smokestack so far down in the water that seawater flowed into the boilers. Another time, an Arco captain sent him out on a tanker main deck in a nasty storm to close a ventilator pipe that had broken open on top of a cargo tank. "The captain turned the ship to the lee, but water came over the deck anyway. I had to jump on a fire monitor platform to avoid being swept overboard."

Cropper is rarely serious in his demeanor, but I did see a weighty expression one time when I asked him about racism. We were up on the bridge wing where Cropper was on lookout duty. He grimaced and looked away at the horizon, as though searching for an answer. "Things have changed over time. There is less of it. But there have been times." He pointed down at one of the winches on the deck and said they were called nigger heads in the old days. "It's been called that a few times around me. I've had to say, yo, man, I don't know what you call it, but to me that's a winch head. I don't take that stuff."

If African-Americans are rare on these ships, so too are women. Carroll's class at the Kings Point academy was the first to include female officer candidates. And for the last two decades merchant ship operators have recruited women so that today some tankers will carry as many as a half dozen at a time. But their numbers have been declining of late. Some claim it is because the conditions are too rigorous, but others say the conditions are too male.

There have been both female success stories and complaints of harassment on Arco ships. The most quarrelsome case involved a radio operator who served with Arco more than eleven years before the company paid her to leave. As a clerk in a Southern California grocery store, and a ham radio operator on the side, she had never dreamed of going to sea before she heard over the ham airwaves one day that Arco was looking for female radio operators. She applied and got the job. She was grateful to Arco for the high-paying position but out at sea she aggravated the difficulties of ship life with her problems, which included difficulties with men, food, and alcohol.

But she bumped along anyway, surviving as best she could, until one day in early 1988 when she decided to protest the graphic pictures of nude women that were plastered on walls all over the ship, and the X-rated videos that were shown in the crew lounges. She complained to company officials in Long Beach that women had put up with this stuff for too long, and to her surprise they acted quickly, issuing a letter to the fleet in March 1988 banning pornography from common areas of the ship. When the letter came out, everybody knew she was the one who complained. She was castigated and ridiculed, and many of the women didn't support her because they felt she had disturbed the balance by which they coexist with men. The radio operator began hearing threats that sounded physical. "I was scared to death out there. I started locking my door." Though she left the company, she keeps in touch with some women on Arco ships and she says things haven't changed enough. "It takes very courageous women to work out there, women who can stand up for themselves."

Up on the bridge this afternoon was another example of women at sea, Jean Holmes, the second mate, whose only addiction is cigarettes and whose reputation is impeccable. She graduated seven years ago from the Maine Maritime Academy where her father is chief mate on the academy's training ship. Among her seven brothers and sisters, three are at sea. A sister-in-law is Maureen Jones, who was the lookout aboard the *Exxon Valdez,* the only person on the ship to realize it was off course before it went aground. (Some investigators say if Maureen had been at the wheel the accident might not have happened.)

Holmes's husband works at a shipyard near Portsmouth, New Hampshire. "He's kind of a paper pusher. He used to work on tugboats himself, but he doesn't like it."

Holmes's freckled face has an outdoorsy look and her brown hair is pulled back in a long, simple ponytail secured by a rubber band. There is a New England reserve about her careful expression, accompanied by a cautious laugh. If it weren't for the cigarette she smokes (swearing all along that she'll quit), she would seem athletic. Born in New Hampshire, she and her family moved to the academy town of Castine, Maine, when she was fifteen. The maritime school where her dad worked didn't appeal to her at first because "the townies didn't like the middies and the middies didn't like the townies." But after a friend went to the academy and liked it, she changed course from her initial plan to study physical education in college. She sailed as a messman on a merchant ship and then signed up at the academy. But after graduating with a third mate's license in 1985, she found it tough getting a job on tankers so she worked as an able-bodied seaman for the first two years. She started sailing as a third mate about five years ago, and now earns around seventy thousand dollars a year.

Holmes says she owes a debt to the women who went before her. They forced the issue on the merchant vessels and convinced the male sailors to make room. "They came to a realization that women are going to be out here for a while." Holmes is careful how she treads in this male-dominated world. She doesn't pick unnecessary fights. She hates pornography, too, but knows that there are better ways to fight the battle without getting the sailors up-in-arms. She fits in by hefting a big wrench on the deck. She seems to have proven herself, and officers like Dean Davis say they admire her. The only question about her, the men tell me, is whether she will stick it out. They've seen too many women fall by the wayside, for reasons ranging from a dislike of sea life to a distaste for confinement with men.

For her part, Holmes plans to take the chief mate's exam this year. Someday, she'll sit for the captain's test, but she is not sure she will be around long enough to actually take command of a ship, since there is something like a twenty-year waiting period for a skipper's job. Things have changed since Carroll made rank.

8

Fire on the Water

*(Gulf of Alaska,
185 miles south of Middleton Island,
January 26, 10 P.M.)*

Ten at night and the watch is going slowly for Dean Davis, nothing but a radar screen to keep him company. The ship has crossed paths with another low-pressure system and the winds are howling again. Even in the dark I can see the ocean argue with the prow. Davis, the man of action, is not one to kill time with idleness. Between rolls the third mate stares out a side window and thinks about emergencies, imagining what would happen if a crew member fell overboard. He would toss a marker over the side and execute a hard-right Williamson turn, a precalculated maneuver designed to bring the ship back to the spot where the turn began. He would call the captain and have the crew get ready with a rescue boat and a resuscitator. Davis says he daydreams stuff like this all the time. He performs these mental drills because, if it really happens, he won't have time to consult a manual or to study the Williamson turn instructions that are posted on the wall behind him. In his mind, he changes the circumstances over and over again to sharpen his reflexes.

The truth is, the chances of finding a swimmer at night in tall waves like this are almost nil. Just about every tanker sailor who has gone overboard in these waters has been lost forever. A mind-numbing refrigeration occurs within minutes and the paralyzed swimmer drifts into a final sleep. But Davis won't give in to fate. He envisions himself slicing a little off the odds of death, just a sliver to give some sailor an outside chance.

I return to the bridge three hours later and Jean Holmes has taken over the watch. She too is engaged in mind games, trying to remember how to administer an intravenous injection using a needle. She is worried about Bob Rich, the first engineer, and his worsening condition. The diarrhea is draining his body fluids and he might need some saline replacement through a tube in his arm.

Holmes is the ship's medical officer, which is a duty handed to all second mates. Two years ago, she took a five-day medical course that included a brief workshop on poking people with needles, which she hated doing. She can always summon the captain, who is the ship's doctor, and he can call an emergency phone service in Maryland where he can get twenty-four-hour doctor advice. Still, everyone knows the chances of surviving a serious accident or illness out here are not great. With luck, if someone is terribly injured, the ship will be in range of a Coast Guard rescue helicopter. With more luck, the water will be calm enough for the chopper to land in the painted circle designated for it on the main deck. In a sea like this one such a rescue would be unlikely. "It's a fact of life, if you are badly injured out here, you will die," said one crew member.

"We are defenseless out here—just like puppies."

It is no surprise, then, that tanker sailors favor accident prevention. Statistics show that each oil tanker can expect at least one major accident every twenty years. They also show that, if you are going to die on an oil tanker, the most likely way to go is by fire. Over the course of a century, well over half the people killed on tank ships were done in by explosions, smoke, and flames.

Crude oil is so explosive the ships that carry it have been called "floating bombs." Although portions of the chemical soup that makes up crude oil are so thick they would smother a lighted match, other parts are gaseous solvents, known as aromatics, that would detonate when a match touched the striking pad.

Even in a small fleet like Arco's, there is a fire victim. The 91,000-deadweight-ton *Arco Texas* was a Chevron tanker when it was struck by lightning in September 1979 in Deer Park, Texas. The bolt of electricity from the afternoon sky caused a thunderous explosion that killed three people on the ship, split the tanker in half, and spilled 630,000 gallons of crude oil. It also detonated four nearby gasoline and oil barges and exploded an ethyl alcohol storage tank on the dock. The blast gave the Chevron ship a new identity, too. The rear end, all that was salvageable, became the stern of a new ship expanded in size from 71,000-deadweight-tons to 91,000 tons. Now the *Arco Texas,* it is our nearest fleet mate tonight, some seven hundred miles away.

Lightning has taken a great toll on tankers, but when you are carrying 114,000 tons of explosive liquids, there are many perils. Fire erupts from collisions, groundings, engine room mishaps . . . and maybe even sabotage. The last thing crew members saw before the 320,000-ton *Energy Determination* detonated was a sixty-five-year-old seaman wandering out in the vicinity of an open tank. They couldn't question the sailor afterwards, for he was shredded and hurled into the Persian Gulf, but he had been threatening suicide for a week and on more than one occasion demanding to be sent home to China. He talked with fellow sailors about setting the ship on fire and just before the blast he wrote letters to his wife, bank, and friends, indicating his death was imminent. Investigators believe he tossed a match or a burning rag into the tank.

Ships started exploding as soon as they began hauling kerosene in the nineteenth century, some on their maiden voyages. Kerosene-ship owners had to shanghai sailors from bars to replace the crewmen who fled when told they were carrying liquid fire.

The situation improved after deterrents came to be better understood. Sailors learned that a tank is most vulnerable when it is empty because the fumes, not the liquid, are what is most explosive. They found ways to control at least one, if not all, of three ingredients of fire—the ignition sources, fumes, and oxygen. Ignition sources, such as fans, pumps, two-way radios, and flashlights, are kept away from the tanks or are designed not to create sparks. And more than one sailor has been fired for crossing a tanker gangplank while palming a lit cigarette.

Fumes can be removed from a tank, but while the dangerous gases are being replaced by fresh air, the contents will pass through a condition known as the explosive range. That's where the hydrocarbon fumes are 2 to 12 percent of the mixture and oxygen is more than 11 percent—a volatile brew that will ignite like dynamite in the presence of a tiny spark. One way to defuse a tank is to avoid the explosive range by keeping the mixture either too lean (having too few hydrocarbon particles) or too rich (having too many). For most of tanker history, that is how tanks were kept safe.

Then came a device called the inert gas system, invented by the Sun Oil Company after Charles Boyle, the fleet manager, saw a crew member burned to death on the tanker *Bidwell* on the Delaware River in 1938. Company engineers devised a system for capturing the gases from the engine exhaust, scrubbing and cooling them in a shower of seawater, and then pumping them into the tanks to displace the oxygen. This inert engine would not explode because it didn't contain enough oxygen. The system worked, and by 1941 Sun Oil had installed it on all Sun tankers over twelve thousand deadweight tons. Eventually the company had the device on more than two dozen ships.

The technology was available to all tanker operators, but few at the time were interested for two reasons: The cost was around two hundred thousand dollars per ship in the 1950s, and some owners were skeptical of its value.

The industry and Coast Guard attitude toward this innovation was illustrated by their reaction to a ruling handed down in 1959 by a federal judge in Delaware. In a case where a World War II–style tanker called the *Mission San Francisco* exploded, Judge D. J. Layton said the owner and operator were negligent for sending the vessel to sea without an inert gas system (known by then as IGS). The judge's ruling would have allowed the families of ten dead sailors to collect sizable damages.

Some Coast Guard safety officers were indignant at the ruling, saying the judge meddled where he didn't belong. Industry officials reacted as though the judge had reached into their wallets. When they appealed, a higher court overruled Layton's decision. The owners saved money, and tankers kept exploding.

Most tanker owners continued to ignore the danger until December 1969 when three brand new super tankers exploded off the coast of Africa in a period of eighteen days. In each case, tanks exploded when they were being cleaned with high-pressure water hoses. The 207,000-ton *Marpessa* burned and eventually sank, the largest seagoing vessel ever lost. The 208,000-ton *Mactra* and the 219,000-ton *Kong Haakon VII* were charred and disabled. Four men died and several were injured.

Led by Royal Dutch Shell, which owned two of the ships, the major tanker companies began an expensive investigation into the causes of tanker explosions. What they found was a deadly hazard contained in a glob of water. During tank cleaning, globs of water tumble toward the floor or fly toward a wall, picking up infinitesimally small charges of electricity the way rain does inside a thundercloud. When the droplets come within a short distance of the steel floor or wall, tiny sparks arc over the gap in their impatient desire to reach ground. No spark is bigger than the static electric shock you would get after walking on a nylon carpet, but it is strong enough to set off a gargantuan explosion inside a tank that contains the right mixture of crude oil fumes and oxygen. Some also say that during the cleaning process steam clouds form inside the tank, emitting tiny lightning bolts.

What made this danger widespread was the construction of new ships with cargo tanks large enough to brew a small thundercloud. Modern ship designers favored big tanks because a ship with fewer partitions costs less and is easier to operate. A typical T-2 tanker of World War II design had around two dozen cargo tanks, none with a capacity greater than four hundred thousand gallons. The *Arco Anchorage* has thirteen tanks, the largest capable of holding nearly four million gallons, or more than a T-2 tanker would carry altogether.

The answer was to inert the tanks.

Even though tanker owners knew that Sun Oil's inert gas system could prevent tank explosions, the maritime world reacted slowly. While it's likely the airline industry would have grounded planes until every one had the device, it would be another decade and a half before it was mandatory on all tankers. Even today there are small tankers that don't have the systems.

Some moved more quickly, but the progress was still limited.

Exxon installed inert gas systems on tankers in the early 1970s, and the world's major tanker owners agreed among themselves to voluntarily install inerting systems on all new tankers larger than one hundred thousand deadweight tons, an arbitrary tonnage threshold based on hunches rather than scientific evidence. With this move, tanker owners had hoped to solve the problem and discourage regulators from requiring inert gas on smaller tankers. Then in 1974 the United Nations adopted a recommendation for inert gas on larger tankers, but it was not a requirement. Meanwhile, the United States adopted a rule requiring inert gas on one-hundred-thousand-ton tankers after December 1974.

But as time went on, more than one hundred people died in explosions aboard a dozen tankers considered too small for inert gas.

What the world needed was a stunning example of the problem. It got one when the seventy-one-thousand-ton Liberian-flagged tanker *Sansinena* sailed into Los Angeles harbor on a clear afternoon shortly before Christmas 1976 to drop off a load of crude oil. The eighteen-year-old tanker did not have an inert gas system, nor did its owners—Union Oil Company and the Barracuda Tanker Corporation of Bermuda—have any intention of installing one as long as they were not required.

The 810-foot-long ship spent the night and most of the next day discharging its cargo of Indonesian crude oil at Union Oil's berth in San Pedro, California. As evening fell, the unloaded vessel was taking on ballast water and venting fumes out openings on top of the tanks (on ships with inert gas this would not happen—the tanks would have been sealed shut). A breeze massaged the harbor, soft enough to stir up the tank fumes but not strong enough to dissipate them. As a result, a vapor cloud formed over the old tanker's deck and became trapped in the space between the mid-deck house where the officers slept and the rear house where the crew stayed. (Old-fashioned tankers had two houses.) The Italian ship captain strolled with a visitor from the mid-deck house to the rear galley over an elevated catwalk, unaware of the fumes below because they are visible only against a lighted horizon, like heat waves on a highway. By leaving the mid-deck house the two men unknowingly saved their lives.

Dinner was nearly done when the breeze shifted direction and a tongue of fumes found its way up a ventilator shaft into the mid-deck house. The fan was on and the gases were drawn up to an open electrical switch that controlled a water pump. At 7:38 P.M., a flash like the discharge of a camera strobe light lit up the space between the houses. Then a stupendous explosion ripped apart the ship and slammed the San Pedro neighborhood with such force that it flattened traffic signs for blocks and shattered all the windows on a commercial street two miles away. Buildings shook forty miles away.

The ship's mid-deck house was hurled 750 feet into the air, taking with it the occupants, a twenty-five-year-old radio officer and a thirty-four-year-old mate. Spinning and twisting end over end, the flying building fell onto a terminal security shack with enough force to drive the seventy-two-year-old guard who was inside some sixteen feet into the ground. Hurled into the air with the house was a section of steel deck, four thousand tons and over five hundred feet long, that crashed onto the adjacent dock. With it went the torn remains of the men who'd been tending the tanks—a twenty-eight-year-old officer, two seamen ages thirty-eight and thirty, and a pumpman and fireman, both fifty-six years old. Another seriously burned forty-four-year-old engine room worker died later at home in Italy.

Nine people were killed, including the security guard, and fifty-eight were injured. Among those were three dozen on shore who were hit by debris and flying glass fragments. In the aftermath, there was so much property destruction over a three-mile radius that six thousand damage claims were filed. Police evacuated over one thousand people and some 260 nearby pleasure boats suffered broken windows and other damage. Almost a million gallons of the ship's bunker fuel was spilled into the harbor.

The investigators said an inert gas system would have prevented the blast since sealed tanks would not have emitted explosive vapors. The crew violated safety guidelines by operating with open tanks during a period of light breezes, but that was often done in a world where oil must keep moving. Wind conditions would have been irrelevant if the tanks had been closed and inerted. As one Coast Guard officer told me, "An inert gas system can cover up a multitude of sins."

Investigators were pretty sure the ventilation fan lit the fuse, but it is instructive to consider the variety of ignition sources they had to ponder: a hot particle of soot from the smokestack, an exposed light-bulb, a cigarette, spontaneous combustion from a stack of rags, a spark from some deck equipment, a toppled ladder, a nearby automobile ignition, a broken flashlight bulb, a gangway telephone, and even the static electricity emitted from someone's polyester clothing.

The Coast Guard could no longer ignore the need for inert gas on smaller ships, especially when one of the agency's cutters was a mile away when the *Sansinena* blew up. Armed with the investigative report, the Coast Guard rewrote the rule to require inert gas on new tankers larger than twenty thousand tons.

The industry also reconsidered the drumroll of ship explosions that were tearing apart the world fleet regardless of size. On the *Arco Anchorage* you can see the inert gas machinery by walking out the back of the house. It is located inside a big white structure that sticks up next to the smokestack nearly as high as the bridge. But if you look at the original blueprints, you won't see it, because it wasn't added until 1977, four years after the ship was launched and one year after the *Sansinena* blast.

At a London ship-safety conference in 1978, the *Sansinena* and other examples carried enough weight that the UN's International Maritime Consultative Organization drafted a treaty amendment requiring new crude oil ships over twenty thousand deadweight tons to have an inert gas system. But nothing was mandatory until 1983.

Meanwhile, the fireworks continued. In the years before the UN rule became law, another 118 people were killed on sixteen ships that exploded without inerting systems. There was even an uncanny replay of the three explosions that started the debate in 1969. This time, two monstrous super tankers were blown apart on opposite coasts of Africa in a matter of hours on the same day, April 3, 1980, but each one sent a different message. The 239,000-ton *Albahaa* had no inert gas system and the six men killed were unlucky victims of an owner unwilling to spend money on a safety device not yet required by law. The other vessel, the identically sized *Mycene,* was newer and was equipped with an inert gas system, but the captain had chosen not to use it. He thought it was malfunctioning, and when the owner pressured him to keep a tight schedule he skipped the inerting process while cleaning the tanks.

For all their value, there are times when inert gas systems don't work. Some thirty tankers have exploded despite having inerting systems on board. Some detonated because the captains didn't use the device and others caught fire when the tanks split open due to heavy weather or collisions. But there are cases where inert gas systems were on during cleaning operations and the tanks blew up anyway. Some experts believe inert gas creates deposits of pyrophoric iron sulfide when hydrogen sulfide gas, contained in the engine exhaust, reacts with rust outside the presence of oxygen. The deposits ignite spontaneously when oxygen is reintroduced to a tank and any fumes present can explode.

Some tanker optimists say the term "floating bomb" no longer applies to oil ships because of inert gas. But Arthur McKenzie, a New York tanker consultant who served with Exxon, says that is one of the most dangerous myths that abound in the industry. Most *Arco Anchorage* crew members agree. "Let me tell you, man, I think about it any goddamn time I open a valve," said one seaman.

The *Arco Anchorage* has an array of fire-fighting equipment, including platforms with water cannons and rolled-up fire hoses spaced down the deck. In an instant, the engine room can be filled with a fire-smothering gas. At one time, the tanker was equipped with chemical fire-fighting foam but nowadays, in a gesture to the environment, the system is loaded with fifteen hundred gallons of a biodegradable foam made partly of pig's blood. It smells so bad, the crew is reluctant to use it during drills, but it supposedly does the job.

On every trip the ship holds a fire and lifeboat drill, usually announced ahead of time. Those I witnessed had a plodding pace about them. The crew was mustered to the deck where a couple of hoses were unrolled and water was sprayed over the side. Crew members were quizzed about their fire-fighting duties and they in turn asked questions of the chief mate. At one drill, a hose leaked pretty badly. At another, the chief steward asked to go inside because he was cold. But when third mate Dean Davis held a seminar to describe how a person crawls through a room on hands and knees to find crew mates trapped in a fire, everybody listened intently. Crew members admitted afterward, though, that the odds are against their controlling a big fire on this ship. It might be impossible, since tankers get so hot the rescue vessels can't get near, and in many cases the fire-fighting equipment is destroyed in the first explosion. Tanker sailors have been incinerated, boiled by steam, and even drowned in escaping oil. Prevention and escape are better bets than fire fighting.

Used properly, the inerting system has minimized the likelihood of the *Arco Anchorage* crew ever confronting a wildfire or detonation. The December 1977 crash off the coast of South Africa of two 331,000-ton sister ships, the *Venoil* and *Venpet,* the largest manmade objects ever to collide on the face of the earth, provides a dramatic example of the inerting system's value. One ship was hauling crude oil and the other was carrying fumes, a potentially lethal mixture. The loaded ship spilled 7 percent of its cargo, enough to pollute sixty miles of bathing beaches, and two crew members were killed when they refused to abandon ship into a blazing ocean. But everybody else was rescued and the smothering virtues of the inert gas prevented an explosion. Courageous sailors and boarding crews were able to bring the deck fires under control.

Even so, oil ships smaller than twenty thousand deadweight tons, and barges that are as large as tankers, still ply the oceans without inert gas since the law doesn't require it. In recent years, more than a dozen tankers of less than twenty thousand tons have exploded.

Jim Atkinson, a sixty-seven-year-old Virginia consultant who is a widely recognized expert on tanker explosions, believes the history of inert gas is a good example of an industry moving sluggishly toward change. A tanker sailor during World War II and a Coast Guard captain until 1979, he was an investigator in the *Sansinena* case and several other major explosions.

"I think this maritime business is one huge accident waiting to happen all the time," he said. "It is not rational. The fault lies with the companies, with regulators, with the people who make the laws, with the naval architects, the classification societies . . . it falls out all over the system."

9

No License to Own

*(Pacific Ocean,
240 miles west of Prince of Wales Island,
January 27, 9 A.M.)*

In one of his mess hall lectures on maritime history, able-bodied seaman Pat Newman links the downfall of the sea captain with the invention of the radio. His theory is that skippers played god when they were beyond the reach of the owner; they could flog a crewman and chose whatever course they wanted. But after Guglielmo Marconi contrived the wireless telegraph in 1895, the landlord could pick up a radio—or, God forbid, a cellular telephone—and chew out the skipper or change his direction. "Now the actual master is Mr. Marconi."

Captain Jack Carroll has four telephones at his desk, some for calling the bridge and engine room and others for calling home—the home office, that is. He can talk to fleet managers in Long Beach any time of the day or night. Occasionally a boss will ring him up, but mostly they send memoranda and other typewritten orders. Newman ought to add the fax and telex to his list of sinful machines. "I love the sea but I resent the fact they are turning it into a bureaucracy," he says.

If it is the bureaucracy Newman describes, then who should be held accountable when something goes wrong? The captain is usually the whipping boy whenever a ship goes aground or collides with another vessel. The tanker owner may pay the cleanup bill, but the tab is usually shuffled off to an insurance company. Occasionally the courts will rap an owner for wrongdoing, but it is a rare moment.

Some say the only way to have responsible fleet owners and shore personnel is to require them to be licensed. If something goes wrong, the U.S. Coast Guard could lift the boss's permit the way documents are taken away from offending skippers, mates, or crew members.

As it is, an owner needs little more than legal tender to put himself and his organization in the driver's seat. Yet the way he spends his money will make the difference between a seaworthy ship and an ill-maintained sinker. Like most skippers, Carroll has little control over the checkbook. From each of the seventeen million dollars Arco spends annually to keep this tub afloat, twenty-three cents goes to crew salaries and benefits; twenty-three cents to pilots, escort boats, and fuel; sixteen cents to maintenance; thirteen cents to headquarters staff; thirteen cents to the bank; seven cents to a bevy of insurance companies; and a nickel is left over for food and incidentals, the only part the captain has much say over.

Carroll can save or spend a little extra on maintenance at sea, but the company has near total control over the important work performed every two years at the shipyard.

The lack of owner licensing also means the honchos can hide from scrutiny. When a newly sold Bahamian-flagged cargo ship was abandoned just outside New York harbor in June 1992, not even the ship's captain knew who the buyer was. Coast Guard officers assigned to the case spent more than two weeks trying to untangle the camouflaged records.

With the unregulated maritime business in a state of near chaos, ships change flags, owners move their headquarters, vessels are purchased and then leased back to the buyer, bankruptcies are rampant, financial backers are cloaked in fancy paperwork, and national origins are irrelevant. A tanker that flies a Liberian flag might be owned by a lawyer in New York, financed by a bank in Hong Kong, and operated by a company in Monte Carlo. It might be classed by the Norwegians, skippered by an Italian captain, and crewed by Taiwanese sailors. The insurer is probably in London, but the keeper of the paperwork might be in Singapore.

Even this ship has unadvertised ownership. Don't let the tall letters on the side of the hull that say ARCO fool you—the real owner

is a group of unnamed investors whose trust is handled by the Northern Trust Company of Chicago and the First National Bank of Chicago.
Arco leases the ship from the owners under a contract known as a
bare-boat charter, meaning, literally, that the ship was delivered to
Arco stark naked—no crew, fuel, food, or other ancillary equipment.
The deal has the tax and depreciation advantages of a long-term auto
lease, but disadvantages as well. Discussions swirl at headquarters
these days around the 1995 expiration date on the lease. Should the
deal be extended even though the tanker will be prohibited from
visiting American shores after June 1, 1998, with its outdated single
hull? Or should the company build a new ship and risk a collapse in
the uncertain Alaskan oil supplies? "Good question," said Arco business manager Frank McCord. "Since that is part of our strategies, we
won't share the answer with you or anyone else."

Deciding what to do about tumbling deadlines is part of the fun
of owning a tanker. And any attempt to typecast the folks who make
these decisions can be as difficult as tracking them down.

National governments, not private companies, own the largest
fleets. Before its breakup, the Soviet Union had the biggest collection,
some 200 vessels, many small ice-breaking tankers. Second on the list
is China with 92. Then comes Brazil (71), the United States (68), Indonesia (47), and India (44). The U.S. vessels are small, too, averaging
only 31,000 tons. The only governments with super tankers in large
numbers are Iran with 33 ships averaging 180,000 deadweight tons,
Kuwait with 27 averaging 114,000 tons, and Libya with 11 averaging
122,000 tons.

American, Japanese, Norwegian, and Greek businessmen com-
prise the majority of private owners. Most American owners are head-
quartered in the United States, but the flag they prefer is Liberian. The
Liberian registry is such a Yankee operation that its main office is in
Reston, Virginia, not Monrovia.

The typical owner could be shown in a snapshot if it were true—
as some people mistakenly suspect—that oil giants like Exxon domi-
nate the picture. Indeed, Exxon, with 60 tankers, has a large fleet. So,
too, does Shell with 46, followed by Chevron (42), Mobil (36), Texaco
(28), British Petroleum (25), Arco (10), and Amoco (10). But taken

together, the world's biggest oil companies, known as the "seven sisters," own only 13 percent of the world's tankers. They prefer to charter someone else's ship, as that protects them from the economic bruising of a prolonged shipping recession. When I say charter, in this case I'm describing something different from the deal Arco has with the Chicago bank. In this case the oil company hires an outsider to supply and operate the boat and the crew. The independent tanker owners who provide these ships are a diverse group: around three thousand oil-carrying ships are owned by around five hundred companies and individuals.

Many independent ships are run not by the owner, but by management companies, much the same way apartment buildings are overseen by property managers. If you want to find some ship managers, just check the buildings along the Avenue of the Americas in New York, Avenue du Metropole in Monte Carlo, and Akti Miaouli in Piraeus, Greece.

Some independent tanker owners sign long-term contracts with oil companies, making their ships near-regular members of the company's fleet. Many others carry single loads of cargo on what is known as the spot market.

Those playing the spot market are hyperactive oil traders who work with telephones glued to their ears, sometimes dealing and re-dealing the same load of oil to different buyers before the ship even makes it to port. A tanker that carries oil on the spot market is like a taxicab, picking up a single cargo the way a cabbie grabs a fare. Once a very lucrative trade, the spot market has lost all its glitter because charter rates are stuck in the basement. Long-term contracts with oil companies aren't so hot, either, so tanker owners are caught in a bind. Many are waiting for the market to improve, limping along with short-term jobs while they barely break even or lose money. They are gamblers waiting for the charter rates to go up.

When these risk-takers buy tankers, they often use a financing method that resembles the game real estate investors play. They obtain contracts to haul oil and then get a construction loan from a bank based on the business they have secured—the same way building developers line up tenants before they borrow money to build. In the best of times this was a sure deal. Anyone who bought a tanker in the first two and a half decades following World War II looked like a genius. With money flowing in gushers, some ships paid for themselves in a couple of trips and were sold for pure profit. Even if they went aground, the scrap steel was worth a bundle. In bad times the road to profit is more circuitous.

For the advanced players, there are complex variations of the financing game where you buy a ship and then lease it back to the seller, all to make huge profits without paying taxes once the vessel is resold. Other times, a single company will own a dozen ships under a dozen company names.

Critics say tanker owners meddle with safety when they play these games because the rules favor deal makers over experienced mariners. "Vessels today are no longer operated by the tried-and-true ship owners, whose roots were at sea, whose profits were good, and who invested money in hiring and training the best people," observed an internal Coast Guard report. The worst of the speculators turn their tankers over to management companies with instructions to make a buck as quickly as possible. When times are tight—as they have been for two decades—that means cutting corners. "Scheduling is everything. Today's adage is to do more with less, make two tankers do the work done by three previously," the Coast Guard report noted.

With charter rates barely covering the cost of operation, money for maintenance is scarce. Arco prides itself as a fleet that doesn't scrimp on repairs, no matter what. McCord, the company's business manager, says it would be unforgivable for an Arco ship to spill oil because the company was too cheap to fix something. "There is never any talk here about scrimping on anything that is safety or environmental," he said. Perhaps. But a Greek owner confessed to Ron Weightman, a Norwegian classification society inspector, that he survived tough times by dividing his tanker fleet into three parts, by age, for purposes of budgeting maintenance. He didn't spend any money maintaining the newest group because they hadn't yet taken enough punishment. The middle group got maintenance, but they did so at the expense of the oldest and rattiest ships, which got none at all.

Weightman declined to identify the candid Greek who ran his

oldest ships into the ground, but if the tanker industry ever opens a hall of fame, there are certain names guaranteed to be there. It's hard to remember what it was like in the old days when tanker owners had identities synonymous with Roman gods. Quiet Norwegians like today's Morten Bergesen just don't inspire the same awe.

At one time or another in the glory days, when oil was cheap and shipping was profitable, at least five tanker tycoons landed on the list of the world's wealthiest people: Daniel Ludwig, Aristotle Onassis, Stavros Niarchos, Y. K. Pao, and C. Y. Tung. They were billionaires above the law, men who consorted with world leaders, made deals with kings, and would have laughed at any Coast Guard officer who handed them a rule book. Ship inspectors and lawmakers quaked in their shadow.

Daniel Keith Ludwig was the strangest and perhaps the most important of the group. He practically invented superships and the speculative method of financing them. He welded, rather than riveted tankers for the first time and moved the house back to the rear of the ship. He broached no meddling and there were times in his life when he could have bought people by the country. But he wasn't ostentatious like some of the other tycoons. He walked from his New York town house to his office on the Avenue of the Americas, and he was an off-the-rack penny-pincher who wore a plastic raincoat. He was adamant about privacy. He granted few press interviews and in the 1960s he stopped talking to writers altogether. One time when a Brazilian government photographer snapped his picture he ordered the negatives destroyed. The staff at his Manhattan office, National Bulk Carriers, Inc., avoided referring to him by name so visitors would not know who he was. A stiff workaholic and a rule-bound perfectionist, he cruelly refused to recognize his only child, a daughter, as his own. Yet he gave most of his fortune to a cancer institute that bears his name.

As for the environment, no one was viewed as a malefactor quite like Ludwig. Not only did he operate oil tankers, he helped pioneer the chopping down of the Amazon rain forest. Born in Michigan in 1897, the son of a real estate investor from a family of ship captains, he didn't manage to become a real power in the ship business until World War II, when he assembled a fleet for the war effort. After the victory, the tankers reverted to his ownership, and gave him the fifth-largest flotilla in the country. He also owned a Norfolk, Virginia, shipyard where he developed labor-saving techniques for welding ships and where he led the postwar drive to build bigger tankers. His Norfolk shipyard turned out tankers as large as the dry docks would allow—some thirty thousand deadweight tons—before he leased a Japanese shipyard where the Imperial Navy's largest battleship was constructed. At a retooled Kure shipbuilding plant, using cheap labor to build tankers at half the American price, Ludwig gave the Japanese a foothold on tanker construction they would never relinquish and one that would nearly sink the American yards.

Ludwig, who had back pain due to an injury from a 1926 tanker explosion, was as penurious with his ships as he was in his personal life. He registered his fleet with "flag of convenience" states like Panama and Liberia where the fees and taxes were low and regulations slack. He hired nonunion crews from the West Indies and cut out shipboard frills like swimming pools and carpets. They used to say his motto was, "If it can't hold oil, it's not on the ship." He became a leader among postwar shipbuilders and prided himself on the quality of ships he operated, but his shipyards in Norfolk, Virginia, turned out three welded tankers in the late 1940s that broke in heavy seas during the 1960s, spilling oil and killing forty crew members.

By the mid-1970s, the efficient administrator was among the world's wealthiest people, worth three to five billion dollars. Starting in 1967, he acquired rights to a piece of the Amazon jungle covering nearly six thousand square miles—half the size of Belgium—and set up what would become the world's largest pulp and paper fiasco. He thought a fast-growing tree from Asia called the gmelina would provide a high-volume wood fiber that could grow in Brazil. But as his bulldozers were mowing down the Amazon rain forest, gmelina trees were found to have difficulty in the thin soil and climate of the Amazon and the Brazilian government pushed him out. By the late 1980s, Ludwig had slipped from some lists of billionaires, partly because he diverted his money to his cancer charity. When he died at age ninety-five, his fleet and his power had been greatly reduced from its former glory.

The other headliners in the postwar tanker boom lost their luster along the way too. Onassis and Niarchos were related by marriage and yacht-based lifestyle, but otherwise they were rivals. No matter how competitive, though, the Greek shipowners operated like a club, making handshake deals that were difficult to track and camouflaging their moves through a series of companies. Two years before he died, Onassis had control of seventy firms and was nearly a billionaire. He played all the angles, registering his vessels with flag-of-convenience states and cutting costs wherever he could. Of course, there were losses. Two of his Liberian-flagged ships spilled nearly nine million gallons of oil within a month's time in 1970 off Nova Scotia and Portugal. Three other ships exploded, killing a total of sixteen crew members. When Onassis died in March 1975 his fleet numbered more than fifty ships, but tough times lay ahead. Today, the remnant of Onassis's fleet includes ten tankers with an average size of 142,000 deadweight tons, which ranks it around twenty-ninth among independents.

Other great tanker barons did not fare much better. After he came out of China during the Communist revolution, Chao Yung Tung built a fleet of 140 ships. When he died in 1982, C. Y.'s fleet was foundering in debt and a decade later it was down to ten ships. His rival, Yue-Kong Pao was the best of the lot and came from a similar background. Y. K.—as he was called—managed to leave behind the largest independent tanker fleet in the world when he died at his Hong Kong home in 1991. His 44 tankers averaged 219,000 deadweight tons. But it had once been the world's largest fleet, period, numbering 190 ships.

Anyone who examines the maritime world will eventually ask the question, who is in charge? The answer is nobody. On the shelves in the captain's office, there are operating instructions from Arco headquarters, and Coast Guard inspection certificates, and documents from the classification society. Everything looks orderly. But the truth is that tankers operate on borderless oceans and pass constantly through different jurisdictions. No single government rules the oceans and no one has full control of the ships or the owners. The international regulation of tankers is much weaker than the system that controls aviation.

The closest thing to a world authority is the UN's International

Maritime Organization, based in London. Unfortunately, the organization and its committees that draft policy are dominated by ship-owning nations. It is little wonder, then, that the IMO is seen as a partisan and ineffective body, operating behind closed doors for the benefit of commerce. Legislation the U.S. Congress passed following the *Exxon Valdez* spill put unprecedented pressure on the IMO to reform. The organization did amend some rules, and some say the atmosphere is different, but others have called for a complete overhaul of the system.

In nautical politics, the world is divided into flag states who have large numbers of ships under their registry, and port states who receive them. Flag states exert the most influence, determining standards for crew size and training as well as ship maintenance and construction in their vast fleets. The most powerful of them include small nations like Liberia and Panama. They offer their flag for a moderate price and since they rarely ask questions about ownership some take advantage of their convenient banners to register vessels under front-company names. And most flag states don't have a government agency that inspects ships, relying on classification societies that are easier to manipulate. At the IMO, small flag states have a powerful voice since a country's vote is often enhanced according to the number of ships it has in its registry.

In recent years, some flag-of-convenience countries have toughened their safety standards and it is interesting to see what happened as a result. Liberia, once considered very lax, saw its tanker fleet shrink from 1,003 in 1975 to 572 today when the rules were tightened. There is an advantage to this, since the Liberian inspectors, who are based in Virginia, now have a higher-quality fleet to deal with. The troublesome rust buckets fled to flags like Malta's, whose tanker fleet increased from 2 to 113.

In December 1988, the Liberian-registered 230,000-deadweight-ton *Pegasus I* suffered an explosion in the bow area while transferring crude oil to another ship in the Persian Gulf. Liberian accident investigators found corroded deck fittings, electrical conduits, and other metals parts, and concluded that a ventilator was left open, in violation of transfer rules, allowing fumes to come in contact with an electrical switch. They recommended the skipper be reprimanded, but before their report was published the ship had switched flags and was flying a Maltese banner off the bow.

Malta is just one of several cheap flags. An official with the ship registration office of the tiny Pacific island nation of Vanuatu once said the only time his country does an investigation or inspection on a ship is when the registree fails to pay his fees.

On the port state side, the United States is the leader. It was a timid leader until the *Exxon Valdez* accident. In the aftermath, Congress passed legislation that required tanker owners to, among other things, place a "certificate of responsibility" aboard every ship declaring who would pay the bill for any spill damages. The new law also allowed spill victims to bill the insurance company directly for damages, a concept known as "direct access." And Congress hiked the criminal penalty for knowingly causing a spill to fifteen years in prison and in some cases allowed for unlimited monetary liability. Since courtroom damage awards in America are higher than anywhere in the world, tanker owners were furious.

Groups like the International Association of Independent Tanker Owners (Intertanko), the International Chamber of Shipping, and the American Institute of Merchant Shipping reacted with brisk lobbying. Tanker owners labeled the United States an outlaw nation and threatened to boycott its shores. Major companies got rid of their tanker subsidiaries to avoid liability. The P & I clubs that insure ships threatened to withdraw from underwriting American-bound tankers altogether.

At a tanker convention in Washington, D.C., the pin-striped crowd acted like street protesters when some key congressional staffers explained the new law. "What happened to representative government?" shouted one British owner. The staffers told the unhappy gathering that Congress was in no mood to reopen the debate over the *Exxon Valdez* legislation. Merchant Marine and Fisheries Committee lawyer Cynthia Wilkerson warned the gathering that restarting the process could produce even tougher laws. "The devil you know is better than the devil you don't know." Congressman Billy Tauzin, a Democrat from the oil state of Louisiana who chairs a House committee that oversees the Coast Guard, apologized at lunch and described how he lost battle after battle in the 1990 session that followed the *Exxon Valdez* spill. "We won one victory when enough Californians left late in the evening." Tauzin warned the tanker owners not to fail if they started a boycott. "Don't bluff us," he said. As it turned out, the threat fizzled.

One lawyer told a gathering of tanker owners that anyone not prepared to spend huge amounts of money better "get the hell out of the business." But tanker owners are gearing up for new battles in Congress. Fourteen tanker-owning nations—Norway, Sweden, Denmark, Finland, Great Britain, Belgium, Netherlands, Germany, France, Spain, Italy, Greece, Portugal, and Japan—meet monthly in a posh room at the Dutch embassy in Washington, D.C., to debate lobbying strategy. They call themselves the "Cotton Club" because the meeting room resembles the famous Harlem nightspot. Norwegian embassy official Janna Julsrud, who was Cotton Club chairwoman in 1992, says the threat of a boycott isn't over. Something like a bad February in Maine might tempt tanker owners to withhold oil. She vows they will not quit until the American law is amended. "This was not a considered, objective piece of legislation. This was an act of revenge. The American public wants tanker owners to suffer. This is overkill."

Others want more reform. Coast Guard Rear Admiral Gene Henn says the industry needs a five-step revolution: Ship owners must heal themselves; the international community must weed out bad classification societies; flag states must set new standards; insurance companies must take responsibility; and port states must band together to "bring the hammer down."

Some of Henn's ideas are taking hold. London insurers recently sent their own inspectors to check some questionable tankers and found that only six of the first twenty-eight were safe, although classification society inspectors had stamped all of them okay. In the face of this embarrassing episode, American Bureau of Shipping President Frank Iarossi—the man who headed the Exxon fleet at the time of the *Exxon Valdez* disaster—accused the insurance companies of harassing tanker owners. He said so many inspectors were coming on board ships they were going to distract the captain someday and cause an accident. Roger Nixon, a leader among the insurers, scoffed at the idea. He promised that they would be doing more tanker inspections if the classification societies didn't clean up their act.

Henn envisions a day when unacceptable standards will result in a flag state losing its membership in IMO and a classification society losing its charter to do business. There is some movement in this direction. For the first time ever, the International Association of Classification Societies is auditing member operations. The IMO has drafted voluntary standards for classification societies, flag states, and port state inspectors. And the Norwegian classification society has expelled more than 150 ships that were considered substandard. But critics say the reform is too little and too late. To date, there is no one with the clear authority to sanction a classification society. Even some shipowners are tired of it. Swedish shipowners recently suggested that tanker owners issue a list of acceptable classification societies and boycott the rest.

For their part, major oil companies have toughened standards lately and when they reject a substandard ship for charter they are sharing their inspection findings with other companies. But the trend will continue only as long as there are more ships available than there is oil to haul. The surplus could be reversed by a war or crisis.

Arthur McKenzie, the tanker consultant who worked forty years for Exxon, has tried to quantify the quality of tankers. Sitting in his New York apartment surrounded by a blizzard of reports, McKenzie has devised a system for rating tankers that he applies to the ships in an annual booklet he publishes called the "Guide for the Selection of Tankers." Each of the world's thirty-five hundred oil ships over ten thousand deadweight tons gets a grade from 1 to 5 (with 5 being excellent). What influences the ratings are a ship's age, the number of times it has changed names or owners, the experience of the owner and manager, the classification society, the flag, and, finally, the number of breakdowns, collisions, groundings, and fires it has suffered. In general, the Danes, Norwegians, and Japanese fared the best in McKenzie's book. Investeringsfond AF of Copenhagen got the highest possible grade of 5, and A. P. Moller, a century-old Danish firm with twenty-nine tankers, had a rating of 4.4. As for the worst, anyone who loves beaches ought to beware of certain Greeks bearing oil.

The Americans get middling grades. The Arco fleet is rated around 3.5, and the *Arco Anchorage* itself gets a 3. By contrast, Keystone Shipping Company of Philadelphia, a family-owned outfit that leases tankers to the Alaska trade, gets a poor 1.4 rating. Industry experts complain that McKenzie's method is imperfect and rough, but the rating book gives a reader a rare means of comparison. McKenzie says the most important factor is fleet management.

Jerry Aspland, the president of Arco Marine, may be to tanker managers what Lee Iacocca is to the automakers. He is either a visionary or a hip shooter depending on how you view him. In a conference room at the Seattle-Tacoma International Airport, Aspland shifted impatiently in his chair and adjusted his glasses when a manager from the state of Washington's newly created Office of Marine Safety asked what state officials could do to hold the line against oil spills. "Keep the heat on. I mean it. You've got to keep the heat on. Keep asking questions like you are doing. I just worry that three years from now nobody will be paying any attention and things will slip back to the way they used to be.

"Over a five-year period we are going to spend six billion dollars picking up oil. I doubt we've spent even one hundred million dollars on prevention."

With statements like this, Aspland has gained a reputation as an atypical tanker manager. It hasn't been easy. In 1985, the year he assumed presidency of Arco Marine, the tanker-owning subsidiary, the parent corporation went through a major restructuring and his employees were handed a heavy pay cut. Then exactly 111 days into his reign, the *Arco Anchorage* struck bottom in Port Angeles harbor, spilling 239,000 gallons of oil.

Yet he has the kind of voice that gets heard among tankermen, legislators, and even environmentalists. A newspaper columnist introduced him at one conference as a man who "put the welfare of Puget Sound ahead of cost." A year later, he was appointed to the marine board of the National Research Council and to the state of Washington's Marine Oversight Board.

He ordered his loaded ships to sail at least eighty-five miles from shore at an annual cost increase of one million dollars each. He convinced the industry to voluntarily obey an eleven-nautical-mile-per-hour speed while sailing loaded through Washington's San Juan Islands. He criticized harbor pilots and goaded them to improve their standards. He started a five-year study of crew operations with the intention of changing the way vessels are organized. He also offered to convert one of his company's tankers into a giant oil skimmer for cleaning up spills.

For all his notoriety, though, Aspland is an unimposing guy, slightly heavyset and slouchy, with the friendly manner of a nice science teacher. But at the Long Beach office where he rules, the people who work for him say they could tell from the beginning he would run the fleet someday. He has determination and guile, and he knows how to play the game. One reason he urges the industry to do things voluntarily is that he wants to avoid further legislation. And he is able to hedge answers with the best of them.

But nobody in the organization misunderstands Aspland's five hard rules: You don't screw with the inert gas system; you don't sail coast-wise inside the eighty-five-mile limit; you don't drink alcohol on a ship; you don't spill oil; and when you are near a port you do not wander outside the shipping lanes.

When Aspland was a toddler his dad worked for a while at a gunpowder plant near San Francisco (he quit the day before it exploded), and then opened a laundry. Needless to say, Aspland knew nothing about ships when he entered the University of California at Berkeley as a chemistry student in 1957. But every time he looks at his big toe—the one on his left foot—it reminds him why he works on tankers. He stepped on a big nail, injuring the toe, just before he entered college and joined the Naval Reserve Officers Training Corps. The toe was healed by the time he took a cadet cruise on a submarine, a trip that convinced him the silent service was his calling. His dream of sailing on submarines was delayed, however, when he flunked out of school. That is when he caught a radio ad for the California Maritime Academy in Vallejo. He had never heard of the merchant marine, but it sounded vaguely like the Navy, and it might have submarines, so he checked it out. He did better in school this time, and won an appointment to the Naval Academy at Annapolis. But to get to Annapolis he had to pass a physical exam and he was rejected when a Navy doctor decided his toe had become arthritic. Still wanting to sail on subs, he applied for a Navy commission when he graduated from the maritime academy. Once again, he had to take a physical exam, and he drew the same Navy doctor. "When I stepped up to the line, he said, 'I know you from somewhere.'" Aspland was turned down again.

So big toe and all, Aspland took a job on World War II–style tankers with an independent company. For six long years starting in 1962 he hauled diesel and gasoline up and down the West Coast, rising in rank as fast as the Coast Guard rules would allow. One day, when he was a chief mate, he stopped into the skipper's office after the captain's wife had died. The man had been laid off by the Union Oil Company just six months before he would have been eligible for a lifetime pension and now he was sitting in his office complaining bitterly about the probate papers he had to fill out following his wife's death. "I looked at him and said to myself, 'Do you really want this? Do you really want to have this situation where you have your salary and no one to enjoy it with?'"

Married by then, Aspland decided to hit the beach to be closer to his wife. "I was bored on the ships, anyway. Going to sea, to me, is truly boring."

Aspland entered California State College in Long Beach in 1968 and obtained a master's degree in business administration, a prerequisite to getting a shoreside job as high-paying as that of a ship captain. After a series of jobs with other companies, he joined Arco, rising through several positions (including manager of safety and health and operations manager) before becoming president of Arco Marine. The perks of the job have given Aspland a pretty handsome life, but if anything goes wrong he is personally and criminally liable. It's a tremendous burden and sometimes he gets scared thinking of the bad decisions his people might make. For Aspland the key to keeping oil off the rocks is not technology but the behavior of people. He bemoans the poor training people get. Only a small percentage of his company's job applicants are employable. The merchant marine licensing system hasn't change much in one hundred years and until it does, he says, the situation won't improve.

Crewmen on the *Arco Anchorage* tell me as we sail south that Aspland deserves much of the credit he gets. The last fleet death occurred in an alcohol-related shipyard accident a decade ago. Each ship has a safety committee and the captain regularly calls safety meetings where crew members are rewarded for attending with cash prizes drawn from a hat.

But every manager has his limits, and on this ship there is evidence of Aspland's blind side hanging on davits just outside the galley where Newman is finishing up his lecture on maritime history and the Marconi radio. I'm speaking of the lifeboats, of course, and so is everyone else on the ship. The type of lifeboats the *Arco Anchorage* has is a source of major concern among the crew members.

There are two lifeboats hanging on steel cables on either side of the poop deck, each one big enough, according to the sign, for forty-eight people. That should be ample for a crew of twenty-four, but crew members tell me they might as well hang Volkswagens over the side. These out-dated rescue boats have open hulls, a joke on an oceangoing oil tanker sailing on northern oceans. What they want on deck are modern lifeboats. These newer boats are totally enclosed cocoons that allow crew members, once they are inside, to eject themselves from the ship automatically. No one needs stand on the deck to let the lifeboat down, and the enclosure will protect them from cold water and fire. The record in favor of covered lifeboats is unimpeachable.

In 1977, the National Transportation Safety Board strongly recommended covered lifeboats for all oceangoing ships (larger than ten thousand tons) after investigating a 1975 tanker collision where many of the two dozen people who died perished because an open lifeboat did not adequately protect them from fire. Liberian investigators similarly determined that the only man who died after a tanker broke in half and burned in the Pacific Ocean was a victim of an open lifeboat.

The International Maritime Organization responded to these cases and others by amending a ship-safety treaty to require covered lifeboats. Unfortunately, the amendment that went into force in 1983 exempted ships built before July 1, 1986, which included the *Arco Anchorage* and hundreds of other tankers.

The *Arco Anchorage* crew members do not hide their disdain for the open lifeboats or the company decision to keep them. "Why do we need covered lifeboats?" said chief mate Svetko Lisica sarcastically. "We've got these new blankets." The blankets are the company's poor substitute for a covered lifeboat. A crewman would don the heavy, fire-resistant blanket over the survival suit that is designed to protect him from cold. Trouble is, the survival suits are already so rigid they are called "Gumby" suits, a reference to the stiff rubber cartoon character. To put a clumsy blanket over the cumbersome Gumby would be inviting disaster on a burning or foundering ship.

So I asked Vu Long, Arco's manager of port engineering, whether the *Arco Anchorage* might be fitted with covered lifeboats at its next shipyard visit. Long was surveying the ship at the time, making a shopping list for the once-every-two-year dry docking. New radars would be installed, he said, and a lot of broken equipment would be fixed. But forget the covered lifeboats—at a cost of $160,000 each, including installation, the company thinks they're too expensive.

Aspland sees no reason for them.

"I do not consider lifeboats a safety issue," Aspland said. "To me that's not safety." He said crew members have brought up the issue for years and he will not budge. Covered lifeboats will be installed on new Arco ships, as the treaty requires, but not on the old ones.

"People today would like us to rebuild the ship. When you want to provide jobs for everyone and stay in the business there are some decisions you have to make. We prefer to spend the money in maintenance so the ships won't sink."

He said a covered lifeboat is only useful if you must abandon ship. "I don't believe that in today's modern world we are going to see many abandonments."

Aspland should read the case of the U.S.-flagged tanker *Surf City,* which exploded accidentally in the Persian Gulf in February 1990. The flames incinerated the first open lifeboat before anyone could get into it. After crew members got into the second boat, the bosun had to stand on the blazing ship to lower it. It got stuck, jerked, and tossed another seaman overboard. The bosun was first seriously burned lowering the boat and then injured jumping off the ship. The man who fell out of the open lifeboat was hurt, too. And five other crew members were also burned because the escape vessel didn't protect them from flames. The NTSB report on the *Surf City* accident once again criticized tanker owners for sending ships out with open lifeboats. All tankers, regardless of construction date, should be equipped with the newer enclosed lifeboats, the report declared.

If Aspland has his limits, he isn't alone among tanker managers. Still, it seems unfortunate that an issue as basic as lifeboats would set a manager like Aspland apart from his officers and crew members. Maybe, though, to some it might not be the only issue. Chief Engineer Jim Vives told me the ship is loaded with safety equipment that is in place only because it is required. "Most of the stuff that's here is only here because it's a regulation, not because Arco cares for my health and safety."

10

The Steam Palace

*(Pacific Ocean,
200 miles west of the Queen Charlotte Islands,
January 27, 10 P.M.)*

C hief engineer Jim Vives is in charge of a subterranean sanctuary. To get to his engine room, you go through one of several doors marked with warnings about ear and eye damage. The hallway is quiet and the door is always hard to pull open, but whenever I step into the noise of the engine room from the calm of the house, I am stunned by the energy of the place. The machinery space—as it is called on the blueprints—is a ninety-foot-high cathedral of machines singing a constant chorus of industrial commotion.

Steel stairways rise in switchbacks, pausing at various platforms where an engineer might bend over a machine to adjust it. Two boilers contain arching steam pipes as magnificent as any found in a pipe organ. The walls of the engine room are also a tangle of ductwork brimming with hellishly hot steam. After it makes two passes through the inferno of the boiler, the steam becomes pure H_2O gas containing not a single water droplet. Such "dry" steam, as it is called, is invisible at 905 degrees Fahrenheit and traveling with such power, it will hit a square inch of steel with the force of a six-hundred-pound hammer. If a pipe carrying this stuff were to spring a pinhole leak, the invisible jet of superheated steam could cut a man in half and then condense into a thick cloud several feet away.

Vives keeps this hazardous place going with a team of seven and a half men—three officers and four unlicensed enginemen plus a wiper who also works part-time on deck. The engine crew seems to be more blue-collar than the deck gang, and Vives brings a tension into the place I could feel the first time I visited. Four years in the Navy right out of high school, a short stint at a shipyard, and then eighteen years with Arco have honed Vives's survival skills and made him a bit crusty. A smallish guy with dark hair who wears the same blue jeans and blue-checked shirt every working day, Vives presents a slight smirk every time I ask him a question. Sometimes he is talkative when I make an inquiry, but more often he is cryptic, or he tosses me a manual rather than an answer. But it is always a good manual with all the information I'd ever need. The engine men tell me not to take his distant and sarcastic style personally because it grates on them, too. Whenever he gets around his men they avoid him and hunker down a bit. Vives is autocratic and a little old-fashioned, like the steam engine itself.

As a steam-driven ship, the S.S. *Arco Anchorage* is one of a dying breed, sort of like the Pierce Arrow car or the nickel candy bar.

Steam ruled the oceans from the nineteenth century to the era just after World War II because the steam turbine was more powerful and reliable than the piston-driven alternative. Shortly after the war, in fact, engineers discovered that carbon and molybdenum steel was able to handle higher temperatures than regular steel; that meant they could build bigger and more powerful steam engines to drive bigger ships. This major improvement helped pave the way for super tankers.

At the same time, however, the piston engine was undergoing some advancements of its own. Diesel engine designers during the 1950s and 1960s perfected the internal combustion machine, so it was more reliable and more powerful than before. Although some feel the diesel engine will never have the torque or beauty of a steam plant, the curve of efficiency reached a point where steam no longer held a distinct power advantage. That's when diesel took over because it provided better gas mileage. When hard times hit the tanker industry in the mid-1970s, it turned to the cheaper-to-run diesel-driven ships and steam never recovered. Only the geriatric American fleet has a lot of steamships these days.

"Diesel Bill" Harrison is irritated that he works in a steam plant because, as his nickname implies, he got his early training around diesel engines. But Arco has nothing but steam-driven ships, and since he works here he is trapped in a steam palace, adjusting valves rather than pulling pistons. He knows his boilers, though. Clambering around the *Arco Anchorage* engine room with his gold earring glistening and his blue coveralls stuffed with tools, the third engineer works easily with his sidekick, engineman Neal Curtis.

Some say men go to engine rooms to hide because it is too noisy to talk. The weather is always the same—somewhere around seventy-five to eighty degrees—and the four-hour watches roll on without a sunrise or sunset to herald their passing. Only the ship's rocking hints of disturbances outside. A clock and a calendar on the wall (with dates crossed off) keep track of the duty tour. For these men, needed repairs are entertainment and a well-machined part is a piece of art. The French Foreign Legion couldn't offer more isolation.

But Curtis says he is here to learn a valuable trade, not to escape. He is an engineman with a hankering to pass the officer's test someday. The deck is a boring place to him, not enough challenge compared to all the moving parts down here. "It would take me years to learn what all those lines are," he says, pointing to the snaky decor.

The thirty-four-year-old engineman is a handsome guy with sandy hair, blue eyes, and a muscular frame. Without self-pity, he tells me the story of a middle-class upbringing that was marred by tragedy. His father worked in an Exxon refinery for some thirty-three years but quit one day when he was offered a better job with a new chemical company. Neal's brother went to work at the same plant and was burned to death in an explosion. His father took the tragedy very hard. Months later, in a funk, dad suggested the whole family take a vacation together in Jamaica. While there, Neal's father slumped over and died of a heart attack. Prior to that, Neal's dad sold his Exxon stock to buy securities in the new company, which turned out to be worthless. It meant hard times for Neal's mother and the family.

Down here in the steam palace he's doing all right. The pay is good, ranging from forty-five thousand dollars a year for an engineman up to some eighty-five thousand dollars for the chief engineer. And the goal is seemingly simple: Keep the boilers hot and the turbines spinning with the minimum use of fuel. Energy conservation is an engineer's passion, something he can judge his talents by at the end of the day. Fuel consumption, logged on a chart, will vary depending on sea conditions and the ability of the engine crew to run the plant efficiently. On an average day, the *Arco Anchorage* burns around thirty-one thousand gallons of bunker fuel. Harrison says cutting something off that number is a competition everybody gets into. "You want to use less fuel than the guys on the shift before you." He got so wrapped up in it, he would go around the house turning off unnecessary lights and other equipment to save two or three hundred gallons of bunker fuel per shift. "I just wanted to see what I could do."

Curtis admires the way a steam engine wastes nothing. The hot surge coming from the boilers drives two turbines, spins the electric generators, powers the cargo pumps, makes fresh water and—nearly exhausted—returns to preheat the water that's going back into the boiler. Everything is linked like a magnificent Rube Goldberg machine.

To see a true hell fire, one need only gaze through the thick glass porthole into the guts of a boiler. The temperature inside is nearly three thousand degrees Fahrenheit. Scores of steam pipes line the walls arching toward the narrowing top of the fire pit. The steam makes its two passes in looping pipes through this furnace before heading down a ten-inch pipe into the first turbine.

The white steel turbines, sitting side by side surrounded by a raised platform, are the muscles that drive the ship, but you can't judge these biceps by their size. The high-pressure turbine, the one that generates the most power, is much smaller than the weaker low-pressure one. The reason is the nature of steam itself—it expands as it cools. The hottest stuff enters the high-pressure turbine in a very compact nine-hundred-degree column. "It's like fifteen hurricanes inside that drum. The power in there is sensational," said second engineer Paul Hogan. By the time the steam reaches the low-pressure turbine, the temperature has dropped by more than half and it is slower, yet the volume is more than twice what it was. The bigger second turbine allows room for the expanding steam while squeezing the last ounce of power from it.

The steel casings of the turbines with all their gauges and throttle controls are what you see from the outside. Inside, steam hurls itself against whirring metal blades that are perfectly balanced because the slightest distortion could cause them to vibrate uncontrollably and to thrash the whirling dervish to pieces. Even when a turbine is shut down, a small electric motor rotates it slowly lest the blades sit too long in one place and warp.

Two drive shafts emerge from behind the high- and low-pressure turbines spinning rapidly at different speeds. Both penetrate a giant gearbox where, inside, a nest of cogs and wheels elegantly reduces the unmatched rotations into one uniform force that comes grinding out the other end to turn the propeller shaft. The shaft, a black metal pipe nearly a foot and a half in diameter, is visible at the very bottom of the engine room near the tail end of the ship. It turns at a speed less than seventy-two times a minute, quite a change from the thousands of rotations the turbines are making above it. The reduction in speed turns the energy into concentrated torque, an investment that gives the giant propeller shaft enough power to churn the ocean.

The five-bladed propeller, twenty-seven feet in diameter, is sometimes called the screw because of the way it turns through water. It pushes us ahead as much as twenty-two feet with every turn, a distance known as the "advance," which varies depending on the resistance the rolling sea puts up against the hull. The chief engineer writes reports every day on the consumption of fuel and the slip of the propeller. The slip is the difference between the distance the ship would travel in perfect conditions and the advance it is actually attaining. Heavy seas increase the slip considerably and cut down on fuel efficiency. Most engineers will skim a little fuel off their reports, although you won't find too many who will admit it. That way, they will have a little extra juice "up the sleeve"—as they call it—in case the ship runs into heavy weather and gets low on reserves. A chief engineer never knows when he might need a little "sleeve" oil in the bunker tanks somewhere.

Bunker fuel is thick and sloppy, the lowest grade of petroleum that comes out of a refinery. As such, it is cheap and it has a high ignition temperature, making it safer to use than the more volatile fuels such as gasoline. Engineers test the bunker fuel when it comes on board to determine its "flash point," or the temperature at which it becomes explosive. The testing device, which looks like an espresso machine, churns and heats the oil while an engineer lowers a small flame into the swirling soup. When the flame pops with a little explosion, the fuel has been heated to flash point. Our current load of fuel popped at 220 degrees, real junk when it comes to boiler efficiency but very safe. The best stuff has a flame temperature around 170 degrees. Anything less than 140 degrees isn't safe because it could explode when it is heated in a tank before it goes into the boiler for burning.

In some cases, ships have exploded and burned because crews used fuel with a lower than safe flash point. Foolish engineers have created extremely dangerous situations by using raw crude oil from the ship's cargo, with a flash point well below 140 degrees, because it is cheaper than refined bunker fuel. The Liberian maritime commissioner warned one Greek ship operator, Magelan Inc., to stop using crude oil as fuel after his investigators discovered illegal pipes on seven tankers linking the cargo intake to the fuel tanks in 1982. Three months after the warning was issued, one of the company's ships, the *Haralabos,* exploded and burned for seven days. Crude oil fumes had ignited in the engine room.

Fires in the engine room are common; an average of three tankers a year are destroyed or severely damaged by them and scores of crew members have been killed. Reasons for engine room fires range from the spilling of preheated bunker fuel onto a hot surface to the breaking of a high-voltage power line.

To make steam and cool hot machinery the ship sucks in seawater from outside, drawing it through a grated hole in the hull. Some salt water is routed to two evaporators where salt is removed by steam distillation to make as much as twenty gallons of pure water a minute, a liquid more pristine than anything you would drink at home. The water must be flawless because contamination would harm the boiler pipes and turbines. Meanwhile, other cold seawater is used raw—undistilled—to chill the machinery. With seawater hovering around freezing temperature in these Alaskan waters, our engines cool more easily and the ship runs more efficiently.

The engine room is also vulnerable to flooding since it sits low in the hull and, unlike the cargo tanks, it is an empty space that can easily fill with seawater. A flooded stern can sink a ship, and some tankers have foundered when the pipe drawing in seawater for cooling has broken and flooded the place. During the Iran-Iraq war of the mid-1980s, the pilots who attacked tankers in the Persian Gulf usually aimed for the engine room.

Yet with all this potential for danger, there are fewer eyes watching the ship's Achilles heel than there were in the past. There were at least three people in the engine room at all times more than a decade ago. Now, on the *Arco Anchorage,* there are two. On some ships, no one is present during the night.

Computer devices that watch over the boiler fire and throttle the turbines have made certain jobs obsolete. Tanker owners have eliminated still other jobs by abandoning seagoing maintenance and saving repairs for times when the ship is in port or in the shipyard. The result is a more ragged operation than a lot of engineers would have allowed in the old days. When Vives took me on a tour of his engine room one day, he complained about the bare-bones maintenance. "Look at that dungeon we've just come through. Officially they'll tell you it's working well. I don't believe so. We're not getting the job done."

A lot of machinery is broken or working badly on the ship right now. The *Arco Anchorage* is equipped with two huge feed pumps that supply water to the boilers—a redundancy that gives it protection against breakdown—but right now only one is working. Harrison explains that the bad one has a leak in its protective packing. "If that packing lets go, you are talking about three-hundred-degree temperature water coming out at approximately eight hundred pounds per square inch. The engine room would fill up with steam. You couldn't see anything. Try to get near it, you'd get burned. You'd never know what hit you." As things stand, if the functioning feed pump breaks down, the ship will be set adrift without power or the ability to stop unless the crew tries using the wounded pump.

In addition, as mentioned before, the steam-driven pump that drives the fire-fighting equipment has been diverted to run machinery that scrubs the inert gas that goes into the cargo tanks.

There are other problems as well. The engineers are having trouble controlling the temperature in one of the ship's two boilers, which means that top power is unattainable. Harrison also shows me a tin temperature gauge, like one you would use for cooking, duct-taped to the outside of one of the electrical generators. This cheap gauge is replacing a broken thermometer designed to protect the generator against overheating. "This is a million dollars' worth of equipment and they give me a fifty-nine-cent thermometer from a drugstore."

Tanker operators point with pride to the duplicate safety equipment on a ship like this. There are double radars, twin steering systems, and dual boilers. If something breaks, there is always a backup to take its place. But there is only one operating propeller and one rudder, a fact of life on most tankers around the world. If the *Arco Anchorage* should lose its propeller, there is a spare bolted to the deck. It could be lowered into place by a crane, but that is a dockside operation more likely be done at a shipyard. Out here it seems that carrying a spare propeller is more traditional than practical. Some cargo ships, passenger vessels, and most warships have dual operating propellers and rudders, and a few critics have urged the Coast Guard to require them on tankers, too. But the idea has not been taken seriously by owners who argue that double propellers waste fuel. While it is true that a single large propeller has proportionately more bite, and is more efficient than two smaller ones, it is equally true that double screws, accompanied by twin rudders, give a ship more maneuverability and allow for a backup in case one system fails.

Most steam tankers, including this one, have double boilers, but in an experiment some naval engineers labeled as irresponsible, the Coast Guard approved the construction of ten tankers and seven other large steamships equipped with only one boiler and no backup. An agency official said American shipyards and shipowners requested the deal in the late 1960s so they could save money in the face of "severe economic and labor pressures," and foreign competition. Always mindful of the shipowners' bottom line, the Coast Guard went along with the idea, saying in one report that the single boiler seemed like a natural development, given the advent of other cost-saving measures like automation and the reduction of crew sizes. "With the rapid escalation of capital and operational costs, the marine industry must maintain the flexibility to be innovative," a 1977 Coast Guard report said. "Therefore, to unnecessarily encumber or prohibit this promising concept would be a tragic mistake."

A number of officers told me the tragic mistake was the Coast Guard's decision to go along with this idea. They say single boilers make no sense, especially at a time when crews are being cut back in favor of computers. Several chief engineers have stated that they would never sail on a ship that had only one boiler. On average, a large vessel can expect to suffer one major mechanical failure each year, and on steamships that problem often involves a malfunctioning boiler. If there is no backup, the ship is vulnerable to drifting onto the rocks. Three single-boiler Exxon ships lost power in Washington state waters in the late 1980s. They didn't go aground, but they did prompt the Coast Guard admiral in charge of the Seattle office to ban them from Puget Sound waters for a while. At the very same time, though, another Coast Guard office was considering reducing the engine-room manpower on those same ships.

When a ship loses power, it lacks not only propulsion but also the ability to steer and stop. When heavy seas broke pipes on the deck of the ninety-thousand-ton Liberian tanker *Braer* north of Scotland in January 1993, seawater entered the fuel tanks and contaminated them. When the boilers and emergency generators failed, probably because of the watered fuel, the tanker became a limp rag that was slammed against the rocks of the Shetland Islands in a storm so violent, it blew oil across the surrounding landscape. The tanker broke up and spilled its entire twenty-five-million-gallon cargo of crude.

If the boiler and emergency generator go lifeless, so does everything else on a ship—lights, power, radars, and radios. The chief engineer on the American tanker *Ocean Wizard* must have felt starcrossed during a 1988 transit from Portland, Oregon, to the Persian Gulf when the starboard boiler failed one day and the other one fizzled the next. The emergency generator was supposed to kick in automatically, but it didn't because it was set for manual operation. When the crew got it started, it died because the diesel engine choked on its own exhaust fumes. So there they sat in a dead and dark ship on the wide-open ocean. It could have been worse had it happened in tight quarters like the Columbia River where the voyage began.

Despite all the muscle down here in the engine room, tankers are notoriously underpowered, considering the tremendous weight they haul. An oceanographic commission in Washington state recommended two decades ago that ships like the *Arco Anchorage* have twice the horsepower they now have so they could stop quickly in an emergency. While there have been proposals to fit tankers with drag parachutes and retro-rockets, presently the fastest way to stop a tanker is to perform a Williamson turn. When a tanker doesn't have room in tight quarters for such a wide maneuver, the captain might perform a "crash stop" in which the engine is slammed into reverse and the rudder is wagged back and forth to create a drag. Such an emergency stop leaves the ship uncontrollable.

Throwing the engine into reverse also puts a tremendous strain on the boilers. The low-pressure turbine is the only one geared to drive the ship backward and it needs a lot of steam in a hurry to reverse the vessel with any authority. The turbine's "astern" element, as it is called, needs half again as much steam as the forward element to produce just two-thirds as much horsepower. Straining to make a crash stop, a boiler is more likely to fail than at any other time.

Even when the tanker is doing routine maneuvers, the boilers strain a bit. One time I witnessed thick black smoke gushing from the stack. Immediately the engineers scrambled to adjust the controls. They are sensitive about exhaust because air quality regulations from Alaska to California ban such outbursts. "One puff and they are all over us," said Hogan. To control the smoke, the company has installed a video camera on top of the stack and a periscope that watches it with mirrors so engineers can see how much soot the ship is disgorging. When the ship is maneuvering during an exit from harbor, the engineers keep a sharp eye on the periscope, making subtle adjustments to the fuel and oxygen mixture so they can avoid air pollution. I was impressed by the way they scrambled whenever they noticed smoke. The ship also carries two kinds of fuel: The cheaper fuel with a lot of polluting sulfur is used for ocean steaming while the cleaner one is used in ports where sulfur emissions are banned.

From inside, the engine room is an impressive place. Standing at the control panel where all the gauges and dials are located, my eye wanders around a mechanical showplace as large as the inside of a warehouse. From the bottom to the top there are seven levels called "flats". They aren't like floors in a traditional building, just steel platforms and balconies set up here and there for access to this or that piece of equipment. The boilers—sitting one deck above the turbines—loom above everything near the stern of the engine room. They reach as tall as a three-story building and have a shiny silver face like some sort of prop from *The Wizard of Oz*. Behind them—at the very end of the ship—is the steering gear room. Inside, two hydraulically driven pistons move horizontally, pushing the rudder back and forth on commands from the bridge. There are two steering gears, in case one fails.

Up another deck is a marvelous machine shop with every kind of drill and lathe a machinist would need to sculpt metal. If they had time, the engineers could reproduce just about any small part that's used on the ship.

But the heart of the engine room is the control panel glistening with old-fashioned gauges, levers, and wheels. Arrows rise and fall to indicate the pressure and heat of the steam throughout the plant. Numbers show the temperature of the fire in the boiler, the fuel in the tanks, and the seawater outside. An intercom delivers commands from the bridge: "Half ahead, full ahead," etc. A dial on the engine room panel reflects whatever adjustments the mate has made with the throttle control at the helm. An engineer keeps watch over the panel, standing near a desk cluttered with the night's necessities: a logbook, a flashlight, a wrench, a pack of Winstons, and an ashtray full of butts. Nearby is a pair of asbestos gloves, protection against the numerous metal surfaces hot enough to incinerate a hand.

To the left is an electrical switchboard big enough to supply a small village with power. The wiring behind the board is out in the open so it can be fiddled with on a moment's notice. Harrison says the 440 volts and 2,000 amps surging through the lines are enough to give anyone the willies. "I go back there to change the lightbulbs and I don't think about it. I just hope I don't touch anything."

The way Vives sees it, the *Arco Anchorage* is a relic for the museums with all its pneumatic controls and other anachronisms. "Turn of the century, the whole thing."

But there is a lot to admire down here, a lot that hasn't been taken over by computers. Once an engineer gets to know a plant like this, the practice of making it run properly can be as subtle as the challenges of a race car. The amount of oxygen being sucked into the boilers can be compared with the efficiency of the steam. An engineman can glance at the panel and see how much bunker fuel, lube oil, hot water, and electricity we are using. At a glance he can even see how many millions of times the propeller has turned since the last time the gauge was set. It's all in the dials.

I worked at a failing newspaper once where the presses were dinosaurs. The key to getting the paper printed every day was a group of pressmen, as old as the machines themselves, who knew exactly where to put the bubble gum to hold everything together. That's the way it is on an old ship. The engineers and enginemen must know the desires of the machine, and they've got to care about it, to love it, to keep it running well. On this *Arco Anchorage* voyage the human element is a little out of whack, like the feed pump. The crew doesn't get along with the engine room boss.

I noticed a difference with Vives right away. When I walked by his office he'd be sitting at his desk doing paperwork. He was rarely in the engine room the way the other chief engineer was when I last rode this ship.

Later, I asked engine room crew members about this and—to a man—they complained that he didn't get involved enough in the day-to-day operation. They are particularly vociferous during this trip because they are shorthanded and need his help. With the first engineer out sick, Hogan and Harrison are trading off six-hour shifts and getting little rest. Crew members have nicknamed the chief Bullwinkle, after a silly cartoon character, and they are very derisive about the fact he doesn't pitch in to take a shift. "The policy of this company is that, while maneuvering, the chief engineer will be in the engine room," said one. "He'll come down twenty minutes, then he'll be gone for three hours."

"I don't work for him. I work for the ship. I just go around him."

With every turn of the propeller on our southbound trip, the mood seems to worsen. A couple of times when Vives wanders through the engine room, his underlings turn to me afterward and make sarcastic comments. They can't seem to decide what bothers them more, his absence or his presence.

Carroll is aware of the dissension, since engine crew members have asked the skipper to intervene. One is even talking about taking the complaint to headquarters. As far as the captain is concerned, the engine room grumbling is one of the biggest problems he faces on the ship. The vessel already has maintenance troubles, he doesn't need a personnel problem with the people who do the repairs. But the skipper is considering the situation with a measured attitude. He says the chief engineer is not making him happy, but it may be simplistic to put all the blame on him. Right now Carroll is trying to nudge the chief engineer toward reconciliation, but he doesn't want to undermine his authority. When Vives gets his annual evaluation, he will learn what Carroll has decided about the dispute.

As for Vives, he is not going to change his ways because a subordinate complains. A pugnacious forty-four-year-old who hails from Philadelphia, Vives has been around the sea long enough to know how the hierarchy works. Vives worked his way up through the ranks from the lowly position of wiper to chief engineer. On the way, he may have lost his desire for hands-on work, but he has never lost his cynical eye or his knowledge of the machine for which he is responsible. He is an unblinking witness to the complacency that has eroded public faith in the tanker industry. He won't discuss his management methods but he pulls no punches when he talks about industry attitudes. He volunteers how, in the past, ships like the *Arco Anchorage* were required to visit the shipyard once a year. Now the Coast Guard says they must go once every two years and if it wasn't required that often, the ship probably wouldn't go. You can't blame that on the chief engineer. Vives says when the industry talks about regulations, it is, "How can we circumvent them to meet our needs?"

"You can't rely on the corporation."

Theoretically, then, we are to rely on the Coast Guard.

11

The Thin Blue Line

(Pacific Ocean,
140 miles west of Vancouver Island,
January 28, noon)

We are in a fog, a vapor so thick I can barely make out the bow of the ship. The water, the steel deck, and the mist fade together in shades of gray as though we are a scene from a black-and-white movie. Somewhere left of us is the northern tip of Vancouver Island, a 280-mile-long wonderland that is wild in parts, heavily logged in others, and very English at the southern tip, where the streets of Victoria clatter with tourist-bearing horse carriages.

We have been sailing off Alaska and British Columbia for nearly three days now, passing, but never seeing, the wildest coastlines in North America. Last night, we dropped south of the richly forested Queen Charlotte Islands, where some of the native people still make their living by cutting trees and netting salmon. Every additional mile the vessel travels, it passes some of the world's richest fishing grounds, not to mention the habitats of whales, otters, sea lions, and eagles.

The Alaskan oil we are carrying has been cooling rapidly as it sloshes around inside the ship's thirteen cargo tanks. The thin hull provides no insulation against the freezing water, so the tepid crude oil is slowly turning cold. Oil actually becomes more destructive when it is cooler. If it spills in a warm ocean, some will dissipate into the air by evaporation. But if it gushes into a cold sea, more will stay on the surface to hit the beaches.

You can't win with oil—it is more explosive when it is warm but more persistent when it is cold.

The ship is bending and moaning, as it has done since it left Hinchinbrook. Although the wind has died down, the seas continue to pound and pitch with a momentum of their own. Every mile of this endless storm we leave behind is a relief.

I sense that the sea is grinding down the crew as thoroughly as it is battering the ship. The chief mate's greenish brown sweater is creased and tattered in its second week of wearing. The chief engineer's blue-checked shirt looks more like an old dishrag. The captain keeps changing his clothes every day, but the spiffy bright colors don't hide the pallor that has crossed his face like the fog that now shrouds the ship.

Down in the galley, volleys of temper are being served up with lunch. The chief steward snaps angrily at the cook when a batch of cookies slumps into a gooey mess on the baking sheet. The baker waves his spatula in the air and whines about the recipe. In the crew mess hall, a seaman's fist gavels the table, rattling some silverware and nerves. By the time I reach the scene, the argument is over. It had something to do with the union again.

Neal Curtis says everybody needs a rest, but "sleep is sure a luxury."

In the officer's mess, Carroll and Lisica are slumped over a couple of plates discussing the day's workload. Some cryptic exchanges between them lead me to believe something is wrong. "Naw," says Carroll. "We're discussing hours. What else?" A couple of crew members—Schramm included—don't work overtime, as is their right under the current contract. Carroll and Lisica must make adjustments around them, an added challenge in these days when no one is supposed to work over the twelve-hour limit. Vives, absorbed in paperwork at the next table, is lucky he doesn't have engine room workers who decline overtime. The ship has trouble enough as it is.

According to the original plan, the *Arco Anchorage* was supposed to be in the Portland shipyard for a dry docking and inspection this month. But as things happen, another company ship has taken its reservation. The dry dock—one of the largest on the West Coast—won't be available for this ship again for another six months.

Back in their offices, Carroll and Vives are keeping lists of broken equipment overdue for repair. Much of the work is too difficult for an overtaxed crew to complete at sea, and some equipment, like the crippled winch on the foc's'le head, need attention right away. A shore contractor has been hired to tackle the job when the ship reaches port. Other repairs have been put off until the tanker gets to the shipyard. Everyone figured it wasn't worth the trouble to patch something now that will be refurbished at the yard. Of course, hanging on for six months will wear down some fingernails.

The company can legally delay the ship's overhaul, but the old hulk's problems just get worse. The girders may be thicker than the ones on a younger ship, but after two decades of pounding this old tanker isn't the vessel it used to be. Every time I walk the deck I see different signs of wear. I noticed this morning that a crane located behind the house was lashed against its moorings with all its wiring ripped out. The captain says the boom hasn't worked properly for over two years. He also told me about the leaky inert gas system. When we crawled into the inert-gas scrubbing tower, a large structure behind the house, fumes stung at our throats. Some crew members already inside were wearing masks as they tried to patch the holes.

The regulators do not care about ancillary equipment like a broken cargo boom when there is so much else to worry about, like a leaky inert gas system or a broken feed pump. As we near the U.S. border, we are reentering the jurisdiction of the U.S. Coast Guard, the federal agency most responsible for assuring that this vessel comes and goes without spilling oil on pristine American beaches. The Coast Guard approved the ship's design before it was built and it boards the vessel annually to see whether it is in acceptable condition. When the tanker is lifted into dry dock this summer, the Coast Guard will be the one to certify if it is fit to return to duty. If we break in a storm, the Coast Guard will be asked to rescue us. If we violate the law, an agency cutter will be the only boat authorized to pull us over. Coast Guard radars will monitor our movements as we sail into port. If we spill oil, the Coast Guard must start the cleanup and oversee its completion. Afterward, the agency will investigate the accident and, if it finds that anyone violated the law, it will prosecute the case. A Coast Guard administrative law judge will hear the evidence and pass judgment. The first line of appeal for a convicted violator will be to the Coast Guard commandant. The Coast Guard writes the rules that govern how this ship operates and passes judgment on any changes. It decides the minimum number of crew members, lifeboats, life jackets, radios, survival suits, and practically everything else that affects safety or navigation.

But the agency is not as powerful as its long list of duties would imply. Having power and wielding it are too different things. I ask Carroll at lunch what he thinks of the "Coasties" and he chuckles softly. "They try hard." The same question posed two years earlier to Robert Lawlor, the other skipper, brought a stiffer reply. "They know nothing about these ships." The Coasties come on board in port sometimes to check paperwork and they will crawl around inside the guts of the tanker when it enters dry dock for an overhaul. But there are green Coast Guard inspectors who ask laughable questions and most have never worked on a tanker, or any other kind of cargo ship. If you are an environmentalist, you worry whether they will give the ships the necessary scrutiny. If you are a tanker crewman, you worry about wasting time answering superfluous questions.

With less than forty-four thousand uniformed and civilian members, the Coast Guard is the smallest military organization in America and in some ways the most overworked. Battered by budget cuts and hamstrung by its own traditions, the agency has two flaws: a military set-up that is inappropriate to duties like ship inspections; and too many tasks with too few people to do them.

Some say that asking a military-style organization like the Coast Guard to inspect the *Arco Anchorage* and other ships is like asking Army tank commanders to oversee the nation's trucking industry. Ship inspectors in Europe are retired ship captains and chief engineers who have years of experience on the vessels they scrutinize and who stay on the inspection job for years. In the United States, however, inspectors are mostly career Coast Guard officers making a stop-off in a busy career. Also hindering a dedicated cadre is the fact that the Coast Guard, like other military services, requires officers and enlisted persons to change jobs every three years. That's fine for the interchangeable world of soldiering, but it creates havoc in a regulatory outfit where experience and continuity matter.

The Federal Aviation Administration permits its civilian examiners time to learn a job in one place. Experts say it takes three years to train a person to examine ships, and by that time Coast Guard inspectors have moved on to another job. More than two-thirds of all Coast Guard inspectors have less than five years' total experience, and that includes the two-year time period they spent in training. Almost none have any background in the merchant marine, so they must learn from scratch.

The job shuffling also affects institutional memory. Most regulatory agencies rely on veteran observers to track evolving hazards and to learn from past mistakes. But it is not unusual when dealing with the Coast Guard to call an office you are familiar with and encounter new troops who know nothing about what happened a year ago.

Officially, Coast Guard officers say the rotating is necessary to assure that officers are trained as generalists, since a small organization can't afford specialists. Informally, they'll tell you a more important reason is advancement and survival. A Coast Guard rule says any officer who is passed over for promotion must retire after a certain period of time. If jobs aren't rotated every three years, there won't be any openings to advance into.

The "up and out" system is so tough that most people are pushed out within twenty years. With fewer and fewer upper-level slots, officers know there are advantages to "staying friendly" with the industry. After all, those who face early retirement will need jobs on the outside and the best place to get them is in the maritime trade.

The agency even encourages this friendliness with a program, more than forty years old, where high-ranking Coast Guard officers take a year off to work in executive slots at companies like Texaco and Exxon. The goal is admirable—better communication—but in an agency where high-ranking officers are thinking about future employment with the people they regulate, this hand-holding raises questions about objectivity.

The exodus from the Coast Guard to industry is constant. In the

Seattle office, for instance, I interviewed a captain in charge of inspections one day regarding tanker and barge safety. Months later, I called back and discovered the same fellow had retired and gone to work for a tug and barge company he once regulated. Another commander I'd talked to about spill cleanup was later working for another barge company. The admiral who once commanded the Coast Guard's West Coast operation went to work for an industry-funded cleanup company. Nowhere in the hierarchy does anyone seem anxious to stop this trend.

Nearly every Coast Guard officer I ever met shows endless tolerance for more work with less pay. How can one question the commitment of an oil-spill boss who stays on the job around the clock, or the bravery of a helicopter jockey who touches down on a rocking tanker deck in a Pacific storm? The issue in the Coast Guard is not dishonesty or sloth, says former White House official Ed Wenk, but organizational culture. "The Coast Guard leadership loves the white-hat image they get for search-and-rescue. They hate to regulate, they hate slapping people's wrists. Until they grow up and accept that regulatory role, which is required by law and the oath of office, they will bend to budget and industry pressure."

The Coast Guard itself acknowledged as much in an internal report where the tendency to "facilitate commerce" at the expense of safety was heavily criticized.

Some say the Coast Guard ought to be split into two parts. One would be a military-style organization that would run the cutter force that rescues people, stops drug smugglers, and halts fish poachers. The other would be a civilian bureaucracy that would inspect ships and investigate accidents.

There, of course, would be the possibility of corruption among inspectors who stay in place too long. Prior to World War II, when the Coast Guard took over inspections, a civilian agency known as the Bureau of Marine Inspection and Navigation did the job and had a reputation for dishonesty—a bottle of liquor or something more in the briefcase would help smooth the way for a successful inspection. Nevertheless, the advantage of splitting the agency would be a clear delineation of jobs and perhaps more resources. As a dumping ground for maritime duties, the Coast Guard, during the 1970s and 1980s, was given more than a dozen new tasks without additional funds to pay for new people. "Doing more with less" is an unofficial motto.

Coast Guard leaders tend to raise their hands whenever a job needs doing. The motive is survival. Ever since the underpaid Coast Guard began life in 1790 as the Revenue-Cutter Service—a maritime tax collector—it has had to fight efforts to dismantle it. Federal power brokers tried to break up the outfit by dispensing its duties to other bureaucracies, including a major effort just before Congress created the modern Coast Guard, name and all, in 1915. The outfit has been able to stave off these efforts by claiming more duties (lighthouse keeping, ice breaking, inspections, etc.). In the federal family the Coast Guard is a runt who must constantly prove himself.

In 1970, spurred by the 1967 *Torrey Canyon* spill in England, Congress passed environmental legislation that gave the Coast Guard the duty to protect American shores from oil spills. Tankers were to be inspected for pollution safety and, when a spill occurred, the Coast Guard was to assure a thorough cleanup. The *Arco Anchorage* was under construction at the time, and between the day the ship's keel was laid and the day it was launched, Coast Guard tanker operations were radically turned from examining lifeboats and engine repairs to concentrating on tanks and cargo systems.

The change in the Coast Guard's attention was accompanied by a growth in its bureaucracy. In 1940, almost half the officers were aboard seagoing cutters rescuing people and fixing navigation buoys. Forty years later, eight out of ten were working at shoreside desks.

A series of tanker disasters in the late 1970s—namely, the *Argo Merchant* spill near Nantucket Island followed by a dozen more in three months—prompted the Coast Guard to add 169 inspectors. Some in the Coast Guard felt additional inspectors were not needed because the shrinking American merchant marine provided fewer U.S.-flagged ships to inspect. But others pointed out that with a deep recession in the industry, owners were more likely to use aging tankers without proper maintenance. Also, more inspectors were needed to handle increasing numbers of foreign tankers arriving at U.S. shores.

In 1979, Coast Guard Commandant John Hayes predicted his

agency would need twice its 45,800-person workforce by 1991 to keep up with the tasks. The General Accounting Office and a House committee agreed that the Coast Guard was in tatters. Both noted the agency was dangerously undermanned; this left the organization unable to do such things as review crew standards on foreign ships because no one had time to translate or analyze the information sent by other countries.

During the Reagan years the agency was forced to trim away 102 of the inspectors, and by 1991 the Coast Guard had fewer people than it did back when Hayes predicted it needed more. Over the decade, the agency saw the portion of its budget dedicated to ship safety reduced by more than 25 percent while resources used to chase drug runners nearly doubled.

The government should have foreseen the outcome of the cuts. An early warning sign was the sinking of an old U.S. freighter named the *Poet* and the loss of thirty-four crew members including the son of a former high-ranking Coast Guard inspector. Congressional investigators concluded the Coast Guard's superficial examination was partly responsible for the disaster. In February 1983, the *Marine Electric,* a 605-foot-long bulk carrier, broke and sank in an Atlantic storm carrying a load of pulverized coal. The National Transportation Safety Board found that the Coast Guard and the American Bureau of Shipping had failed to detect crucial corrosion problems. But some in the Coast Guard didn't want to hear this. Retired Coast Guard Captain Dominic Calicchio, one of three officers appointed to conduct the Coast Guard investigation, says his superiors asked him to remove comments from his report criticizing Coast Guard and ABS inspections. Fortunately, he declined to pull his punches.

Retired Coast Guard Captain Rene Roussel, former head of marine safety in Seattle, says inspectors saw their job as a dead-end assignment and they wanted out as soon as possible. "There were guys saying, my God, what have I done? I've given up my career." It got so bad Roussel says the Coast Guard academy wouldn't allow inspection department recruiters to talk to students on campus. Turnover was so extreme among inspectors that, the year prior to the *Exxon Valdez* accident, the Coast Guard planned to graduate thirty-nine officers from its inspection training program but only seventeen of them stuck it out to the end. At one time, the inspection department was missing half of its required personnel.

To understand how this affects inspections on a ship like the *Arco Anchorage,* I visited a shipyard in Portland, Oregon, home of the largest dry dock on the West Coast, when our sister ship the *Arco Fairbanks* came in for an overhaul. When the empty tanker arrived— weighing one-fifth of what we do today as we roll in waves—the shipyard bay was lowered into the river to allow the vessel in, and then was raised with the ship in its grip. Supported on two hundred blocks like a beached whale, the hull emerged with few barnacles attached because the Alaskan water is too cold for them.

Everything was opened up inside, not so much for the inspectors but for hundreds of workmen who swarmed over the place to revamp the equipment with the help of the crew. The *Fairbanks* skipper said his crew, which stays on the ship, hates the loss of privacy. "We don't usually lock our doors out at sea, but you've got to here." Also the ship, so tidy at sea, got filthy as the turbines and boilers and generators and pumps were disassembled.

I clambered into a center cargo tank to get a mole's-eye view of the task facing an inspector, something I'd been unable to do on this trip because of all the seawater washing over the deck. A simple hatchway through the main deck led to a ladder, sixty-eight rungs to the bottom. Feeling as though I had entered a gymnasium through a skylight in the roof, I noticed there were no smooth walls in there, but abundant rafters, floor joists, and beams that are all exposed. In the dark at the bottom, I tightroped across a gloomy manmade cavern on the back of a knee-high steel beam—one of many ribs holding the ship's spine together. The hole I had entered was now seven stories above me, a patch of light in the heavens, like a hole sawed through the surface of a frozen lake. The floor under my feet was laced by longitudinal beams three feet apart, each one identical to the one I was standing on. They extended the entire length of the ship, but I could see only as far as the next bulkhead. Deep I-beams coursed up the walls and arched over the ceiling. These stiffeners look like the dividing walls inside a car battery when they are represented on a drawing.

The space I was standing in was ninety feet long and forty feet wide, but it was only half of the tank the inspector would examine. The other half was obscured by a massive wall dividing the tank lengthwise. The big bulkhead has holes in it so oil can circulate among both halves of the tank, but is solid enough to stop oil from sloshing on a rocking ship. Without this baffle, the crude could roll in waves with enough force to break out a bulkhead or make the ship unstable.

A good inspector knows where the weak points are in this huge place, but looking for cracks in here is like searching for a pencil mark on the wall of an unlit cathedral. Even with the help of a flashlight, there are thousands of crevasses to consider. By one industry estimate, an inspector who tackles a super tanker will be eyeballing seventy-four acres of steel and considering eighty-five thousand pits as well as thousands of cracks to sort out the real problems from superficial ones. He must also look for trouble spots in 750 miles of welds—enough to stretch from Seattle to San Francisco—and climb around thirty-five thousand feet of ladders.

Crawling on hands and knees with a ballpeen hammer, the inspector taps the steel and listens for a healthy ring or a sick thud. If some area seems suspicious, he can bring in more sophisticated X-ray equipment to check it over. Sometimes, a lot of steel must be removed and replaced on an aging ship.

The upper reaches of a tank are especially difficult. They can be inspected two ways: by building expensive scaffolding or by inflating a raft inside the tank and slowly filling it with water, which is risky since the inspectors can get trapped between rafters at the top. No wonder tops are the least-examined portion. Actually, by some estimates, no more than 20 percent of the steel on a tanker gets checked at any dry docking. A truly thorough job would take one thousand hours of work, but the Coast Guard gives it around eighty hours. Often the companies make the job more difficult for inspectors by bringing in ships that have wax and oil all over the tanks, but Arco ships arrive in the Portland shipyard well cleaned and ready for inspection because it is a firm corporate policy.

If oil tankers were all the inspectors had to worry about, it would make the job easier. But scrambling around the shipyard on bicycles, they must also contend with container ships, chemical carriers, off-shore barges, offshore oil rigs, passenger vessels, and other marine machines. By one government estimate, the Coast Guard's staff of around 250 inspectors is responsible for thirty-six thousand vessels. When I visited the shipyard in 1989 I found a staff of three inspectors who had just survived a visit by ten tankers, a cargo ship, and a barge—all at once.

The Coast Guard is also expected, once a year, to inspect every foreign-flagged tanker that enters U.S. waters. The short examination, which averages thirteen man-hours, focuses on the ship's documents, since there is usually no time to thoroughly examine the hull. In September 1990, two Coast Guard petty officers overlooked the small foreign-flagged *Contessa*'s crumbling, rusted deck and declared everything in order after a thirty-minute inspection of the ship's papers. Three weeks later off the coast of Oregon the corroded *Contessa* was forced to jettison eighty-one thousand gallons of its diesel fuel cargo after springing a leak and swamping in seas not much rougher than the ones we are rolling in today. When the nearly sunken hulk was towed to port, inspectors found a deck so wasted they could practically put their fist through it.

The assumption is that the country where the ship is registered will do a more complete inspection job. However, many places, like the small Caribbean nation of St. Vincent, which registered the *Contessa,* have no Coast Guard and instead rely on industry-financed classification societies, the equivalent of a city turning over building inspection to a nonprofit organization financed by general contractors.

Since there are no international licenses or standards, the quality of classification society and Coast Guard inspectors varies. Some societies like the American Bureau of Shipping use full-time employees, but others employ freelancers who could be either experienced mariners or out-of-work real estate salesmen.

The same is true of marine accident investigators, whose work is as vital as inspectors' because they uncover the destructive lessons of history. But an international dearth of qualified maritime forensics has all too often left the industry no more informed or wiser after a mishap than it was before. Dick Tracy never left the beach, for instance, when the Norwegians botched their investigation of the June 1990 fire aboard the tanker *Mega Borg,* a highly publicized accident that killed four crew members and spilled four million gallons of crude oil into the Gulf of Mexico. The Norwegian investigators couldn't identify the exact cause because bad weather and a lack of ventilation hampered their examination of the hull's interior, so back on shore they leafed through the scant data they had and made an educated guess. Then they quietly allowed the owner to tow the ship to Pakistan for scrap, the equivalent of the police letting a motorist haul his car away from a fatal accident scene before the investigation is done. When the Norwegians had second thoughts, they sent a Pakistani surveyor to examine the ship but by then it was too late; the vessel had been cut to pieces on a beach fifty miles from Karachi.

Closer to home, an ex–Coast Guard investigator, Gregory Tompkins, told me he quit his job after four years because he realized how poorly trained and incompetent he was. The forty-two-year-old college graduate, a civilian, had been happy during the twelve years he worked in a Coast Guard office registering ships, before the service made him an investigator during a reshuffling of jobs at the Seattle base. He attended a three-week class at Yorktown and was supposedly ready to go. But in November 1989 he was investigating a fatal collision between a freighter and a fishing boat when he realized he didn't know what to ask of the witnesses. " 'Geez, you guys hit this boat. What happened?' I didn't have any real navigational expertise to draw on."

Some people are trying to improve the low standards in the maritime industry in the wake of recent tanker accidents like the *Exxon Valdez* in Alaska, *Mega Borg* in Texas, *Aegean Sea* in Spain, *Braer* in the Shetland Islands, and *Maersk Navigator* in the Malacca Strait.

The Nautical Institute of London—a six-thousand-member organization that promotes ethics and professionalism—recently set up an anonymous reporting bureau known as the Marine Accident Reporting Scheme (MARS) for sailors who would like to blow the whistle on safety problems. Modeled after an aviation program, it allows crew members who spot trouble to report what they see without retaliation. Their anecdotes, with the names of ships removed, are published in a Nautical Institute magazine so others can learn from them.

Maritime investigators are also taking tentative steps toward worldwide coordination. In 1992, they formed an organization known as the International Marine Accident Investigators Forum. Canadian investigator Brian Thorne said friends in the aviation world were shocked they had never done this before.

Meanwhile, on the inspector front, the Coast Guard is adding 120 examiners. And Coast Guard headquarters has established a SWAT team of highly trained "traveling inspectors" who can fly at short notice to any site where a tough inspection problem arises, like suspicious cracks in a hull. Inspectors are also taking more frequent rides on merchant ships to see how they operate.

Problems, however, continue to haunt the inspector corps. The training program is still not turning out enough graduates to fill the open slots, and the three-year job rotating system continues to take its toll. Roussel, the retired marine safety captain from Seattle, predicts the corps will end up in the same condition it was in a few years ago. Like the post–*Torrey Canyon* era, the next few years will bring new tasks and not enough resources or personnel to handle them. "They'll be thin again. Actually they are thin right now. It's just that they are so happy to have new bodies."

Meanwhile, as specks of sunlight break through the fog, Carroll stays in his office on the *Arco Anchorage* and types a computer list of maintenance troubles, which he will send to headquarters at the end of his tour. Probably the most thorough and important inspection a ship gets is the one done constantly by the crew. Trouble is, some captains and engineers hedge on their problems, not putting them on paper, as if a broken temperature gauge is a personal failure. Carroll says if he doesn't identify the ship's problems, they won't get fixed and he'll wallow in them. No regulator is going to help if he doesn't help himself, not in this system anyway.

An Arco headquarters engineer told me that while he cooperates with Coast Guard inspectors, he would consider it a personal failure if a Coast Guard officer found something Arco didn't already know about, like a Boy Scout showing a soldier how to fight. Trouble is, that is not the attitude on all the fleets around the world. And there are a lot of nooks and crannies that can hide trouble on a ship like this.

12

Nooks and Crannies

*(Pacific Ocean,
120 miles west of Vancouver Island,
January 28, 3 P.M.)*

The afternoon sea releases its grip on the main deck and the fog has lifted. No spray crosses the railings and the rollers that pounded our ship for a thousand miles are a polite ripple, as though the angry ocean saw civilization coming, straightened its tie, and started acting like a lake.

The pipes and railings that were surrounded by water a few hours ago are now drying in the sun, so Captain Carroll releases us to the out-of-doors. No one will drown in these conditions, but no one will relax, either. Work crews wander from the house to the main deck like paroled sinners, everyone with a list of chores to do. The sunshine is welcome, but a cold breeze convinces me to tuck my face deeper into my zipped-up collar. The raw weather and threat of another storm permit only short bursts of tinkering, so anyone who isn't asleep or working inside is mustered to the deck where the railings, pipes, and winches crave attention. Newman, a bucket of paint in one hand, shades his eyes against the rare sunshine and studies the gray steel for patches of rust. "All this fun, plus six bucks an hour." Third mate Dean Davis, a bucket of tools in one hand, saunters up to a rusty-looking mechanism on the right side of the deck and starts disassembling it. He is after a broken cargo-tank dipstick that has been measuring oil with a mind of its own.

Eric Nalder

The deck looks much like it did before it faded underwater a few days ago. I check for debris, since a crewman told me he once found a shark slapped against a breakwater after a storm, but I find none, and like the crew, I have things to do. I've got an appointment with pump-man Daryl Akery for a tour of his hidden domain, the pump room. Akery's job, as we near Washington state, is to assure that everything in the pump room is safe and in good working order for our discharge at the refinery. We won't off-load for a couple of days, but the tedious process starts now.

A pumpman is a well-trained deckhand responsible for the plumbing that moves the crude oil around, and for the winches that haul in the cables. Anything that breaks on deck and down in the tanks is his to worry about. "We are the fix-it men on the ship." Akery just joined the ship in Valdez and is new to the job. He is a replacement for the other pumpman, Dennis Meehan, an introverted but well-liked worka-holic who departs for vacation as soon as we reach Cherry Point. Meehan is a valued crew member, but he has avoided me most of the trip, and his shyness has become a fulcrum for joshing. The captain and the chief mate sent down an order one day instructing him to speak to me. He complained so vociferously the pranksters started giggling before they admitted it was a gag. In contrast to Meehan, Akery is a jocular good old boy from a small town in the center of Missouri not far from the Ozark Mountains. A friend of Meehan's, Akery tests you with a cocky manner at first but when the banter simmers down you are a warm handshake away from a friendly midwestern conversation. He was a wild man in his day, in fact he had a two-county reputation, but a two-year marriage and a nineteen-month-old daughter have given him something to yearn for. Now, after six years with the company, it is a struggle for the thirty-two-year-old man to go to sea. "I'm just starting to realize it's hard being away from home."

Akery has a pumpman's personality: before he feels right, his callused hands need a tool to grip and a broken gadget to repair. He was an able-bodied seaman before, but did not like standing bridge watch or steering the ship. "You've got a tanker nine hundred feet to eleven hundred feet long. They start swinging and you've got to know what you're doing." Better at mending things, he tried the engine room

[164]

for six months and then started apprenticing with the other pumpman.

As we stroll onto the main deck, heading for the pump room tour he promised me, Akery chats with a soft Missouri drawl, his boyish face topped by a bright red baseball cap and the oil-stained hood of a navy blue sweatshirt jutting out of the back collar of his blue coverall. Well padded against the cold, he has more to do today than show me around. The place we are going—his domain—has been sealed off for days because of the pounding seas and he wonders whether anything is broken.

The entrance to Akery's pump room is a small cavelike door in front of the house. We step in and peer down a ten-foot-wide shaft that is pierced in the middle by a ladder that drops at least sixty feet to the first landing. Everything is painted stark white, including dozens of closely spaced pipes that run side by side down the walls. Staring into a monochrome pit with so many parallel lines falling away from me, I start to feel dizzy.

Gripping the ladder tightly, I descend into the heart of the ship's cargo operation, a throbbing junction of the pipe works where huge pumps will soon push the oil ashore. Wedged between the cargo tanks and the engine room, this canyon of a place is where the explosive crude oil comes as close as it ever gets to the heat of the power plant. Although susceptible to fire, this room cannot be safeguarded by a blanket of inert gas, since people like Akery must be able to breathe fresh air while they work.

Being so vulnerable, the room is designed with such features as lights that are explosion-proof and a ventilation system that changes the air content every few minutes to evacuate any fumes that might collect down here. Everything is painted white so that the pumpman can spot a leak wherever one occurs. A dab of oil will noticeably stain this surface.

The steam-driven pumps at the bottom of the pump room were idle when we loaded cargo in Valdez because the force of gravity brought the oil down a steep hill and onto the ship. But when we get to Cherry Point every ounce of the 35-million-gallon cargo must go uphill to get off the ship, and to do so it will be sucked through this room by four pumps sitting side by side along the back wall. Just one of these powerful pumps can drive 260 gallons of oil over the side of this boat in a single second, hurling it up a twenty-inch pipe with a force equal to 120 pounds per square inch. All four of them can empty the tanks in less than twenty-four hours.

Although the muscular turbines that drive the pumps are located inside the adjacent engine room, their drive shafts breach the wall into the pump room so they can power the pumps. The solid wall between the pump room and engine room assure that the heat of the turbines never comes in contact with the explosive crude oil surging through the pumps.

When Akery and I get to the bottom of the ladder, the pumpman squats next to one of the pumps and runs his finger over a gasket and joint, looking for signs of leakage. Akery says if he finds a crack, he can't weld it because doing so would set off an explosion. Epoxy must do the job until the ship gets to the dry dock where crude oil can be drained out of the system. Because so many parts of a tanker are near the explosive cargo, a lot of broken stuff gets patched with epoxy.

Next, Akery strides across a steel catwalk to a main valve to examine a chain that secures a faucetlike handle. The two ends of the chain are joined by a stamped metal seal, a guarantee that no one can disturb the handle without breaking the seal. Cargo is secured this way against theft or illegal dumping. The captain of the ship, with permission from shore, is the sole person authorized to break the seal and dump the cargo at sea, a desperate act performed only if the ship is foundering or threatening to break up, as happened a while back in the case of the rusted-out tanker *Contessa*.

Akery glances around the room, his eye stopping here or there, examining the general condition. "Your thing out here is constantly checking everything." He especially doesn't want a pump bearing to freeze up because it could overheat and ignite the cargo, or the pumps themselves to start running without oil inside them because they would choke up and delay off-loading.

Akery must also concern himself with the way the ship's valves are lined up, so when we unload our cargo the oil flows in the right direction through thousands of feet of pipe. Make a mistake and oil can go into the wrong tank, spill on the deck, blow out a valve, rupture a line, or explode. "You can fuck up fast on this job."

When Akery completes his inspection, we climb the ladder to the deck where he huddles with third mate Davis over the housing that contains the broken dipstick tape, which needs to be hauled out of the tank and taken inside for repairs. The wind is bitter cold on the hands, so, fully bundled, I stand behind the two men to provide some shelter.

I would have explored the main deck more on this trip had the ocean not claimed it for so many days. Now like a beach at low tide, it stands dry and ready for inspection. Ahead of me, the deck looks like an unburied sewer project. The great platform of the forward hull is dominated by four 20-inch cargo pipes that carry oil lengthwise down the deck and four equally large manifold pipes that run crosswise to the sides of the deck and are linked to the cargo pipes by valves. Adding to this weave of pipe are several smaller conduits, bundles of them in several sizes, coursing the deck alongside the larger pipes.

Upkeep on this ductwork is troublesome since it soaks in brine for much of its life. And these are not simple tubes of steel, but arteries connected by complex valves and interrupted by expansion joints that accordion with the change of temperature and the bending of the ship. Valves and expansion joints rust, and the seals inside of them get brittle, so they must be constantly repaired. And the pipes corrode where water sits at the bottom, so the crew must pull them apart and rotate them.

Second mate Jean Holmes, having just finished a tour of duty on the bridge, has joined the other crew members who hit the deck when it opened up. She and Newman are attacking a pipe joint with a hammer, chisel, and grab bag of other tools. Holmes grunts as she tugs at the stubborn ring. Corroded by rust and gummed up by a worn gasket, the ring around the joint feels as though it is welded in place. Newman gets impatient and grabs at the hammer Holmes is using. "Gimme that thing. Lemme try from here." Rank has less privilege out here when you are doing dirty work on deck.

While they grunt and hammer, I wander toward the bow, thinking of the unseen cavities under my feet. While the cargo tanks are the largest portion of the ship, they remain shrouded in mystery on a loaded voyage like this, cauldrons of poison no sailor may enter. Not only does the dense blanket of crude oil keep the bulk of this creature off limits, it obscures the noises produced in the tanks, which insulates tanker crews from signs of trouble. Coast Guard reports describe cases where a groaning tanker broke a rib or a plate while sailing through heavy seas, but the captain took no defensive action because he could not hear the sharp report of cracking steel deep in the hull. Adding to the unseen risk below are pipes running the length of the ship—more of the big ones we see on deck, and just as burdened with valves and expansion joints.

The designers created many perils when they installed such huge tanks on modern oil ships: the mini-thunderstorms, the muffled damage, and the larger-than-ever oil spills.

I jokingly thought of this tanker as a giant oil can with a propeller before I got acquainted with it, but now I see how complex a contraption it is. Besides ribs and pipes hidden from view, there are remote-controlled tank-cleaning guns hanging from long pipes near the tops of the tanks. These devices scrub a gymnasium-sized void with robotic shower heads, slowly lowered under the command of a computer. An oil can that cleans itself is no simpleton.

Sloshing beneath my feet is sufficient crude oil to make gasoline for three thousand automobile trips around the world, but the unrefined gunk we are carrying won't power any automobiles until it has been turned into a clean solvent like gasoline. This crude carrier is a "dirty" ship in the vernacular of the trade as opposed to a "clean" ship that carries refined products like gasoline. The industry probably regrets the terminology these days, but the truth is that crude oil, with all its complex molecules, can be as dirty and persistent when it clings to the walls of the tanker as it is when it stains a rock on the beach.

When our dirty ship pumps its cargo ashore at Cherry Point, thousands of gallons of the black, sticky crud will stick to the walls and rafters on the insides of the tanks. If it were left there, it would make the ship more difficult to inspect and it would represent a considerable loss of profits. To clear the architecture of this "clingage," the sealed tanks must clean themselves, by remote control, even as the ship is unloading.

What is surprising is the detergent of choice for scouring these foul innards. After the advent of inert gas reduced the risk of explosions in tanks, researchers made a rather odd discovery: The cargo itself is a better cleanser than water or anything else.

The spherical sprinkler heads hanging from the roof spray the walls and ceilings with high-pressure jets of crude oil, the same crude that is clinging to them. The technique—called crude-oil washing—was impossible until inert gas became standard. A mist of crude oil is far more explosive than a tank full of steam, so a good supply of oxygen in the tank would be disastrous.

Crude oil does such a good job as a solvent, the cleaning operation takes only a little over two hours. But efficiency is not the only benefit. The biggest advantage to using oil to clean the tanks may be that the clingage is simply pumped ashore with the cargo. Back in the days when water was regularly used for tank cleaning, the water-clingage mixture was stored in tanks and then dumped overboard after the ship got to sea. The practice of dumping oily water overboard was reduced by treaties two decades ago, but, before it was discouraged, tankers would disgorge some three hundred million gallons of oil into the oceans annually. One veteran of the East Coast trade said ribbons of black oil would stream behind the ships. "It was a dirty trade."

However, modern tankers like this one still jettison some oil overboard. The need arises because ballast water is carried in dirty cargo tanks on unloaded northbound voyages. For the most part, the oil that contaminates the ballast water settles to the top and is skimmed off as cargo and pumped ashore. But some residue remains. Under current law, a tanker like this one can dump as much as one gallon of oil overboard for every fifteen thousand to thirty thousand gallons of cargo the ship carries. No more than a dozen gallons can hit the water per mile and a tanker that plays this game must be fifty miles from shore. Although each ship must keep a record of the oily waste it dumps overboard, regulators have no way of monitoring the practice other than checking the paperwork. Violators are tough to catch. When suspicious tar balls and oil slicks drift ashore, chemists can identify a sample by its characteristics—fingerprinting it, so to speak—but rarely does this detective work result in a polluter being brought to justice. Even if a captain is honest, the machines that monitor the oil dumping are notoriously unreliable. Nevertheless, while the regulation is poorly enforced, most experts do believe it has sharply reduced the chronic oiling of the seas.

I winced some the other day when Jimmy Doyle, the utility, tossed the galley garbage overboard. Although a common practice on all ships, I thought as I watched the sacks drift in our widening wake that the ocean is still regarded as a limitless dumping ground.

There are times when the tanks need more thorough cleaning than crude-oil-washing, like when the *Arco Anchorage* goes to the yard this summer for repairs. To scour the innards before dry docking, the captain will anchor the ship in some protected harbor and for two weeks crew members will set up portable sprayers to hose down the walls with hot water. The black chunks of wax that come off like asphalt must then be scooped off the floor and disposed. In some parts of the world, this dangerous work is done by children and low-paid laborers, but in this case the crew will muck out the last piles of goo.

There are also times during unloaded northbound voyages— when a ship is free from roiling seas—that crewmen will crawl inside to inspect the steel or to do extra cleaning. That didn't happen on our last unloaded sailing because the ocean never permitted it. But on a previous trip crew members were working in the tanks when seas jolted the ship unexpectedly, forcing them to cling to the ladders like mountain climbers in a storm.

As with plenty of other tasks on a tanker, the cleaning can be quite perilous. The caverns must be aired out and then tested for any remnants of poisonous gas. An officer and at least one other person will descend the ladder first, wearing a breathing mask and oxygen tank. Air pumps are set up to ventilate the place and a lookout "angel" will stand watch at the hatchway to assure that no one is injured or overcome.

Once a tank is certified "gas free," more crew members go inside without oxygen tanks and use mops, scrapers, and buckets to muck out the junk that collects in the bottom. It is filthy duty, sinfully dank, and hated by everyone. Sometimes it can be fatal. Even in tanks declared "gas free," pockets of poisonous fumes hide in leftover gunk or collect in corners. Once disturbed by a mop or hose, the vapor will waft free. A man who sailed with a different company in these waters told me how, while working on a cleaning crew, he got dizzy when a pocket of gas was freed from the mouth of a pipe at the bottom of a tank. He tried climbing the ladder to escape but as he neared the top, gasping for air and losing focus, he realized he would not make it. Staggering to a landing about fifty feet above the floor, the fifty-seven-year-old seaman unbuckled his belt and then rebuckled it to the stanchion just before he fainted, a trick he learned from a training film. Otherwise he would have tumbled to his death. "I've held onto that belt and I'm going to have it framed." The lookout who was supposed to watch from above had wandered away, but a mate happened to look into the tank and called for help. Three men including the guy who tied himself to the ladder were treated at a nearby hospital for chemical poisoning. A doctor told the men, if they had not been found in another ten or fifteen minutes, they would have been dead. That tanker, owned by a Texas company, was a sloppy operation that obviously didn't learn a lesson quickly; another man was similarly "gassed" on the same ship a year later.

But even in a better fleet like Arco's, crude oil fumes pose constant hazards. Aside from the short-term danger of asphyxiation, some researchers believe there is the long-term risk of cancer. One study showed an unusual number of cancers among Coast Guard inspectors who have spent a considerable amount of time crawling around inside cargo tanks. Such news has some tanker sailors wondering whether a disease-causing time bomb ticks aboard the ship. When Carroll's daughter was born with a birth defect, he thought of the time he was gassed as a cadet, and of the hours he'd spent working unprotected by breathing apparatus down below. The doctor assured him there was no connection, but some worry that crude oil fumes will someday lay low the tanker sailor the way coal dust annihilated the miner.

Companies like Arco take extra precautions against oil-emitted poisonous gases such as benzene and toluene. On the tanker deck, for instance, when the ship is loading or unloading crude, crew members are told to wear filtered breathing masks. The company takes the safety measure seriously enough to order men to keep their faces shaven so the masks will fit properly.

A tall exhaust pipe near the bow releases tank fumes a safe distance from the deck, but the winds sometimes push them back down. This underlines the need for masks, but the rule is not strictly obeyed. During the early stages of loading in Valdez, I noticed that most deckhands were not wearing their masks, but had them draped at half-mast around their necks. When I asked Newman why the crew wasn't wearing them, he replied that the plastic mask is too warm and cumbersome to work with. But near the end of loading, as the oil level rose to the top of the tanks, the fumes got thicker and everyone put on their masks. The place looked like a World War I battlefield.

The townspeople in Valdez told me they, too, are concerned about the noxious fumes venting in their direction from the tankers across the bay. Although the Alyeska Pipeline Service Company has denied it, some scientists say the Valdez terminal is among the ten worst benzene polluters in the country, giving the town a bathtub ring in the air. Despite Alyeska's protests to the contrary, an independent study showed that 90 percent of the community's benzene—equal to levels in Dallas—comes from the oil terminal and the tankers. Alyeska will probably have to follow the example now being set at the California refinery docks, and install equipment to capture and treat the benzene gases coming off ships like the *Arco Anchorage*. Arco is also experimenting with a gas recovery system installed on the newly outfitted *Arco Fairbanks*.

As the afternoon wanes toward a January sunset, the bosun hikes down the main deck to the foc's'le house with a bucket he wants to stow. The foc's'le house is as much the bosun's storage shed as it is a dike raised in defense against the oncoming waves. Tacked onto the bow, it is a ten-car garage in the ship's front yard, a thirteen-foot-tall afterthought that catches whatever junk a sailor can't find a place for. It would be roomier if the middle were not dominated by a casement that holds the stowed anchor chain. But like garages everywhere, the remaining space is filled with rope, chain, tools, and canisters—everything twenty times beefier than the stuff I keep at home, understandably so, since tanker work demands Texas-sized dimensions. Small against the darkening sky, the bosun finishes his work and heads back to the house, just as the weather puts on a winter grimace.

As night falls and the ocean takes a last swipe at us, the captain closes the main deck again. Winds are crossing the rear quarter of the ship and we are rolling some, not as bad as the ride we took outside Hinchinbrook but treacherous enough that I brace myself as I climb the stairs to the bridge. Gazing out the wheelhouse window, the scowling line on the far horizon and the ocean's monochromatic blackness make me wonder what the mood is like below the surface, the part I cannot see. The ocean's skin is a simplified place where the water and sky draw a line. Underneath the opaque waves there throbs a three-dimensional world of gill breathers who swim in canyons unimaginably deep. More than one hundred feet below the bridge, the bottom of our hull breaks into this watery environment, but barely dents it, given the enormity of the ocean. Even so, the long frigate I see from the bridge is a blimp when it greets the fishes. Like an iceberg, most of this ship is underwater. Although the oil we carry is lighter than water, it has enough mass piled high in the tanks to sink the hull until it reaches a balance between the molecular weight of the cargo and the density of the water outside. According to the laws of physics, there should be one hundred tons underwater for every fifteen that rise above.

The condition of our sunken hull is anybody's guess right now. The company hires divers once a year to check the underwater health of the ship. There are even times when a tanker captain will unbalance his ship by emptying rear ballast tanks and filling front ones so the ship will stick its rear end out of the water for inspection. But except when a vessel goes to the yard, the crew never sees the bottom, or the rudder and prop. And it is such an important part of any ship.

Keeping an oceangoing machine clean and efficient is a constant battle with rust and other corrosives. The tanker below water is a box with a very flat bottom. The lower forty feet is painted red with a special substance designed to kill the barnacles and other creatures that cause corrosion and slow down the ship.

Hitchhiking electricity will also encourage corrosion, so the outside of the hull is laced with tiny electric wires that carry a low amount of voltage designed to neutralize and remove any static electricity that builds up on a ship's hull as it slides through the ocean.

Also under the tanker's midsection are grated holes, known as sea chests, which are the openings where pumps suck in seawater to cool the engines and fill the ballast tanks. There are two sea chests, one located on the bottom of the ship where it won't suck air if the vessel rolls from side to side; and another is found slightly to the side where it won't suck mud when the ship crosses a shallow bottom. When I was in the shipyard, I stuck my head inside a sea chest and got the creepy sense of a fish about to be guzzled by the machinery.

When the ship goes into the yard, corrosion on the hull and crud in the sea chests aren't the only cleaning projects that face workmen underneath the hull. Back at the rear of the ship is the five-bladed propeller, which, if one could see it as the tanker passes through the water tonight, would look like a piece of brass jewelry hanging from the ship's tailbone. When I was in the yard, workmen were polishing the screw to a bright sheen, not to impress the fish but because a propeller free of pits and rough spots will spin the water more freely and give the company 2 to 3 percent savings in fuel. The savings are enough that the company will hire divers to polish the blades in years when the ship isn't going into the yard.

Behind the screw is the eighty-ton rudder, roughly rectangular in shape and as tall as a four-story building. We have a spare propeller bolted to the main deck, but there is no spare rudder. If something should happen to this one, we would be effectively without steering, not as impossible an event as one would think. The stock that holds the rudder in place is thick, but the combined forces of the ocean and the momentum of the ship put tremendous pressure on the huge flap, and some have fallen off.

Throughout the night, the rudder is getting commands from the ship's autopilot as the tanker keeps its straight line. But by 6:10 A.M., halfway through Svetko Lisica's early morning watch, we are ten minutes away from the biggest turn of the trip. Our instruments tell us that we have a little over three nautical miles to go until we reach the spot on the ocean where we turn left for the final westward leg of our trip into the Strait of Juan de Fuca. Our heading is 123.5 degrees— south and west—and our speed is 13.7 nautical miles an hour. The ship feels busy.

Down in the engine room the weary boys test the gear, a Coast Guard requirement before we enter Washington state waters. They check the steering equipment and as a test they put a load on some of the other big machines. The dials on the instrument panels tell them everything is in working order.

Up on the bridge, Captain Carroll is awake—a little sleepy-eyed, but conscious and holding a steaming cup of coffee. He feels a little fresher, he says, and attributes it to the fact he slept better last night than he did the previous two nights. Good thing, because we are entering areas of heavy traffic and sailing closer to shore, perils worse in some way than the heavy weather of the open ocean. As Carroll talks about his preparations for this trip into inland waters, he comments that he must check with the Coast Guard by radio and assure that all the radars, radios, and navigation tools are in working order. It is all very routine, and Captain Jack knows what he is doing, but he explains that somewhere in the back of his mind there is always a little wariness when he navigates a busy waterway. "You can be a good guy or you can be a bad guy. But if you go on the rocks and spill oil, your kids will hear about you, and your wife will hear about you, and your friends will hear about you."

13

Steamrolling an Ant

(Pacific Ocean,
50 miles west of the entrance
to the Strait of Juan de Fuca,
January 29, 6:30 A.M.)

Captain Carroll is smiling. Not a smirk, mind you, just an Irish grin. Early in the morning of our fourth day, after we make our big left turn toward the mouth of the Strait of Juan de Fuca, we are on a final run to the refinery. As the helmsman points the ship toward Buoy Juliet, the marker identifying the doorway to Washington state, the radio chatter increases in frequency as wanderers from all corners of the globe report their positions. Carroll is pleased about a radio conversation he overheard a few minutes ago.

"Remember that other ship, the *Prince William Sound,* the one that turned left when we were coming out of Hinchinbrook? She's seven hours behind us now."

Carroll won the race. The other ship, by taking a shortcut over rougher and shallower water, was slowed to a crawl by the heavy seas. Carroll's choice to go right, on the long route over the hundred-fathom curve, was a good one. He can't pin it to his chest, and it won't be recorded on any performance evaluation, but a young captain likes the feeling of a first-rate decision. It was with an educated guess that he turned the ship to the outer ocean, away from the tempestuous shallows. But it was a professional toss of the dice, an odds-on winner in a game too often lost by amateurs. It had the mark of good on-the-job schooling, of years spent paying attention to the better plays of other captains. As a result, the *Arco Anchorage* is leaving the ocean today, mostly intact, nicely trimmed, pretty much on schedule, and in good hands.

The captain gets about two minutes to enjoy it all before Willie Herbert walks onto the bridge and announces he's got a medical problem. A hernia, or some such problem that was operated on when he was a boy, is giving him trouble. "Let's just take a look at those balls," says Dr. Carroll, as he escorts the cook-baker back into the chart room. Crouching under the light as Willie drops his drawers, the proud athlete who attended a prestigious academy and worked his way up to the vaulted position of ship captain must now stare into the naked crotch of a man who epitomizes the bad name given to sailors. Carroll doesn't want to think about where Willie has been with his privates, he just wants to get the examination over with. Maybe this is why captains earn so much money. "Willie's got enlarged balls," the skipper declares afterward, as Willie strolls back downstairs. "He'll see the doctor in Port Angeles."

"Now there's another unfit for duty for me. Is it me? Did I cause this? No. But it'll go on the record against me." First there was the woman who wrenched her shoulder, then the guy who got carpal tunnel, then the worsening condition of the first engineer, and now Willie with oversized testicles. What's next? Maybe the bridge of a ship should be the setting for a television sitcom.

But the captain's worries about the crew are soon forgotten as more pressing matters lie ahead. We are entering one of the busiest shipping lanes on the West Coast, and compared to the open ocean, this is the freeway on Labor Day.

The ship's radar shows targets ahead of and behind us. One is probably a small fishing boat. The other, we know from its radio report, is a container ship gaining on us from behind, much faster afloat than the *Arco Anchorage* and stacked to the eyebrows with boxes from Japan. Another vessel carrying empty containers is also coming up from the stern. A squadron of swift Canadian Navy ships plays war games to our left. "You know when you've got a Navy ship on your radar screen," the third mate once told me. "They won't say a word over the radio, but all of a sudden the dot on the screen will take off like a bat out of hell." Coming toward us, but still a long distance away, is the black silhouette of a U.S. Navy Trident submarine, a surfaced gunslinger carrying enough ballistic missiles to destroy a country. Just in front of the sub, also coming our way, is a Russian freighter. It's just another day in the neighborhood.

The Strait of Juan de Fuca is a convenient back door to America, cutting horizontally into the nation's upper-left-hand corner. Two friendly nations, the United States and Canada, argue politely over vessel traffic control and pollution in this moat that separates them. Those who value aesthetics see the strait as a nature preserve and those who value commerce see it as a shipping lane. Beauty and the beast live side by side. About ten thousand vessels of all sizes pass through here every year, more than one an hour around the clock. The Coast Guard radar screens that watch over it get so jammed during hot fishing seasons, they appear to have a case of measles.

To the south of us, we get our first glimpse of the Lower 48 as the Olympic Peninsula becomes visible through a mid-morning haze. A dark bluff overhangs a village, shadowing it so the details of the buildings are barely visible in my binoculars. Most residents are descendants of an American Indian tribe whose ancestors paddled wooden canoes from their pebbled shoreline a century ago. Now the tribal members fish in aluminum boats and log with chain saws, both powered by gasoline engines. They worry, too, about oil spills and are petitioning the government for a powerful tug to be stationed at their village to control any tankers that might lose power.

To the north, invisible from my vantage point, are the outer reaches of Vancouver Island, where virgin trees still grow and roadless shorelines make a final stand against the cities and towns encroaching from the east.

The seas are calm and the air is on its best behavior. But the strait has a quick temper. "Don't come here in a small boat unless you've got your ass tied to the deck," said one crewman.

Between here and the refinery dock at Cherry Point are 110 miles of water and probably three or four locations where statisticians predict there will be a major oil spill someday. Buoy Juliet—or J Buoy for short—is one of them. Port Angeles and the Rosario Strait are two others. We will be passing by all of them. Still, these waters are safer than some. The 600-mile-long Strait of Malacca, separating Malaysia and the Indonesian island of Sumatra, is a choke point for cargo ships heading to Singapore and for Persian Gulf tankers sailing to the Far East. Ships run into each other with such regularity in the Malacca Strait, there is talk of banning tankers altogether. That's an unlikely move, though, since most of Japan's petroleum squeezes through the slot. The Houston Ship Channel, a shallow, muddy passageway, is ranked number one in this country for collisions partly because ships must perform a maneuver known as "Texas Chicken" to pass each other in the narrow channel. The limited sailing space means that entering and departing tankers must meet nose to nose and then, at the last possible moment, each one turn sharply right, seeming to bounce off the banks and passing each other less than one hundred feet apart. The pilots say it is a crazy but necessary game until the channel is widened. Spills are so commonplace in the channel, some Texas officials worry the public has become inured to them. Other high-risk shipping lanes include the Strait of Gibraltar, the Strait of Dover, the Strait of Hormuz, the entrance to the Red Sea, the lower Mississippi River, the entire Gulf of Mexico coast, the Delaware River near Philadelphia, Nantucket Sound, the Arthur Kill waterway in New York and New Jersey, San Francisco Bay, and the waters around Long Beach, California. Some have taken limited action to protect such high-risk areas. Following the breakup of the tanker *Braer* in the Shetland Islands, the British government asked the tanker industry to reroute loaded ships away from several hazardous waterways that provide access to an oil terminal at Sullom Voe.

Although computerized radars and vastly improved navigation systems have cut back on collisions, they have not been a complete solution. In 1991 alone, oil ships were involved in six major mishaps, including a smashup with a passenger vessel off the coast of Italy that killed 141 people. There were two fiery collisions in the Strait of Malacca in a four-month period in late 1992 and early 1993, including one that killed 21 sailors.

The hazards are a kaleidoscope in crowded waterways, some with an offbeat flavor. Submarines, for instance, cruise underneath tankers to hide from sub-chasing airplanes. The Navy for security reasons won't discuss the tactic, but *Arco Anchorage* crewman Marvin Cropper remembers an American sub surfacing next to his tanker off Connecticut and the sub captain telling his tanker captain he had been traveling underneath him for a long time. "Think of what would happen if it came up, you know, right through number three center tank." In 1984, a nuclear-powered Soviet submarine did just that. It surfaced into the belly of a Soviet tanker while sneaking out of the Strait of Gibraltar. Both vessels limped away without reporting the extent of damage.

Although they don't prowl this side of the Pacific, modern-day pirates are a hazard in places like the Strait of Malacca. Traveling in speedboats, and armed with automatic weapons and machetes, the pirates can quickly board a low-slung tanker that has little protection other than water cannons. With 130 attacks in 1991 alone, the International Chamber of Commerce established a regional piracy center in Southeast Asia to report pirate movements the way others would forecast the weather. The loaded tankers are juicy targets because they are slow, they sit low in the water, and the captains carry lots of cash. In one case, a forty-five-thousand-deadweight-ton Bahamian tanker drifted out of control for fifteen minutes in a busy shipping lane east of Indonesia's Bintan Island after seven buccaneers tied up a mate and crewman on watch. Later in the same area, another band of cutlass-wielding pirates set fire to a Cyprian-flagged chemical tanker and stabbed the third officer in the chest, leg, and arms.

In these West Coast waters, however, the number one peril is an obstacle known as the commercial fishing vessel. Carroll carefully notes the location of each one as we enter the strait. Big ships are predictable, and for the most part they will stay in the traffic lanes, but you never know about a boat chasing a school of fish. Run over a net and you could end up paying the fisherman as much as thirty thousand dollars for the damage. The nets also tangle in the ship's rudder and propeller. As the thin filament works its way into the shaft it can cut the lubrication seals. Usually the damage isn't serious, but there have been instances of small lube oil spills and of malfunctions. To combat this problem, Arco has installed Ninja-like knife blades around the rim of the ship's propeller shaft to shred the nets before they can tangle in the machinery.

Then again, from the fisherman's point of view, the deep-draft ships are like so many elephants stampeding around them. "They don't give a damn about us," said one. Shrouded in darkness and surrounded by heavy seas, some fishermen install sheets of metal on their highest radio masts to assure that they will make a good impression on a hundred-thousand-ton ship's radar. But in the outer seas, where the rollers rise as high as apartment buildings, a fishing boat is in constant danger of disappearing from the leviathan's electronic view.

The result of this peril was demonstrated by an encounter between the tanker *Golden Gate* and the fishing boat *Jack Jr*. on Labor Day evening in 1986. Two days before the incident, Jack Favaloro, a fifty-six-year-old Italian immigrant, took his seventy-three-foot fishing boat (named after his son) on a voyage from San Francisco to rich fishing grounds seven miles west of the Point Reyes lighthouse in the Pacific Ocean. It was a routine outing for Favaloro and his two crew members, Vincenzo Ingargiola and Thomas McCarthy.

The tanker *Golden Gate* was also on an ordinary run to Washington state when it left Martinez, California, on Labor Day carrying a partial load of crude oil. It was windy and foggy on the Pacific when the sixty-two-thousand-ton oil tanker sailed under its namesake, the Golden Gate Bridge. Some say the ship was in no shape to proceed at full speed, around fourteen nautical miles an hour, into a fog bank, especially with the transmitting and receiving tubes inside both radars nearly worn out, making them less sensitive to small objects on the water. The collision-avoidance system was turned off because it had been sounding false warnings. But skipper David Hilger, thirty years old, a graduate of the same Kings Point academy that Carroll attended, was a confident guy, almost cocky. He had been master for only six months, but like Carroll he was a fast-rising star in the Keystone Shipping Company fleet.

Some say the captain should have posted a bow lookout in such poor visibility, as anything beyond fifteen hundred feet was obscured by fog, and anything closer than five hundred feet was shielded from view by the bow of the ship. Two fishing vessels had already crossed the tanker's bow, and one was less than a third of a mile away. But even as the fog deepened, Hilger didn't slow the ship or post a bow lookout.

Standing orders prohibited crew members from slowing a Keystone ship without the captain's approval, and Hilger saw no reason to do so. "Maybe coming into Houston, yeah, you'd damn well better slow down. Out at Point Reyes? No. None of the other ships slowed down that day either. No one ever slowed down in the fog, unless there were ships around them, and I mean close, dead in front of them." Captains like to keep the pace and they trust their radars. "Bigger drunks than Hazelwood go on up to Valdez, too," he noted.

Hilger said the seas were too rough to post a lookout on the bow. He could have assigned a lookout to the wing of the bridge, but instead he sent the crewman below to wait on standby. He said crew cutbacks force tanker captains to use fewer people on the bridge—"a bigger accident waiting to happen." But Hilger, too, went below to complete some paperwork, leaving the chief mate and helmsman alone. "If the captain was on the bridge every time you had fog on the West Coast, you would never sleep."

The veil thickened as the *Golden Gate* steamed toward the *Jack Jr.* Favaloro had a net streaming out behind the boat and the engine was shut off. Wearing blue jeans, a T-shirt, a blue work shirt, and a nylon vest, Favaloro was not prepared to go for a swim in cold water, nor were his two companions.

On the *Golden Gate* bridge, chief mate Peter Lieb figured a dot he saw on the radar screen was a false reading caused by waves. He marked the spot with a grease pencil, and didn't see it again as the weakened radar made another five sweeps.

Unaware he was making no impression on the *Golden Gate*'s radar, the skipper of the *Jack Jr.* radioed the big ship bearing down on him from a half mile away, asking whether the crew could hear or see him. The chief mate on the *Golden Gate* took the call, looked at his radar again, adjusted its sensitivity, and saw nothing closer than a dot representing a passenger ship five miles behind him. Because the chief mate didn't know the *Golden Gate* was the ship Favaloro was worried about, he identified himself over the radio as "a ship" and kept steaming. The fisherman called out on the radio again, warning the approaching ship that it was getting awfully close. The *Golden Gate* officer radioed back that the fisherman ought to "stay put," but he still had no idea where the *Jack Jr.* was located.

Four seconds later, the fisherman cried out on the radio: "You're going to hit us. Change your course. What are you doing, man? Jesus Christ. Oh, my god. Mayday. Mayday. Mayday." Favaloro and his two crewmen were never heard from again.

No one on the tanker heard the impact, including the chief mate. William McGivern, the former U.S. attorney in San Francisco who investigated the case, said that makes sense since a tanker that hits a boat a thousand times smaller is "like a steamroller going over an ant." But even if the crew heard nothing, McGivern doesn't buy Hilger's claim—which he sticks to today that he didn't realize immediately afterward that his tanker had run over something.

When Favaloro cried out the last time over the radio, the chief mate on the tanker turned hard right and called the captain to the bridge. He looked over the side for debris and didn't see any. But four men working on the stern did see pieces of broken white wood and an orange object they thought to be a life vest. One of them reported this to the captain, but Hilger did not inform the Coast Guard of the debris sighting until the next morning. "There was no reason to report that they saw debris, at least over the airwaves. I wanted to make sure their story was right. Debris is always on the water." However, Hilger did contact company headquarters by satellite telephone that night to say he may have hit a fishing boat and that workers on the stern might have seen life jackets in the water.

The *Golden Gate* steamed ahead for fifteen minutes following Favaloro's final transmission. When the Coast Guard raised Hilger on the radio, he seemed puzzled. "He basically played dumb," said McGivern. The Coast Guard asked the *Golden Gate* and the other ships in the area to search for survivors because they wouldn't last long in the cold water. The tanker turned and searched for more than two hours before the Coast Guard released it to continue its voyage. Five days later, Favaloro's body was found by a passenger boat four miles from the accident site. The other bodies were never recovered.

McGivern believes it was a case of hit-and-run, but Hilger says he didn't know he had hit a boat until divers found a fishnet tangled in his tanker's prop four days later.

A little more than two days after the accident, the *Golden Gate* steamed into the Strait of Juan de Fuca, past our current location, and picked up a pilot at Port Angeles. Two Keystone lawyers and two Coast Guard investigators got on with the pilot, which is when Hilger realized "it was the big shit." Instead of cooperating, the company told the captain and crew to say nothing to the investigators. Hilger made no public comments until he spoke to me in 1992. Even when Coast Guard officers served subpoenas, the skipper and his lawyers wouldn't turn over logs, charts, and other documents. "The master of the *Golden Gate* claimed he did not know the whereabouts of the ship's documents," the Coast Guard report said.

When investigators found scratch marks on the *Golden Gate*'s hull and remnants of the *Jack Jr.*'s net in the propeller, the FBI opened a criminal investigation. A grand jury indicted Hilger under a seldom-used federal law that makes it a felony punishable by up to ten years in prison for a captain to cause someone's death by misconduct or negligence. "I found it unbelievable," Hilger said. "What about a physician who kills someone on the operating table? He doesn't face that."

McGivern felt Hilger was negligent in six ways—sailing with worn-out radar tubes, leaving the bridge in the fog, not slowing down, not posting a lookout, not trying immediately to rescue the fishermen, and not reporting evidence like the debris seen by the workmen. "I thought we had a good case," McGivern remarked.

But while some expected the case to set a precedent by defining maritime negligence, it died on a technicality. The appeals court said Hilger was indicted in the wrong court (San Francisco), since maritime law says a person who commits a crime on the high seas will be tried either where he is arrested or where he lives (or in Washington, D.C., if none of the above apply). Hilger was living in New York. McGivern asked his Justice Department colleagues back East to re-indict Hilger, but they did not think they could prove negligence. Keystone paid sizable damages to the families of the dead fishermen, but the criminal case was dropped.

Life did not go badly for Hilger after the accident. Keystone paid his salary while he got a master's degree at Harvard University. By the time I talked to him, Hilger was running a video dating service in Manhattan and trying to syndicate a cable television mating show he calls *The Game of Love.* "It turns out that I'm creative." He kept his skipper's license, "in case I ever want to skipper the good ship *Lollipop.*"

Passing Buoy Juliet this morning, Captain Carroll has no intention of ending up like Hilger or Hazelwood. Both his radars are in good condition, and although we are making good time—fifteen nautical miles per hour—there is no fog. Third mate Dean Davis is with him on the bridge, as are a helmsman and a lookout. In traffic, your asshole gets tight, says Carroll, but it ought to. Better a tight asshole than a loose ship. The easygoing attitude of the open ocean has left the faces of these men, and I sense their concentration as I watch the quickening of their pace. I was agitated myself a while back when I saw my first driftwood, a sure sign of land. I even thought I could smell the scent of civilization. Carroll depresses the talk button on the ship's two-way radio and talks to the closest thing there is in the maritime world to an airport traffic control tower, a maritime traffic coordinator.

In a darkened room on the fourth floor of a Seattle waterfront building, a Coast Guard petty officer stares at a dot the *Arco Anchorage* is burning on his radar screen. He can't quite hear Carroll's arrival report over the radio so the traffic coordinator asks the skipper for a clarification. "Seattle Traffic to *Arco Anchorage,* you are coming in very weak. If you have high power, go to it."

Carroll repeats his arrival message, telling the Coast Guardsman the name of his ship, his location, destination, and speed. If there is anything seriously wrong with his vessel, he should report it now, but the broken feed pump and the crippled inert-gas pump aren't worth mentioning. The radar operator repeats Carroll's cryptic message in a bureaucratic monotone. "We understand that you are loaded with Alaskan crude oil. Your arrival is 1350 for the pilot station. Seattle to *Arco Anchorage,* your radio sounds very weak compared to other ships in the area."

Carroll makes a few adjustments, for he wants to avoid any problems caused by a malfunctioning radio. But even if he did have a lasting communication glitch, the Seattle Coast Guard station would not stop him from sailing. As marine traffic "coordinators" they do not have the regulatory power of their brethren, the air traffic "controllers." As with everything else in the maritime world, it is very different from aviation. Where a traffic controller can tell a pilot how fast he can fly and at what elevation, nobody easily tells a ship captain what to do. But the hope is that a little advice from traffic coordinators might prevent accidents like the collision of the *Golden Gate* and the *Jack Jr.*

A quarter-century ago, ship traffic coordinators were unheard of. An experiment in Rotterdam in the late 1950s showed for the first time that a harbor advisory service could cut foggy-weather accidents four-fold. The Dutch system was copied by a few other ports in Europe and Asia, but did not catch on in America until 1968 when Coast Guard officers began keeping track of ships in San Francisco Bay by taking the radio reports from ships and moving models around on a table to represent their positions. The Coast Guard didn't pry money out of Congress for a radar system to spot the ships on their own until 1971, when a collision between two Standard Oil tankers under the Golden Gate bridge caused an oil spill and a lot of public ire.

The Puget Sound Vessel Traffic System was born a little more than a year later. It, too, was a tabletop operation at first. Even today, the Coast Guard spends less money on its vessel traffic systems nation-wide than the Federal Aviation Administration spends on a single tower operation at the Seattle-Tacoma International Airport.

Twenty years ago a study recommended that vessel traffic systems (VTS) be installed in twenty-two harbors in the United States, but by 1989 only eight were actually in place, including Puget Sound, Houston-Galveston, San Francisco, Prince William Sound, Berwick Bay, Louisiana, Sault Ste. Marie, Michigan, and Louisville, Kentucky. In 1988, the Coast Guard turned a deaf ear to protests from the National

Transportation Safety Board and others, and shut down its systems in New York and New Orleans because of budget constraints. Shortly after the New Orleans system was scrapped, a tanker spilled nearly a million gallons in the Mississippi River in an accident that might have been prevented by operating the New Orleans VTS.

Investigators say a neglected traffic system in Prince William Sound also contributed to the *Exxon Valdez* disaster, since the wandering Exxon tanker slipped away from Coast Guard surveillance because of ill-maintained radar equipment and complacent operators. Afterwards, Congress allotted more money to upgrade the Coast Guard radar systems in Prince William Sound and Puget Sound.

Although there were problems in the past, Canadian and U.S. traffic coordinators are doing a better job of meshing the directions they give the ships in these neighboring waters. Carroll made contact yesterday with a Canadian Coast Guard station located in a small fishing village on the west coast of Vancouver Island. Tofino Traffic, as it is called, handles all incoming ships—whether they are headed for the United States or Canada, until they enter the Strait of Juan de Fuca where Seattle Traffic seamlessly takes over.

Carroll welcomes the traffic coordination system, and like his boss, Aspland, he wishes for better equipment and tougher rules. Carroll likes the more assertive Canadian operators. "They are always right. They force captains to repeat the commands. They'll yell at the guy." Seattle Traffic does a good job describing conditions, Carroll says, but they don't push hard enough. "They won't move the fishing boats out of your way."

To be fair, Tofino Traffic has an easier job than Seattle Traffic. The Canadians monitor a couple of radars out on the open ocean. From a grim-looking building above the Seattle docks where the Coast Guard keeps its cutters and icebreakers, Guard Captain Chet Motekaitis oversees the largest and most complex marine traffic advisory system in the world. Covering more than twelve hundred square miles, Seattle Traffic has twelve radar sites that watch a variety of activities including container ships barreling into Puget Sound, tankers lumbering up Rosario Strait, fishing boats massing around a salmon run, tugboats pulling a flotilla of logs, sailboats tacking around a race course, and

Navy ships conducting maneuvers. Cutting through all this craziness, usually on a perpendicular path, is a ferry system as bustling as any in the world. Each type of vessel must report in and each creates its own special problems.

The Coast Guard radar operator who is talking to Carroll right now is 125 miles from the *Arco Anchorage*. He sits with a half-dozen other people who are monitoring a dozen radars under a seven-foot ceiling that compresses the forty-by-thirty-foot room. Motekaitis needs two dozen employees to properly run this video parlor operation twenty-four hours a day, but for now he has a staff of only half that many, and they are all working overtime.

Packing crates sit unopened in one corner of the room, evidence that new equipment is being installed. But the old equipment the guy is using now is stuff air traffic controllers haven't seen for decades. As the radar operator watches the *Arco Anchorage*, he records its position on a little slip of paper, which he posts next to his radar screen. Paper collects there like confetti. Inside the packing crates is the solution to his problem—new machines that will keep track of everything by computer and show ships moving down the waterway on pleasantly colored electronic maps. If an operator wants to know what a particular ship is doing, he can touch a button and get information on the direction and speed, plus an estimate of the time it would take it to converge with any vessel in its path. (It is much like the CAS system we have on the *Arco Anchorage* today.) In the meantime, the equipment sits in crates while the Coast Guard makes the necessary upgrade to its radar towers. Other improvements may follow. Someday, automated weather stations may give Coast Guard operators constant condition reports, something they must get now from the ships. And in the future vessels entering the harbor may carry transmitters that will provide Seattle Traffic more complete data than is presently available through radar. Just such a system is newly in place in Prince William Sound.

Equipment, however, is not the only answer. As with most changes in this entrenched profession, mariners are reluctant to accept the power of traffic cops. Some in the industry argue that captains and pilots know better than a shoreside controller such things as how many miles the vessel needs for an emergency stop or what point on the compass it should steer to. It has also been argued that a captain better understands the complex relationship between safety and the schedule. In the last two decades several studies have recommended mandatory traffic control and speed limits, but the Coast Guard, ever mindful of industry objections, has ignored them all.

Motekaitis, the commander of Seattle Traffic, worries more about the old-fashioned skippers who scoff at his operation than he does about the critics who want tougher rules. As such, he isn't a proponent of mandatory controls, but instead would like some cooperation. To court the old salts he offers a helping hand rather than a hammer. There is a twenty-five-thousand-dollar fine for grossly violating vessel traffic system regulations, but Motekaitis prefers to send violators a letter reminding them to play by the rules. "There's a lot that I could do, but along with the authority is a responsibility to use that authority in a prudent way." He says mariners will go along with him if he can get them to see the value of his system, not if he punishes them. "Very few folks out there want to go bump in the night."

Coast Guard traffic coordinators are slowly gaining acceptance, partly because of successes. Recently a loaded tanker leaving Port Angeles found itself nose to nose with a southbound freighter. The eavesdropping Coast Guard radar operator realized the officers on the two ships had misunderstood each other, and intervened to avert a worldwide headline.

Even with traffic coordinators, though, these waters are anarchy compared to highways onshore. For example, the strait is a divided passageway—with eastbound and westbound lanes of one thousand yards in width—but the rules say, if a ship leaves the lane, or changes direction, the lane rules no longer apply. And motorboats create their own brand of havoc, all of them driven by people who are not required to hold an operator's license. The ability to drive a speedboat sans permit and to sail on the sidewalks are inalienable rights in these waters—something like owning a gun.

Fortunately, there are rules and courtesies that apply to the biggest of vessels. Ships meeting each other must exchange information to assure they pass safely. English is the required language, though foreign officers are often not fluent. A Chinese cargo ship hit a fish processing boat near here, in fog, because the crew could not understand what the Coast Guard radar operators were saying. In an emergency, everyone is supposed to know "Seaspeak," a simple list of key words that work well over a scratchy radio. Davis says with the risk so great for misunderstanding, the less you say to a foreign boat the better. "With a foreign vessel, you give a heading and you say I'll pass you green-to-green or red-to-red [referring to the color of the lights on each side of the ship]. That's all you want to say."

Actually, all radio talk is brief since the frequency bands are limited. One should save philosophical discussions for the marine telephone.

14

At Least One Way Out

(Strait of Juan de Fuca,
January 29, 10 A.M.)

The bosun is a picture of concentration as he steers the ship. He stares straight ahead while he chats with me in a distracted manner, sometimes pausing in mid-sentence. There is nothing directly in front of us right now, but another crewman is telling stories of his encounters with small boats. He and the bosun agree that weekend mariners make the sea lanes, uh, very interesting. A sailboat in San Francisco Bay nuzzled the side of the crewman's tanker because the amateur yachtsman wanted a closer look at the big ship. Windsurfers play in the bow wave, and motorboaters cross the ship's path, as though a tanker could stop on a dime, which it could do if the dime was a mile in diameter. I ask Carroll what he would do if he had to choose suddenly between hitting a sailboat or running aground. "I've thought about it. I don't know. One thing I always try to do is leave myself one way out, at least one way out."

The cargo ship *Great Land* is closing on us, doing some twenty-one to twenty-two knots in contrast with our fifteen. Carroll glances at the radar screen, which serves as his rearview mirror, to assure himself that the *Great Land* will have room to overtake us on the side closest to shore. Carroll moves the *Arco Anchorage* as far toward the middle traffic lane as he can because he wants the cargo ship nearest to the beach where its load of empty truck trailers would do less damage than our load of crude. "If he shits the bed, I can go to port [to the left] and get out of the way." Chess moves like that are the survival techniques of inland sailing.

The mate writes the word "arrival" in the logbook, marking the time we left the Pacific Ocean. Though nautical record keepers say the ocean's edge is the start and finish of a voyage, we have a lot of water to cover between here and the refinery.

From this point on, the nature of our trip changes. During our ocean voyage we sailed more than a hundred miles from land, but in the next day and a half we will come as close as a few hundred yards of shore. To reach the refinery at Cherry Point we must cruise through one of this country's most valued and striking waterways; we passed one federally protected marine sanctuary a few hours ago and are bellying our way toward another one. There are portions of this high-priced neighborhood that are ridiculously vulnerable to a ship carrying oil, but it is the only road to Cherry Point.

In the olden days a captain knew he was going aground if he heard the sound of the surf, since that meant it was too late for his sailing ship to escape. However, a modern oil tanker with a belly fifty feet deep in the water will run aground long before anyone hears the surf. For that reason, a tanker captain must know exactly where he is at all times.

Carroll gets quick and easy advice from an array of sophisticated machines that help him navigate and pilot his ship. (By definition, you "navigate" on the open ocean and "pilot" close to land.) The tanker has sensors on the roof that gather data from the heavens and others on the keel that bounce sounds off the bottom of the sea. Each device feeds information to a receiver that sits on or near the chart room shelf. The receivers are metal boxes that rest side by side, competing for the honor of telling us our latitude, longitude, speed, distance traveled, the time to the next destination, and the topography of the ocean floor.

For centuries, ships relied on celestial navigation and dead reckoning to find their way until just a third of a century ago when one improved navigation device after another came into being. With names like loran, SatNav, and GPS, each of the new systems is present today on the good ship *Arco Anchorage*. This committee of dull-colored boxes is, in the vernacular of the trade, a redundant navigation system—meaning there is at least one machine in reserve if the primary one craps out. They are not pretty, but as long as they are in working order, Carroll can get a readout of his location in clear digits.

On a trackless ocean, with no street signs, a captain is constantly looking for imaginary intersections expressed in horizontal lines of latitude and vertical lines of longitude. (At the equator, the lines are sixty nautical miles apart, and are divided into minutes, which are one nautical mile apart.) With his experience, a blindfolded Carroll could conjure by memory a mental picture of latitude 48 degrees, 14.2 minutes north and longitude 124 degrees, 01.2 minutes west—which happens to be our current position in the Strait of Juan de Fuca.

But like any good captain, Carroll has been trained to mistrust his memory, to insist that his oil ship be guided not only by eye and instincts, but by the immaculate objectivity of science. So even when the crew sees a familiar landmark on shore, they must confirm where they are by employing the science of "triangulation." The sextant triangulates by scoping the angle to a couple of stars and then calculating mathematically what the third corner of that triangle would be. Modern machines do the same with radio beams and computers, eliminating the sailor's cumbersome calculations, not to mention the problem of clouds obscuring the skies. No longer do sailors need beams of starlight when they have devices that measure the length and angle of radio beams coming at our ship from land-based antennas or satellites. These tools have shelved the sextant, and they constantly update the degrees and minutes of our everchanging latitude and longitude.

The first automated system to come along was the post–World War II loran, which relies on radio beams transmitted by land-based antennas scattered around the United States and Canada. Right now, our loran receiver is tuning in to a Coast Guard antenna located on a high plateau above the Columbia River and to two others in opposite corners of the state of Nevada. The sites were chosen for altitude and remoteness, which cut down on interference. Trouble is—although the name loran is derived from the words "long range navigation"—it is a short-ranged system that cannot help a ship much more than a thousand miles from shore. It is also easily disrupted by static interference, so the federal government plans to dismantle the system around the year 2010.

SatNav, the next generation, is a system of five low-flying satellites whose radio beams are measured by the receiver on the ship that takes advantage of a phenomenon known as the Doppler effect (the apparent change of frequency that occurs in a radio beam as it travels through space—akin to the change in pitch you hear in a passing train whistle). Unfortunately, the low-flying SatNav satellites serve only a portion of the globe at any given time and they are subject to error.

GPS—the Global Positioning System—has revolutionized navigation and brought a sophisticated guidance device within reach of Joe Six-pack. Much more reliable than anything in the past, GPS, deriving information from a complex of high-flying satellites, can tell people where they are, which way they are going, how fast they are traveling, and how long it will take them to get to their destination. Under optimum conditions, with help from an accurate land-based receiver, the GPS system on the *Arco Anchorage* can establish our location within the width of a city street. So ubiquitous is this technology, it is spreading to the cabs and cabins of long-haul trucks, buses, delivery vans, airliners, ships, and even private automobiles. Handheld receivers the size of a sandwich are now advertised in magazines for the price of a good stereo system.

The history of GPS has an odd parallel to the history of the sextant, since both required the invention of a good clock to be truly accurate. The sextant, a small telescope mounted on a protractor, was better than any previous star-, sun-, or moon-measuring system, but its accuracy was questionable when mariners had no way of knowing the time of day at the all-important Greenwich meridian. European rulers offered massive rewards for a reliable ship's clock, and the bounty paid off in 1766 with the invention of the windup timepiece.

Modern scientists needed something of astounding accuracy when they conceived of a navigation system that takes readings off satellites whizzing around the earth at a distance of eleven thousand miles once every twelve hours. Miscalculate the time by nanoseconds, while triangulating a position off an object traveling that fast, and you could end up in Idaho rather than the Strait of Juan de Fuca. The key development was the atomic clock, a chronometer that parses time down to a billionth of a second using the pulsating atom. Once invented it made GPS possible.

The Defense Department conceived of the GPS system for warships, planes, and rockets in 1973, but in 1985 the Defense Department made the system available to civilians around the world, free of charge. (Using codes, the Pentagon keeps the most accurate version of the system to itself.) GPS is constantly spawning new technology. When the *Arco Anchorage* goes to the shipyard this year, an electronic chart, another GPS-based device, will be installed on the bridge. Using it, the crew will be able to watch the ship's progress as a dot on a video-screen map.

The closer we get to terra firma, though, the more Carroll and his officers will rely on the good old radar. The radars give the officers a constant picture of the surrounding land, a rough map that is amended on the screen every time the beacon makes a new sweep. Every five or ten minutes—without fail—a mate is required to check our position on the radar screen and transfer that information to a paper map in the chart room.

Whether we are relying on radar or GPS, it would be poor timing to have an electronic breakdown in inland waters like these. And if a hot wire should suddenly poke out some portion of our electronic eyesight, the crew does not include technicians trained to do surgery on them. As we head east down the cavernous underwater trench that is the Strait of Juan de Fuca, the radio officer George Peloso—the closest thing we have to a shipboard microchip man—strides onto the bridge holding a steaming cup of coffee in one hand and a sheaf of messages in another. He is savoring the good weather, and expecting no trouble. Though his white beard gives away a hint of advancing years, his hair is dark brown and the eyes look younger than his sixty-six years. He started with Texaco in 1953 and never missed a day's pay in thirty years, an unusual record in an industry so marked by strikes and laid-up ships. But tanker trips are rare for George now. Although his current three-hundred-dollar-a-day contract with Arco arose when the regular radio officer got drunk, there won't be many more summonses to the deck of a tanker. Radio officers like Peloso are a vanishing breed. With modern communication devices as easy to use as a telephone, the Federal Communications Commission gave Arco permission recently to dump its radio officers so long as the ships go no farther than 150 miles from land. In other countries, regulators are allowing ships to drop the radio officer regardless of how far the ships sail. When Carroll is on vacation next time, he will attend a brief radio course that will allow him to become the ship's radio officer when he returns. When he comes back there will be no one like Peloso, and the company will pocket the old guy's unused salary.

To Carroll, the loss of a radio officer means more work, and he might not be able to sail over the one-hundred-fathom curve exiting Hinchinbrook because it is too far from shore. But the skipper worries less about losing his radio officer than he would if the company was cutting a mate or an engineer.

To Peloso, and a fair number of others, this attitude is a mistake. He agrees that maybe the radio officer is no longer needed to send messages, but he could fix a gizmo that breaks. Granted, many members of the engine room crew are clever enough to repair electronic devices, but the computer age is rapidly leaving them behind. No one on the ship is specifically trained to troubleshoot the more complex software and hardware that hums inside the radars, collision-avoidance systems, or GPS receivers. If it is true, as some people say, that the computer is becoming as important to ship safety as the radio, then Peloso wonders why the radio operators could not be converted to computer techs rather than dumping them overboard. The salty sea air and the vibration of the ship constantly tamper with high-tech devices. Why not have someone trained to stay ahead of the trouble? Peloso doesn't blame shipowners alone for this oversight; he criticizes his fellow radio officers for miring themselves in the traditions of their job rather than retraining themselves for the future. But Peloso also asks, why are the regulators not worried about modern ships that are one failed microchip away from disaster? The answer is—like everything else in this competitive maritime world—that the issue will not reach the table until there is a well-timed disaster.

On the other hand, the more I watch the *Arco Anchorage* bridge operation, the more I realize these crew members don't blindly trust machines. They know that even a paper chart can fail them. A tanker spilled oil in Alaska's Cook Inlet when the captain relied on a chart that did not show a boulder that had moved on the bottom because of heavy underwater currents. The passenger vessel *Queen Elizabeth II* hit submerged rocks off Martha's Vineyard in part because the bumps weren't included on the map.

Teamwork and training among crew members are higher priorities to Carroll than the machines and maps he uses for guidance. As the Olympic Peninsula slips by on our right, the pulse quickens in the wheelhouse and I see the clockwork crew in action. The mate checks the map more often. The lookout glances over my shoulder at the water as we chat. The captain paces the bridge like a baseball manager in a tight ninth inning. No need to give orders when these tasks are ingrained in a sailor's memory. And this routine won't change even when the ship gets its newfangled electronic chart at the next shipyard visit. The mates will still pencil their position on the paper chart every ten minutes or so, and the captain will peer at every passing landmark. Verification keeps the officers alert, and the ship off the rocks.

Carroll has tuned this squad as well as he can in the short time he has been in charge. When he took over the ship he posted thirteen standing orders. "1. A deck officer is to be on the bridge at all times when the vessel is underway or at anchor. 2. Both radars shall be in use at all times when underway or at anchor ..." And so on. Yet Carroll leads by example, not fear, and he expects his mates to act without supervision. As near as I can tell, the three mates waltz adroitly without the dancemaster on their case. Davis visits the radar screen automatically, and when Carroll asks for a speed change or something else out of the ordinary, he replies with a simple "yes, Cap." There are no elaborate discussions over the orders of the day, and Carroll seems relatively comfortable with his high-paid partners.

Even so, fleet manager Jerry Aspland and others in the industry are taking a close look these days at the way people operate on the bridge. Using the Coast Guard estimate that human error was the cause of 215 out of 369 American accidents involving tankers during the two years ending the 1980s, Aspland believes that changes in "bridge management" are absolutely essential. While machines have changed, the watches, routine, and pecking order that govern the wheelhouse remain significantly unaltered since before the days of Captain Bligh. The Coast Guard fiddled with licensing requirements a few years ago, for the first time in four decades, but it wasn't a revolution. Unlicensed seamen no longer hold their documents for life, as they did before the *Exxon Valdez,* but must renew them every five years. There are also required drug tests, and driver license records are checked for drunken driving tickets whenever an American sailor renews his documents.

But the *Exxon Valdez* spill focused more attention on inebriation than on competence. A third mate can still qualify to be a master in nearly half the time it takes an Army second lieutenant to reach the rank of major. When he or she does get an unlimited master's ticket, a captain is qualified to drive anything from a small passenger vessel to a half-million-ton tanker. Airplane pilots are checked out and licensed for each type of aircraft they fly, but in the maritime world one unlimited license is good for all. When officers are tested, the Coast Guard examiner doesn't even sail with them to see how they do their job. Everything relies on a log of the person's experience and on a multiple-choice test.

Some critics charge that when men like Aspland focus on human error they are ducking questions about the equipment (i.e., double hulls). But Aspland says nothing affects safety more than teamwork and training. A bad decision can drive even a double hull onto the rocks with enough force to split it open. To put this to a test, Arco is conducting a long-term study of bridge operations. And, in the meantime, the company's operating instructions say each officer must know every job on the ship, including the captain's. Mates must be willing to challenge the captain if he is wrong and captains must listen and explain themselves. In the old days, the old man might have flogged an uppity mate, but Aspland hopes twenty-first-century management will go the other way and reduce the possibility of error.

Not once did I see a mate question the captain's judgment on the *Arco Anchorage*. But in support of Aspland's point of view, I noticed while reading accident reports that ships too often go astray when neither bad weather, bad equipment, nor bad luck could explain the mishap. Manmade misfortune requires no help from nature. Today, for instance, the skies are slightly cloudy but visibility is nearly perfect. The water is doing little more than rippling and we will soon pick up a pilot for our approach to the mill town of Port Angeles.

But in conditions nearly identical to these, in broad daylight on a summer afternoon, the Greek tanker *World Prodigy* ran into well-marked rocks, making Rhode Island's shoreline another victim of human error. The thirty-thousand-ton ship was only three years old and equipped with every navigational device a captain would ever need as it approached a Rhode Island pilot station in June 1989 carrying eight million gallons of Bulgarian heating oil to the city of Providence. The forty-four-year-old Greek skipper was more experienced than Carroll and he was sailing a smaller ship that could turn and stop more quickly than this one.

Yet when he slammed into the rocks, it was a textbook case of bridge management blunders.

Captain Lakovos Georgudis and his crew were relative strangers, the captain having been there for only four months. He had only six hours of sleep before he climbed the stairs to the bridge at 5 A.M. the day before the accident. Then he stayed there with nothing more than catnaps for thirty-six more hours, all because he didn't trust his officers to guide the tanker through patches of Atlantic fog and an armada of fishing boats.

Entering Narragansett Bay around four o'clock on a sunny Friday afternoon, Georgudis slowed his ship to meet his Rhode Island pilot. He was accompanied on the bridge by the chief mate, a helmsman, and a lookout—a complement similar to what we have on our bridge today. But at 4:15, he sent the lookout below to help the bosun rig a ladder for the pilot. At 4:22, he sent the chief mate downstairs to calculate the ship's draft and trim on the control room computer (the owner's agent on shore was demanding the calculations before his office closed for the weekend).

That left the captain with a relatively green twenty-nine-year-old deckhand at the helm as the tanker approached a shelf of rock shallow enough to rip three feet off the ship's hull. The visibility was great, but the groggy captain was using a British map that didn't show certain marker buoys and he was mistaken about the spot where he was supposed to meet his pilot. Then, worried that the chief mate had not returned with the calculations for the main office, he went back to the chart room himself to do the figuring on a pocket calculator. That left the young helmsman in charge, with no one checking the ship's position. No one noticed the buoy on the left side of the ship that should have been on the right. The pilot—heading toward the ship in a boat—noticed the tanker's predicament and radioed a warning to move left, but Georgudis told the helmsman to steer a meager ten degrees, when he should have ordered a crash stop. By then, the ship was going aground.

Early the next morning near Newport, Rhode Island, a man watching the oil spill cleanup from a state park remarked to a reporter that guys like Georgudis "ought to hang." When investigators asked the captain how he had grounded his ship on Brenton Reef he replied, "That's my big question."

You would think this would send a message to all fleets of the world about bridge management, but it didn't. Shortly after the *World Prodigy* grounding, the International Maritime Organization endorsed money-saving experiments where ships would sail with only one person on the bridge at a time—an all-purpose officer pinch-hitting as his own mate, lookout, and helmsman. Fortunately, in these waters, the Coast Guard is considering a rule requiring two people on the bridge at all times.

But an international treaty that set better standards for watch-standing languished in the U.S. Congress for more than a decade because politically well-connected companies that run fleets of boats carrying supplies and people to offshore oil-drilling rigs in places like the Gulf of Mexico feared the standards would force them to hire more crew. The treaty—first proposed by the U.S. Coast Guard—was ratified only after the influential boat-owners were assured it would not affect them.

Obeying good watchstanding practices, we slow down to meet our pilot near Port Angeles. We are passed in the strait by a Navy Trident submarine going the other way. Over the radio, we pick up an officer on the sub who is forcefully telling the Russian freighter ahead of him to stay the hell out of his way. The Navy guy's voice booms with irritation and the Russian, speaking in broken English, sounds apologetic. It's a bitch driving a boat loaded with nuclear weapons down a crowded waterway.

Driving a tanker is not much more fun, especially when it is going slow. Cropper is turning the wheel, and the ship is responding glacially, since the water pushes less forcefully on a rudder moving slower than ten knots. Go much slower than six knots and you can't steer much at all.

There are at least four ways to control the rudder on this ship. One is the steering wheel, which sends a signal to a switch downstairs that moves a steering gear piston that moves the rudder. Another is a little black handle next to the steering wheel that will send a similar signal to the switch downstairs. A third system is the autopilot. And if all else fails, an engineman could steer the ship by flipping the control switches down in the steering gear room himself. And in a final desperate move, the engine room crew could ratchet the rudder around by hand—a very slow process.

Right now, down in the rear of the hull, both *Arco Anchorage* steering gears are up and running. Each machine—the size of a big generator—has hydraulic rams that can swing the rudder from one side to the other in twenty-eight seconds. Coast Guard rules say both machines must be functioning whenever the ship is near shore—a belt and suspenders approach. Only out in the ocean is the ship allowed to run on one gear at a time.

While the redundancy close to shore may sound reassuring, some researchers say it does more harm than good. National Transportation Safety Board investigators have discovered that, when two steering gears run simultaneously, and one malfunctions, the bad one will fight with the good one and both will be paralyzed. The result, documented in several accidents, has been a tanker with a mind of its own. The NTSB recommends that only one steering gear system be operated at a time, but the Coast Guard has been reluctant to change the rule. As with all things in the maritime industry, it will take time to sort this out. Rules and traditions die slowly.

The best we can do on the *Arco Anchorage,* I guess, is to pay attention to where we are going. Of that, we got confirmation only this morning. A captain on a coastwise tanker like the *Arco Anchorage* never knows until the last day whether his destination will be changed, to feed some other region's craving for oil, before he reaches port. We didn't know last night—absolutely for sure—whether the company would keep us going to Cherry Point or reroute us to Panama. As it is, the schedulers have made one alteration in our itinerary. Before we steam to Cherry Point, the ship must anchor at Port Angeles where it will take on bunker fuel and allow a crew of contractors to work on our busted winches. Our stop in Port Angeles is necessary because another ship is taking up our place at the Cherry Point dock, and spending more time there than expected. Port Angeles, located some sixty-three miles from the entrance to the Strait of Juan de Fuca, has a nicely protected harbor where a lot of ships and tankers pick up fuel or make repairs. Pulling into the gas station is also an opportunity for crew members to go on a furlough. The pulpmill town isn't much, but it is bigger than Valdez and closer than the communities around Cherry Point, which are a thirty-dollar cab ride away from the refinery. Newman says a stop in Port Angeles is a respite from jail. "Make a phone call, do a little shopping, God forbid, have a little brew."

15

Why a Fender Bender Killed
Four Thousand Birds

*(Port Angeles,
January 29, 1 P.M.)*

W e are near enough to Port Angeles to read tall words on the sides
of buildings. Before we enter the harbor, the pilot boat nestles
up to the side of the ship effortlessly and two Port Angeles pilots
ascend the ship's ladder. A senior pilot is teaching a younger guy how
to handle a tanker. Striding toward the house, the older fellow looks
grandfatherly in a comfortable red sweater and gray fedora hat. The
younger man, in a white shirt and tie, could be selling insurance as he
hands the captain a newspaper and chats briefly about the condition
of the ship.

The pilots order the *Arco Anchorage* to slow down to four knots
for its final approach to the harbor. The port is protected by Ediz Hook,
a long jetty whose name is derived from its curving shape. A Russian
cargo vessel and a worn-looking American oil tanker are visible inside
when our ship reaches the end of the hook just east of the harbor
entrance. The mill-town smokestacks smolder in front of a spectacular
hedge of mountains. The ridge rises so impatiently behind Port Angeles that a brief drive takes tourists to a mile-high viewpoint where
untracked wilderness unfolds in one direction and glittering seascape
in the other.

The mile-wide harbor is tricky, though, because 40 percent of it,
the portion closest to town, is too shallow to accommodate a tanker

loaded this deeply. To avoid going aground, the ship must execute a J-shaped turn to stay in the north end of the harbor where the water is deeper. The senior pilot is giving the junior guy some advice about all this. "Never put your nose into Ediz Hook. Put your nose on the tip or just east of it." As he says this, the current plays games with our course. The helmsman is steering 145 degrees, but the ship is making 155.

As we slide past Ediz Hook, I can't help but smile as the radio picks up some talk from a northbound Japanese ship, the *Matsukaze*, which is reporting its position on the Pacific Ocean just outside the strait. We have heard radio reports on this trip from some hall-of-fame tankers, including the *American Trader* that recently spilled oil, the *Golden Gate*, which ran over a fishing boat, and the *Thompson Pass*, which cracked open at Valdez. But the *Matsukaze* popping up on the airwaves is something special, especially as we enter Port Angeles harbor.

In April 1988 the *Matsukaze* was barreling the same direction as it is today when the lone officer on the bridge sat down on the captain's chair and fell asleep. At Whiskey Creek Beach, seventeen miles west of here, the ship missed a dogleg turn and sailed straight onto the beach at a speed exceeding fourteen nautical miles per hour. The impact was like an early morning earthquake as twenty thousand tons of steel, corn oil, cottonseed oil, lube oil, tallow, and bunker fuel punched ashore. A huge boulder ripped the keel open the way an angler's knife slits the belly of a fish, and the stone jammed so hard into the stern, it was carried back to Japan with the vessel before it could be removed.

Yet the sliced tanker spilled absolutely nothing, not an ounce of the ship's cargo or fuel. The reason was simple: The *Matsukaze* is protected by a double bottom consisting of a layer of steel on the outside, a vacant space and then another layer of steel surrounding the cargo itself.

Such was not the case two and a half years earlier when this ship, the *Arco Anchorage,* touched a rock on the bottom of Port Angeles harbor at a speed slower than an old man's walk. When the ship's plating broke open, oil was spilled and four thousand birds died and a generation of clams was heavily damaged. All this happened because the *Arco Anchorage* has less than an inch and a half of steel to protect its cargo from the sea. There is no double bottom, like the one on the *Matsukaze*.

So every time the *Matsukaze* pulls into the Strait of Juan de Fuca, it makes a solid argument for double hulls. And every time the *Arco Anchorage* enters Port Angeles harbor it provides a hearty "amen."

It was December 21, 1985, the shortest day of the year, when the *Arco Anchorage* made its fateful turn into the mill-town harbor following a three-day voyage from Valdez. The situation was practically identical to the one we face today. The captain was informed by radio a few hours earlier that the Cherry Point refinery dock was busy so he would have to drop anchor in Port Angeles for a short layover. The weather was what we see today: calm seas, a forty-degree temperature, unnoticeable wind, and a slight haze that didn't hide much from view. There was nothing in the air or the water to make a sailor dread this approach, just an ordinary maneuver four days before Christmas.

Captain Robert Sullivan was youthful like Carroll, although he had more years in the captain's suite. The only change in routine was the early arrival of the pilot, Robert Leson, who was filling in for someone else and had extra time to spare. The *Arco Anchorage* was dogging along at six knots in a smooth sea so the sixty-five-year-old pilot had no trouble climbing the rope ladder to the tanker deck. The crew had never seen this pilot before, but he had a credible bearing about him and a professional composure. The chief mate said he was so quiet, he was boring, yet he gave his commands with great authority.

What they didn't know was that Leson had been involved in ten reportable incidents in an equal number of years as a pilot, grounding three ships and bumping several docks. His dossier was so checkered that the state pilotage commission reprimanded him twice and later changed its procedures for reviewing pilots' records. But pilots don't wear their records on their sleeve and no one on the *Arco Anchorage* knew what they were dealing with that day. Leson himself had a very different view of his past than others did. Fifty years on ships, starting as a lowly deckhand, made him feel as though he knew a thing or two about the sea. He believed his unhappy record as a pilot was little more than the pilotage commission harassing him for others' mistakes. He dismissed his critics as armchair mariners who are "never there at three o'clock in the morning when these things come up." A pilot, he once said, "is paid to take chances."

Sullivan was under the impression, of course, that pilots would not take chances with his ship. As he turned the controls over to Leson that day, the captain stood back and watched the pilot with trust. Some investigators say the ship was in trouble almost immediately. They believe the tanker's final approach brought it too close to the outer edge of the harbor, a move that necessitated an unusually wide J-turn to keep it on course. Whether that was true—or whether the problem was the swift currents, as Leson would later claim—the pilot ordered a sharp increase in propeller speed to give the rudder more turning power as the ship rounded the bend into the mile-wide entrance at Ediz Hook.

Trying to stay near the north end where the fathoms are generous, Leson told the crew to hold the accelerator at a relatively fast forty-five RPMs, during the sharp twenty-degree turn. But a vessel skids as it turns, and moves mysteriously with the currents and quirks of the local waters. The *Arco Anchorage* was turning in the direction of safe waters but sliding slowly toward the shallow shelf at the south end of the harbor.

The captain was getting nervous by this time, but still made no comment to the pilot. Even the third officer, standing on the bow waiting to drop anchor, felt queasy. "It was not a beautiful approach," she would later say. Yet the closest thing to an outward expression of alarm came from the helmsman, who repeated the pilot's commands with a louder voice than normal, as if to subtly plead with Leson for reconsideration.

A tanker crashes at a slothful pace, not at blinding speed like a car; the accident is usually well under way by the time anyone on board realizes what is happening. In the case of the *Arco Anchorage,* the pilot had time to put the engines in full reverse, but instead he ordered half power because he was under the impression the *Arco Anchorage* boilers couldn't handle the pressure. Someone once told him this ship's engines had a tendency to die, or even to explode, when the turbines were thrown into full-speed reverse. He could have asked the captain whether that was true, but he didn't.

With the propeller grinding backward at half speed, the ship finally slowed down and came to a stop. Then it began moving slowly backward and to the left, toward the shallows. At slow speed, a ship with one propeller will always drift—or "walk"—in the direction the propeller is turning. (Double screws on other types of ships overcome this tendency because the props turn in opposite directions, canceling each other out.)

As the vessel slowed, the captain felt more troubled by the ship's position. The Fathometer indicated there was plenty of room underneath the hull, but any mariner knows that the depth sounder is measuring the bottom under just one portion of the 900-foot-long hull. There was plenty of water underneath the depth sounder, but 125 feet forward the vessel was going aground.

"Are you happy with the spot?" the captain asked the pilot as the ship slowed almost to a stop. Leson responded that he was content with the location and Sullivan ordered the anchor dropped. The chain got hung up in the winch for nearly a minute until a crewman hit the brake, to loosen it, with a hammer.

Even though the ship was moving sideways at less than two miles an hour, it would have taken more than a 15-ton anchor to stop it. Only the power of two locomotive engines pushing with all their might would have halted the momentum of this 120,000-ton mass. Experts say the tanker's belly slid over a huge boulder and kept moving across it for several minutes. The first victims were some ratfish and dogfish squashed underneath. The steel plates on the bottom of the ship—one and five-sixteenths inches thick—were pushed upward some six inches with a force of a half-million pounds of pressure, until the metal could no longer take the strain. With an instantaneous rending like a popped balloon, the hull ripped apart, opening a forty-foot crack in two cargo tanks.

Up on the bridge, the crew heard a sound like three muffled gunshots. The captain and crew looked at each other with an expression of frozen puzzlement. Somebody asked whether a door had slammed. Someone else wondered whether something had been dropped on the deck. It was wishful thinking. The skipper ran to the window and saw mud frothing up from under the ship. Then he saw the oil, thousands of gallons of oil, erupting from under the left side of the ship like a thick black milkshake. The captain knew in an instant that his career might be slipping away. He ordered the pumps started to suck oil from the ruptured tanks. It was a good move. Only 4 percent of their contents entered the water. The remainder stayed inside when the level in the tanks reached equilibrium with the level of the water outside.

The beginning of cleanup, however, was all too typical chaos. It would be another three hours before any containment booms were available to surround the mess quickly spreading from the *Arco Anchorage*. The 239,000 gallons that escaped the ship was small by world standards, but plenty enough to do tremendous damage to the harbor's environment. Dungeness Spit, east of town, is a wintering spot for over a hundred thousand waterfowl. At one time or another, every species of migrating bird in North America visits here. Also in the path of the oil were the breeding grounds of commercially valuable crabs and clams.

The captain and his crew scattered to the pump room and down to the deck to do what they could. Left alone, the pilot checked the ship's position, already thinking of his defense in court. The captain returned and asked the pilot why he had guided the ship so deeply into the harbor. "I wanted to stay clear of traffic," he said. With that, forty-five minutes after the accident, the pilot left the ship and the mess to the captain. Leson watched his career go down the drain on the evening news. "It spoiled my whole week."

Arco spent eleven million dollars on the cleanup and accepted a thirty-thousand-dollar state fine. Leson retired and appealed a thirty-thousand-dollar fine levied on him. Although he lost his case on appeal after appeal, Leson insists to this day that the ship hit a deadhead log, not a rock, and that he was framed by Arco and the Coast Guard.

For his part in the accident, Captain Sullivan was neither fined nor charged with any violation, but the company demoted him to chief mate. He rose in rank again, and was demoted again, when he and another pilot drove the unloaded *Arco Juneau* into the side of the Carquinez Bridge near Vallejo, California, in February 1988.

There are a lot of questions that could have been asked following the *Arco Anchorage* grounding. Shouldn't the captain have spoken up earlier? Shouldn't the state pilotage commission keep a trouble-prone pilot like Leson away from oil-carrying ships? Probably.

But there was one simple truth tragically lost in the debate: The ship would not have spilled a drop of oil if it had been equipped with a double bottom like the *Matsukaze*. That fact was not mentioned by the Coast Guard in its final report.

Experts have debated for decades how well tankers are protected by double layers of steel. Tanker consultant Arthur McKenzie likes to take his argument from the kitchen; he argues that proportionately, the steel skin of a single-hulled tanker would be as thin as a cellophane wrapper if the tanker were shrunk to the size of a bread loaf. "Would you feel safe carrying oil in a plastic bag?"

The argument over the need for double bottoms became very public in 1967 after the *Torrey Canyon* hit the rocks in a grounding so violent that the ship would have spilled oil even if it had had a double bottom. The disaster, however, taught the public an important lesson. Once millions of gallons of oil get in the water, you can't clean it up. If double bottoms would prevent other spills, the public was all for it. Nevertheless, single-hulled ships like the *Arco Anchorage* kept rolling out of the shipyards as foot-dragging, greed, obfuscation, and a public-be-damned attitude prevailed.

Even after hundreds of spills where a double bottom would have made a difference, some tanker people view the double skin with great skepticism. They cite real and imagined difficulties with salvaging and operating the ships and some feel the unwashed landlubbers have no right interfering with their business.*

---

*In the beginning, the debate focused on the "double bottom," not the more complete shroud known as a "double hull." A double-bottom ship the size of the *Arco Anchorage*

As I peeled through mounds of reports written after the *Torrey Canyon* spill, I came to realize that all the proof ever needed in favor of double bottoms was gathered during the first three years of the 1970s by a small group of Coast Guard officers working on the eighth floor of Washington, D.C., headquarters. One was an Illinois-bred engineer named Jim Card, a meticulous technician who seemed destined to make admiral when he graduated in 1964 among the top ten of his U.S. Coast Guard Academy class. He was a junior-grade lieutenant on a West Coast cutter when the *Torrey Canyon* hit Seven Stones Reef in England. Then in 1970 he earned dual master's degrees in naval architecture and mechanical engineering at the Massachusetts Institute of Technology and joined a Coast Guard bureaucracy, called the Merchant Marine Technical Division, where the main task was finding errors in shipbuilders' blueprints. However, when a rash of tanker accidents inspired a new emphasis on environmental safety, Card and six other men in the technical division began work that was to leave them at the center of the tanker debate for decades to come. Along with Card, there was supervisor Henry Bell, who two decades later would help write one of the most devastating reports the Coast Guard ever published on the subject of tanker safety. Another top officer, Gene Henn, would head up and profoundly change the agency's safety and inspection program following the *Exxon Valdez* spill. A third, William Benkert, would lead the Coast Guard effort to mandate double bottoms in the early 1970s, and then switch sides to head an industry organization firmly opposed to the idea. And Card's coworkers—Virgil Keith, Joseph Porricelli, and Richard Storch—would coauthor a landmark report on the safety problems plaguing the tanker industry.

In 1971, the group issued a report, "Tankers and the Ecology," in which they used data taken from fourteen hundred spills, fires, explosions, hull cracks, engine failures, and collisions to argue that double

---

would have a layer of steel, a nine-foot space, and another layer of steel between the bottom of the cargo tanks and the sea. A double-hulled ship would have a similar protection up the sides as well. A double bottom protects against groundings while a double side is defense against collisions.

hulls, inert gas, stronger ships, clean ballast tanks, vessel traffic systems, and improved ship controls would help prevent future spills. One wonders if anyone was listening.

At first, the answer seemed to be in the positive. A meeting of the United Nations' International Maritime Organization (then called the International Maritime Consultative Organization) was set for the fall of 1973 in London. On the agenda was a provision that would require double bottoms. Bell wanted to take strong evidence to London because tanker owners were firmly against the idea, partly because double-bottom ships cost 5 to 30 percent more than single-hulled ships, and partly because a double-bottom ship carries less oil than a single-hulled vessel. Bell asked Card to determine whether a double bottom would have prevented previous spills involving single-hulled tankers. Card's task was immediately made more difficult by the sketchy state of Coast Guard investigation records. He had to search shipyard repair records and painstakingly reconstructed how rocks had penetrated each tanker bottom.

The process took months, but Card produced a report strong enough to withstand scrutiny. It showed, very clearly, that in twenty-seven out of the thirty tanker spills, no oil would have escaped the ships had they been equipped with double bottoms. A total of over three million gallons would have stayed in the tanks. Many of the accidents he reviewed were hauntingly similar to what would happen to the *Arco Anchorage* in 1985.

Unfortunately, few owners were impressed, and the double bottom was rejected. Despite the lack of international action, some in Congress wanted the United States to go it alone, to require that oil ships visiting American shores be equipped with double bottoms. The Coast Guard at first seemed to support the measure, when the commandant gave notice in January 1973 that the agency was considering a double-bottom regulation. But under pressure from the industry and a Republican administration reluctant to buck the owners, the Coast Guard snapped an about-face and supported a weak alternative.

To insure against future initiatives, the industry went on a counteroffensive against double bottoms by gathering support from key members of Congress. One was New York Congressman John Murphy, chairman of a committee that oversaw the Coast Guard, who told the agency to ignore the "ivory tower experts who would use this issue . . . for a few days of political gain." Murphy would later be convicted in federal court of accepting bribes from federal agents posing as oil-rich Arabs in a case known as Abscam.

Card, Bell, and others continued their work, but industry intransigence took its toll. Keith and Porricelli left the Coast Guard and together formed a consulting firm, based in Annapolis, Maryland, that later lent a strong voice to the state of Alaska's case against Exxon following the *Exxon Valdez* spill. To Keith, the arguments in favor of double hulls were simply good science. "You can't beat the laws of physics."

Storch grew tired watching the moneyed and powerful ignore the laws of physics and left the Coast Guard and the capital for a career as a University of Washington engineering professor. He thought someone, maybe the insurance companies, would understand the difference between the minor cost of double hulls and the major expense of spills, but he grew disillusioned with the ability of reason to make an impact on the system. "I don't think there was any strong resolve on the part of anyone, including the Coast Guard, to push it very hard."

Despite what appeared to be a defeat on the issue, double-bottom advocates kept the debate alive. And then in 1976, Jimmy Carter was elected president, and the single-hulled tanker *Argo Merchant* spilled nearly eight million gallons of fuel oil off Nantucket Island, all in a month's time. In subsequent months, fourteen more tankers spilled oil. The public was up in arms, and the new administration was inclined to do something.

The double-hull debate revolved around three issues:

Salvage: Opponents claim a double bottom fills with water in an accident, making the ship harder to control. Proponents say the heavier ship is easier to rescue because it stays in place.

Operations: Opponents say fumes from leaking tanks collect in the space between double hulls making them susceptible to explosions. Proponents say you just fill them with inert gas. Opponents say sailors will get lost cleaning the honeycomb maze of a double hull. Proponents suggest making double bottoms easier to enter.

Cost: Opponents say building double hulls is too expensive; proponents say it would add less than half a penny to the price of gasoline at the pump.

Two outspoken men, William O. Gray and Arthur McKenzie, stepped into the fray, representing some of the greatest expertise in the industry. Although they spent much of their careers in the same tanker division at Exxon, they are like bookends in the double-hull debate; Gray is the most noted opponent of double hulls, and McKenzie is the top advocate.

Gray doesn't look like the distinguished son of a chemical company executive who grew up in Greenwich, Connecticut, but more like a Nebraska farm kid, with a lanky frame, a large friendly face, and a dominating set of ears. After getting degrees in mechanical engineering and naval architecture from Yale and the University of Michigan in the mid-1950s, he did stints as a naval officer and a ship designer with Bethlehem Steel. But when the American shipyards hit their decline, he joined Exxon and soon became one of its most innovative engineers.

Exxon was the dominant force in the tanker industry, and other companies often followed in its wake. Yet after Gray convinced the company in the late 1960s to build five large tankers with segregated ballast tanks (located where they would protect some of the cargo tanks from collisions), the senior management abandoned the idea when the tanker magnate Daniel Ludwig announced the construction of much bigger ships than Exxon's. "Geez, can't you do that, too?" said one. The company ordered Gray and his colleagues to redesign the Exxon vessels without segregated ballast so they could hold more oil. Although Gray was disappointed, he bit his tongue and for years guided the company adroitly through many public relations storms. McKenzie, who describes Gray as a friend, calls him "the Rommel of the oil companies." While at times critical of tanker operators, Gray's vast knowledge and skill made him one of industry's best public relations weapons. He has been especially adroit in arguing there is simply no proof that double bottoms and double hulls work well enough to be mandated.

McKenzie is not cowed. Born on a sailboat in Maine more than seventy years ago, he seemed destined to be involved in the tanker business: his father, a onetime missionary, was a tanker captain; his brother, cousin, and a couple of uncles also served on oil ships. McKenzie served more than a decade aboard Exxon tankers (then called Standard Oil of New Jersey), but after World War II ended he took a series of shoreside jobs with Exxon because he disliked the mucking out of tanks and the cramped ship life. He oversaw tanker operations, worked on the ice-breaking *Manhattan* project, set up a noted ship-handling school in Grenoble, France, and helped devise the method of cleaning tanks with crude oil rather than water. When he retired from Exxon in 1974, Gray took over his senior nautical advisor job.

McKenzie became interested in double bottoms after talking to a Coast Guard officer who was headed for the 1973 London conference, and by the time he retired from Exxon he was an avowed advocate. He has become so involved that today his name is synonymous with the debate.

Many double-bottom proponents felt their time had come when President Carter presented Congress with an environmental package that included a proposal for mandatory double bottoms. In February 1978, another treaty conference was held in London to take a second look at the unratified 1973 agreement. The Carter administration saw it as an opportunity to make the case for double bottoms again, and so did people like McKenzie. But once again the IMO trotted out Gray's favorite compromise—ships would be built with segregated ballast tanks located in places where they would protect some, but not all, of the cargo tanks. Double bottoms and double hulls were rejected, and even existing ships were exempted from segregated ballast. Today, a decade and a half after the London conference, fewer than 40 percent of the world's oil tankers have segregated ballast tanks. As for double hulls, less than 15 percent of the world's tankers have them.

Some double-bottom advocates blamed the head of the U.S. delegation, then-Admiral Benkert, for presenting a lukewarm case. "Sometimes I wonder if the U.S. Coast Guard is really a subsidiary of the oil industry—you certainly mouth their ideas and proposals," said George Reinhard, in a letter to Benkert following the conference. But Benkert, a hero in the Coast Guard who has a mountain in Antarctica named after him, told me in an interview shortly before he died that he did the best he could. "We busted our ass." He said Card's studies, without follow-up research, did not provide enough information to build "a strong, overpowering statistical case." He ultimately did admit he had not been an advocate of double bottoms. "All this stuff costs money. I could build you a tanker tomorrow that would be risk-free from the standpoint of spills. Somewhere in here there should be a happy medium." Maybe chemical tankers need double hulls because chemicals hurt people but, "We have not seen fit to approach crude oil, or other types of petroleum products, in the same vein because the risk isn't there for people."

When Benkert retired five months after the London conference he became president of the American Institute of Merchant Shipping, an organization of shipowners that had opposed double bottoms.

The reforms that did come out of the London treaties failed to stem the tide of oil spills. One month after the 1978 conference, the *Amoco Cadiz* dumped sixty-eight million gallons of crude oil off the French coast, the worst tanker disaster ever. More spills and more hand-wringing followed, but for over a decade the battle for double hulls was lost. The economic pall that hung over the troubled tanker industry left no one in the mood to spend extra money for safer ships. And with the government budget cuts of the 1980s, the revolution that began on the eighth floor of the Coast Guard's Washington, D.C., headquarters was shelved. For a decade, the world paid little attention to tankers. There were spills, but they didn't happen in the right place.

Then came the March 24, 1989, grounding of the *Exxon Valdez* on Bligh Reef. Ironically, like the *Torrey Canyon,* it was a grounding so violent it would have pierced a double bottom. Yet it once again showed the public, with television clips of dying otters and birds, how hopeless it is to clean up oil once it gets into the water. When subsequent studies indicated the tanker would have spilled less oil with a double bottom, the debate heated up again. Adding to the controversy was a series of additional spills, including the February 1990 accident where the tanker *American Trader* ran over its own anchor off Huntington Beach, California. In that case—a clear argument for double bottoms—the Coast Guard captain in charge of the cleanup was none other than Card himself. "It makes you wonder," said Card, who attained the rank of admiral shortly afterward.

In 1990, the U.S. Congress passed a law requiring tankers entering U.S. waters to have double hulls on a gradual schedule that ends in the year 2015 and the International Maritime Organization followed suit with a similar provision worldwide. To achieve passage, however, Congress left room for future disasters. The generous schedule means the single-hull tankers stay afloat for a long time. Also, the double sides required on the new ships will be too thin to withstand the impact of most major collisions. Studies have shown that a double side must be extremely wide—maybe twenty-seven feet on this ship—to buffer against the extreme force of a run-in with another ship. Something that beefy would take up two-fifths of the overall width of the ship, displacing too much cargo space, in the view of shipowners.

There had to be trade-offs. But even more important, the law gave opponents one more chance. It said double hulls would be required only if the National Research Council did not, in a subsequent study, come up with a better alternative. It was a matter of pride for the tanker industry to find one.

"If I am going to commit suicide, at least I should have the right to choose my own weapon," said London-based tanker owner Phillip Embericos.

Gray, who left Exxon in 1987 and joined the Skaarup Oil Corporation in Connecticut, was appointed to the all-important National Research Council board that was assigned by Congress to determine whether the double hull or an alternative would prevail. Other members were: Henry Marcus, an MIT professor; David Bovet, a naval architect and author of an early Coast Guard double-bottom study; J. Huntly Boyd, Jr., a naval architect and noted salvage expert; John Boylston, a ship manager and designer; John Burke, an oil company tanker executive; Thomas Hopkins, an economics professor; James Hornsby, a former Canadian Coast Guard official; Vojin Joksimovich, an expert on risk; Sally Ann Lentz, an environmentalist with Friends of the Earth; Robert Loewy, an engineering professor; and Tomasz Wierzbicki, another MIT professor. Marcus was chairman and Gray was vice chairman.

The board looked at a number of alternatives: ships with double sides and no double bottoms; tankers with double bottoms and no double sides; protectively located segregated ballast tanks; smaller tanks to reduce the size of spills; a flexible membrane that is like an inner tube inside a tank; a vacuum system that prevents a spill the way you stop water from flowing out a straw by putting your thumb on top; and a practice where tanks are loaded only as high as the sea level outside (the oil stays inside a punctured ship because it is in "hydrostatic balance" with the heavier water of the surrounding ocean). Only one proposal, however, emerged as a possible alternative to double hulls. The final research council report said an innovation known as the Intermediate Oil-Tight Deck warranted further study and should not be rejected outright as a substitute. Otherwise, the report said, double hulls were the best idea.

The mid-deck tanker, as it is called, has a double side wide enough to protect against collisions but no double bottom. To prevent a spill in case the bottom is punctured, the design relies on the "inverted jar" principle. If you fill a jar with oil, and submerge it in water upside down, the oil won't leak out even if you remove the lid because the heavier water pushes upward, keeping the lighter oil inside.

To create the same effect, a mid-deck tanker is built with cargo tanks divided into upper and lower halves by a sealed barrier known as the middle deck. When the ship is loaded, the lower tank always rides completely below the waterline. If the bottom of the ship is ever punctured, the submerged lower tank would act like the jar and keep most of the oil inside. The upper tank is not affected. And because the mid-deck tanker wastes no space on a double bottom, it can have wider double sides.

Gray especially liked the idea because a ship with such wide double sides is a lot like his favorite double-hull compromise of the past, protectively located, segregated ballast tanks.

But others, like McKenzie, saw the mid-deck tanker as unproven technology since no tanker of such a design had ever been built or tested. He believed it was a red herring tossed out by the tanker industry to foil the double-hull requirement. Gray nearly admitted as much when he said to me, "I'm not just in favor of the mid-deck tanker. I'm anti-mandate for the double hull."

Gray and Marcus were the only two research council board members strongly in favor of the mid-deck alternative. The others disagreed in varying degrees, mostly because the idea was untested. The mid-deck design survived the research council review because Gray argued so fervently for it. By getting the council's nod, the mid-deck design was thrust into the international limelight.

After the research council report was issued, I learned that the debate was tinged at the last moment by a sticky controversy. When the board was drafting its final report, Marcus revealed that Gray's boss—Ollie Skaarup—had given Marcus's department at MIT a $120,000 grant shortly after Marcus was appointed to the study panel. Some board members were concerned not only because Gray and Marcus were the only two who strongly favored the mid-deck design, but because Skaarup had recently signed a joint venture with a Japanese shipping firm, Mitsui OSK Line. Another Japanese company, Mitsubishi Heavy Industries, was then in the forefront of advocating mid-deck tankers. "They suggested, therefore, that I was carrying the ball for the Japanese companies," said Gray. "I felt mad and sick." The panel quizzed the two men at a meeting in early 1992 and the council's marine board staff director, Charles Bookman, investigated. He concluded there was no connection between Skaarup and Mitsubishi and therefore no conflict of interest. "We decided this was an appearance problem, not an actual problem," said Bookman. "I don't think Bill [Gray] had anything to do with the grant. Hank [Marcus] has had a long association with Ollie Skaarup. He knows him well." Said Marcus, of the flap, "I view it as a non-item."

Later, however, Skaarup and Mitsubishi would collaborate on a joint study that said the mid-deck tanker design is more effective, in some accidents, than a double hull.

What was important to Gray in the research council deliberation was that the mid-deck tanker idea had survived its most rigorous hurdle, emerging as a counterpoint to the double hull and keeping the debate alive. If you believe Gray, he was championing an alternative that might save the world from spills caused by collisions. If you listen to critics like McKenzie, it was a last-ditch effort to stave off the double hull and other reforms imposed after the *Exxon Valdez* disaster. Shed doubt on one part of the package, and the whole thing, including liability provisions, might unravel.

When the IMO agreed at a 1992 meeting to accept the mid-deck tanker as an alternative to double hulls, it seemed as though Gray and the other mid-deck advocates had gained advantage.

But McKenzie and the other double-hull advocates were not sitting still. Other researchers, some friendly to McKenzie, including his son, soon demonstrated, using models in test tanks, that the unproven mid-deck tankers would spill oil whenever the bottom is pierced because a ship will rock back and forth, discharging the cargo as it is agitated. And the whole idea depends on the notion that the middle deck will remain intact. Wary of untried notions, and influenced by these studies, the Coast Guard rejected the mid-deck tanker as an alternative, thus effectively killing the idea—for now.

Despite the double-hull legislation, there are several unresolved safety problems. Some experts worry that the steel on the new double-hulled tankers will be rationed between the inner and outer hulls, making both of them weak. The result could be another rash of buckling and cracking ships. McKenzie feels new tankers should be built 30 percent beefier than they are now.

Scary, too, are the prospects of explosions because the Coast Guard and the IMO standards do not require the owners to fill the buffer spaces between hulls with inert gas. William Chadwick, chief inspector with the Liberian registry, says his organization sent out an official warning to owners of double-hulled ships, saying that not inerting the void spaces is like playing with fire. Inevitably, there are going to be cracks and leaks of fumes, and then all that is needed is a source of ignition. Chevron official Tom Wyman counters that his company will prevent trouble by using good maintenance procedures. But for Chadwick history suggests that not all owners will be so responsible.

Arco fleet manager Jerry Aspland sees another problem with public perception: that the citizenry will assume all is well now that the law says the tanker industry must build double-hulled ships. As he told one public gathering, "Do not walk away from it now."

As he sails the *Arco Anchorage* into Port Angeles harbor today, Carroll pays close attention to his position in the harbor, staying well clear of the south end where he understands the price of a fender bender.

The *Arco Anchorage* has cut an easy wake into a glassy smooth harbor and the ship's single hull is well clear of any rocks. The tanker comes to a stop and the pilot gives his okay to drop anchor. Carroll gives the order to release the hook. His command comes out of the walkie-talkie that chief mate Svetko Lisica is holding in his hand as he stands at the bow looking over the railing. He tells the bosun to release the anchor, and the bosun pulls a rusty handle. An incredible cloud of red dust fills the air as tons of steel chain clatters down the hawsepipe with the sound of a metallic thunderstorm. The anchor hits the water with a slow splash and when it reaches the bottom the chain keeps going for a while. The bosun explains that the anchor itself is not what will hold us in place. The chain is a lot heavier than the anchor, and it does most of the work.

I wander up to the captain's office and remind him of the accident that took place here more than five years ago. I ask him about double hulls and like most crew members he is ambivalent. Most say the double hull is not good enough, that it would not prevent many types of spills, including those caused by collisions. Carroll says the value of double hulls depends on conditions—the weather, the speed, the load, and the skill of the crew. Sure the *Arco Anchorage* would not have spilled oil in 1985 if it had had one, but the *Exxon Valdez* would have dumped cargo regardless. If his ship had a double hull, Carroll says, "I'm not going to drive it any differently."

16

Pooping in the Wind

(Port Angeles Harbor,
January 29, 4 P.M.)

C arroll leans back in his chair, puts a steel-toed running shoe on the
desk and cradles the back of his head with his hands. As the ship
drifts in a slow arc around the anchor, I can see the snow-capped
Olympic Mountains in the porthole behind him. The afternoon scenery
changes a tad as we talk and so, too, does the mood. We are discussing
the single most expensive ecological disaster in history—the nearly
three-billion-dollar cleanup that Exxon paid for in Alaska. The captain
draws in a breath and looks at the ceiling, as though he could find
something up there to erase the idea. Spills are not something a tanker
captain likes to dwell on, but he must consider the danger every time
he sails. He could ring up an Exxon-sized tab tomorrow night making
a wrong turn in Rosario Strait.

Studies say the "worst-case scenario" in these parts is a grounding involving a tanker the size of the *Arco Anchorage* in the narrowest
portion of Rosario Strait, a spot we must pass through more than
halfway between here and the Cherry Point refinery. If that happens,
and the ship dumps the same percentage of cargo lost by the *Exxon
Valdez,* it would release seven million gallons of crude oil, enough to
devastate the area and overwhelm any cleanup effort. Since most oil
remains in the tanks, it is unlikely the ship would dump its whole load
of thirty-five million gallons. The thought is hardly consolation, how-

ever, because after you've chucked at least a million gallons, the amount of oil doesn't matter. Everything is black, ugly, and hopeless as far as the eye can see. Birds, sea otters, whales . . . every poor creature that uses the water surface can fall prey to the muck. Death is a pretty good bet for the panicked bird who tries to preen oil from his feathers, only to have it slide down his throat. A sea mammal whose well-groomed fur loses its insulating power finds himself in the unfamiliar grip of the water's icy temperature. An oiled beach is a morass of undulating tragedy.

Most of us watch these scenes with horror, but it is a detached sort of horror. For the tanker captain, it is the sight and smell of a career going down the drain. Although Joseph Hazelwood avoided prison, he did not regain his career. The last time I checked, he was working as an assistant in the law firm that defended him and doing occasional work as a freelance ship inspector. He briefly got a job as an instructor at a New York maritime academy, but was let go when subsequent publicity created embarrassment for the school. The captain of the *Torrey Canyon,* Pastrengo Rugiati, lost his license and livelihood and never sailed again. Many others have gone down in disgrace. Some say the next American tanker disaster will be so expensive it will take down a company as well as a skipper.

When the governors of the coastal states saw the astronomical cost of the *Exxon Valdez* spill, they assigned committees to inventory areas like this one so they would know ahead of time how much money to charge a company like Arco in case of a major spill. Like a home-owner listing possessions for a future insurance claim, the committees counted birds, whales, otters, sea lions, clams, oysters, and crabs. The map they made of the Port Angeles area is dotted with marine mammal territories, rich fishing grounds, sensitive beaches, Dungeness crab habitats, clam beds, and bird sanctuaries. Carroll must sail through this Monopoly board tomorrow night without going to jail. As he does so, he can contemplate the fact that Exxon spent forty thousand dollars on the attempted rescue of each and every one of five thousand oiled sea otters found in Prince William Sound. Add to that price the loss of two hundred harbor seals and four hundred thousand birds. By some estimates, Exxon spent nearly three hundred dollars for every gallon spilled cleaning up the mess, compared to an average one hundred dollars a gallon spent on previous disasters.

Environmentalists say the way to stop carelessness is to place a high price on it. The owners and insurers say it isn't the high price of negligence they worry about, but the astronomical cost of inadvertent error. Arco is a big company, but unlike Exxon it is not among the world's largest corporations. It could not afford an unlimited tab for damaging these surroundings. Carroll wonders whether the folks at headquarters realize the thin line they walk on.

"We're the boat people," he says. "We're different from the bean counters back at headquarters. They sit there and do their work and don't realize their entire future depends on us. The boat people can take this corporation down in one move.

"If I run this ship aground, the bean counter in Dallas will lose his job. I know that. Everybody on this boat knows that. We cannot afford to spend the kind of money Exxon spent in Alaska. If we fuck up, Arco is gone."

In a sense, Carroll's job is simple. For his salary, he must avoid calamity and bring home the oil. Even people who hate oil tankers need fuel for their cars, factories, and furnaces. They would raise hell if he spilled any and they would be furious if he didn't deliver. Around 85 percent of western Washington's oil arrives from Alaska aboard ships like his. Carroll brings a load down here once every eight days on average; the *Arco Anchorage* carries a bigger portion of this region's petroleum than any other vessel because it comes here so often. When we pull into the Cherry Point dock tomorrow morning, shortly after midnight, we will pump enough crude oil to the refinery to produce 14.5 million gallons of gasoline, nearly 9 million gallons of jet fuel, nearly 8 million gallons of diesel, 1.6 million gallons of refinery gas, 1.2 million gallons of butane, 1.2 million gallons of coke, 1.2 million gallons of other products including heating oil, and 200,000 gallons of propane.

Our load will give the region slightly less than a two-day supply, something like a 10-gallon fill-up for a million and a half cars. Just behind us will come another tanker loaded with the region's next fix.

To a land addicted to oil, tankers must sail constantly, regardless of wind and sea conditions. They must find their way to refineries that are tucked behind chains of islands and located next to bird sanctuaries. The oil docks and refineries of Washington state are located in the worst possible place for tanker access. They were built at a time when convenience to the pipeline serving the major markets was more important than environmental safety, and now it would cost billions to move them.

Tomorrow night, on the last leg of our voyage, we will sail through the San Juan Islands, a place so treasured, the federal government is setting the surrounding waters aside as a marine sanctuary. The tanker will travel as close as half a mile from underwater obstacles and shorelines in the Rosario Strait, a waterway famous for swift current, dense fog, heavy winds, and thick boat traffic. For anyone's money, the Cherry Point run is the worst possible path for oil tankers, yet it is the state's busiest tanker thoroughfare, with more than five hundred ships going through every year.

The oil industry said in 1977 the odds of an oil spill in this region were only one in a hundred years, and the amount would be roughly 107,000 gallons. By contrast, a British Columbia statistician named Brian Pinch said the chance was more like one in ten years, and that the volume would be around 206,000 gallons. Pinch proved the better prognosticator when the *Arco Anchorage* dumped 239,000 gallons into Port Angeles harbor in 1985. The oil industry estimate was off by ninety-two years and half the oil.

So what happens if the Coast Guard's worst nightmare comes true, and seven million gallons spill in Rosario Strait? The chances of cleaning it are none whatsoever. Zero. Forget it. No amount of contingency plans, equipment, personnel, or technology will sop up that much misery. No one has cleaned up more than half the oil from any major spill and the best you can expect to recover in most cases is 15 percent. Once a spill exceeds a million gallons, only a fraction will ever be scooped up.

The horror of an oil spill cannot be captured by a single picture the way a photo can show a fire consuming a building. When a rescue worker plucks a dying bird off a tarred rock, one barely discernible from the other, he cannot see the slick smothering an undulating generation of waterfowl behind him. A photographer once likened it to

Vietnam: "every day, a new body count." A feature writer saw similar parallels: "Helicopters drone across the sky, boats beach on shore, men land, size up the situation and depart." A hopeless war against a ubiquitous enemy.

Oil industry officials bragged in the old days that they could handle any catastrophe. In 1975, a Shell Oil Company refinery manager told a Washington state legislative committee that the equipment then available in the Puget Sound region could just about wipe up a 4.5-million-gallon oil spill in a single day. No sweat, if you tossed in the Navy, Coast Guard, and Canadian equipment, the day and night crews could attack eight million gallons.

Reality has this inconvenient tendency to foil such wild claims. When the *Arco Anchorage* went aground in Port Angeles harbor, it took hours just to get containment booms ready, since someone had forgotten to tie the sections together beforehand. In 1988, when a barge spilled 231,000 gallons off the Washington coast, cleanup crews were so ineffective, the muck spread up the coast as far away as British Columbia and down the coast as far as Newport, Oregon. Spills were getting out of control that were one-thirtieth the size of those the Shell man was so confident he could corral.

What really deflated oil company puffery, though, was the pathetic response to the *Exxon Valdez* spill. The night the tanker hit Bligh Reef, and for two days afterward, the calm weather and smooth sea conditions were perfect for a cleanup but the contingency plan the oil terminal operators had boasted about for years was worthless. The plan called for Alyeska, the terminal operator, to have a cleanup barge at the spill site within five hours, supplying important items like containment booms. It took three times as long because the barge was under repair and equipment was buried under snowdrifts. A tugboat carrying equipment necessary to pump oil off the stricken vessel didn't get there for nearly twelve hours.

The world watched an abject failure unfold in slow motion. By the time Exxon had sufficient equipment on hand, a storm had blown in with winds of over seventy miles per hour. The gales drove the oil ashore with such force it was splashed against the sides of trees forty feet above sea level. Techniques such as chemical dispersants and burning might have worked earlier when the water was calm, but now they were hopeless under such stormy conditions. And the skimmers that scoop oil off the water's surface were equally useless. From that point on, as the Alaska Oil Spill Commission said, "Crews were doomed to chase a spill they would never contain." They did what they could, skimming a few barrels, protecting a few sensitive areas with booms, and saving a few otters and birds in hastily assembled wildlife rescue centers. But mostly they counted bodies and watched the oil spread.

The hopelessness of the effort was dramatized by tape recordings obtained by plaintiff's lawyers three years after the spill. On one, Exxon public relations man Don Cornett tells Alyeska vice president Bill Howitt during the cleanup, "Doesn't matter if they are really picking up a hell of a lot of oil at this point. It makes a real bad impression on the public without any activity going on."

Howitt later replied: "So it behooves us to have everything flapping in the breeze that we can, whether it's catching oil or not?"

Cornett: "Yeah, absolutely."

Howitt: "Of course we're pooping in the wind here, but that's classified."

Some say when Exxon could not skim oil, it sponged up human anger with dollar bills. The Prince William Sound fisherman who had howled so publicly about the destruction of their fishing grounds in the first days of the spill were a prime target. The cleanup contractor leased boats from fishermen for hundreds and even thousands of dollars a day. Those who succumbed to the temptation were called "spillionaires," and if the money stopped their grousing, it was all part of the plan. As Cornett told Alyeska president George Nelson on tape: "I would encourage you to take the three noisiest fishermen down there and hire those suckers and load 'em down with something, and have them drive it around Prince William Sound." Nowadays, with the catch suffering, many of the fishermen are going broke.

Carroll was on an Arco tanker sailing the Gulf of Alaska when the Exxon tanker went aground. He didn't hear the news until he settled in for his 10 A.M. coffee break the next day. As the days crawled on, and the oil continued to spread, Carroll was as frustrated about the cleanup effort as the general public. He could feel the heat of public opinion crawling up the necks of every tanker sailor. He could imagine the comments he would hear back home. To Carroll and the other Arco crew members, these were ass-dragging days for the oil ship boys.

And with the cleanup efforts going nowhere, the Coast Guard closed the Port of Valdez for four days, even though the slick had drifted away from the tanker lanes. Empty tankers, including several Arco ships, stacked up at anchor in Prince William Sound waiting to get a load of oil from the pipeline. Oil company executives like Arco's Harold Heinze began to worry about another kind of crisis—a major energy shortage on the West Coast. Heinze knew that West Coast refineries like Cherry Point operate on a thin backlog, with maybe a five-day supply of crude oil available in storage tanks, under the best of conditions. "There is not a lot lying around." As head of Arco Transportation, Heinze sent an urgent message to company lobbyists to tell President Bush he didn't have much time, that the port must be reopened or the nation's Pacific Coast would go dry. "In my estimation, it came pretty close."

Valdez was reopened and the oil began to flow. But to the public this concern over the oil supply just underlined the perception that oil companies worry more about keeping the tankers rolling than they do about safety. Heinze was right, of course; tankers must rumble out of Valdez like clockwork or the freeways in Los Angeles come to a screeching halt. But it smacked of greed when the nation's television sets were tuned to pictures of oiled otters and dying birds.

If the *Exxon Valdez* fiasco renewed public cynicism about oil companies, it also provided a textbook example of the risk we take whenever we carry petroleum on water. No amount of Exxon money could erase the public's perception that cleanup crews are helpless once oil is spilled. Some spills that followed the *Exxon Valdez* disaster just hardened the popular view. Two years after the *Exxon Valdez* spill, when a Chinese freighter ran over a Japanese fish-processing boat, causing a spill of one hundred thousand gallons of fuel oil near the entrance to the Strait of Juan de Fuca, many were amazed at the pathetic response.

The skimmers were slow to arrive and once they got to the site they were ineffective. Oil hit the beaches and birds were killed. The environmental toll was small compared to the *Exxon Valdez,* but some wondered, if these guys can't corral a spill from a fishing boat, what the hell are they going to do with a tanker?

Good question, said Martin Keeley, an environmental activist from Point Roberts, Washington. "A whole lot of memos have been passed around the various government offices in both countries, lots of meetings have been held, and lots of consultants have been paid fat salaries. But the bottom line is that we are still not ready to cope with an oil spill."

At least after the Valdez experience, oil company officials don't have the gall to claim they can control an eight-million-gallon spill. Bill Gray, the former Exxon official, says in the time he has been in the oil industry he hasn't seen any real progress. "Despite an awful lot of money and some pretty creative ideas thrown at the situation, it has been very disappointing."

Historically, every time a spill has caught the public attention, companies and governments spent big bucks on cleanup research and equipment. Noted scientists who specialize in the field, like Ottawa's Merv Fingas, find themselves in great demand. "Everybody goes out and dusts a few cobwebs off their plans and buys a little more equipment," Fingas said. And each time there is little progress. "Things get better," he said, "but not miraculously better."

The task is an enormous one. Anyone who has tried to scoop drops of vegetable oil off the water in a boiling saucepan has experienced something akin to recovering spilled petroleum in a tossing ocean. Out on the open water there are three ways to do the job: skimming, burning, and treating the oil with chemicals or biological agents.

Whatever method is chosen, the first challenge is to contain the oil with a floating dam, known as a boom, made of a material roughly similar to that found in a life preserver. In most cases, the boom arrives too late and is never ample to necklace a spill much larger than, say, one hundred thousand gallons. But even if sufficient quantities of boom arrive on time, they have intrinsic weaknesses. No boom is strong enough to contain a wave of oil a foot or more thick, like the one that poured out of the *Exxon Valdez*. And even if it is strong enough, oil will slide right under a boom if the water current is moving perpendicular to it at a speed greater than one nautical mile per hour. Finally, booms are all but useless in waves higher than six feet. Fingas says booms are useful with smaller spills, but when it comes to major disasters, "Booms are at their limit."

Trouble is, oil must be contained by booms if a skimmer is to have any chance at picking it up. There are many different models, but they are all designed to separate oil from water and scoop it up. Some skimmers collect the stuff on a conveyor belt, others screen it out using a weir, while a few sop it up with strands of oil-attracting rope. Cleanup crews in Prince William Sound found that even dredges normally used for sucking mud from the bottom of a shallow harbor can easily be converted to skimming by turning their suction pipes upward so they attack the slick from underneath. They also tried sewer-sucking vacuum trucks mounted on barges.

Like booms, though, all skimmers have major weaknesses. They, too, are easily defeated by wind and waves. They get jammed with driftwood and other junk that collects in the oil. And most don't have large enough storage tanks to handle a big spill, so they need ready access to ample barges. Also, no single skimmer is good for every type of oil. Some are adequate for thick crust but will fail if faced with a thin sheen. To cover the gamut would require keeping an impossible variety of machines on hand.

On top of all these problems, skimmer operators have trouble just finding a slick. A sheen shows up nicely in the sunshine, but not in the darkness, fog, rain, and waves that are more typical of the sea. To be truly effective, a skimmer operator must locate not just the slick but the thickest portion of the oil. Airplanes with special infrared lenses, and some types of radar, are useful, but it is difficult to coordinate them with the skimmers. Researchers hope the global-position satellite system will make the job easier.

Fingas said a great deal of research could markedly improve the effectiveness of the everyday skimmer. After a series of spills hit

American shores in the wake of the *Exxon Valdez,* hundreds of entrepreneurs heard the call, believing they could build a better oil trap. Some mailed hasty sketches to the Coast Guard while others dispatched slick brochures. One inventor claimed his miracle machine could have peeled off the *American Trader* spill in California before anyone noticed. "It never would have made the papers." Committees were formed to sort promise from absurdity, and there were hundreds of ideas to consider.

Even Arco Marine President Jerry Aspland got into the act. He proposed converting one of his company's seventy-thousand-ton tankers to a giant skimmer that would lap up a two-hundred-foot-wide swath of ocean in one sweep, pulling in twelve times more oil and water than any other cleanup vessel now in operation. He dubbed it "Big Gulp." He was pretty miffed when others in industry showed no interest in his proposal, because, among other problems, the ship couldn't operate in shallow water and it would be costly to replicate. Aspland figured, though, that "people don't have vision."

Whether it is because industry has no vision, or designers have no ideas, oil has so far eluded the invention of the ultimate spill machine. Some scientists say the most hopeful technique is burning the oil. Sometimes a large portion of a spill is burned off when a stricken tanker catches fire, as happened recently with the *Mega Borg* in the Gulf of Mexico and the *Aegean Sea* off the coast of Spain. But purposely setting a spill on fire is seldom attempted. Some twenty-five thousand gallons was burned away from the *Exxon Valdez* spill, but it was a minor experiment. The technique is rarely used because it requires ideal conditions and quick reflexes: The slick must be floating on calm water, and it must be no thinner than thirty sheets of typing paper (three millimeters). Fingas says that in order to burn a major spill there must be a couple of dozen boats and a lot of fireproof boom present for an attack that has to happen within the first day, since the more flammable portions of the oil will evaporate quickly.

Of course, there is always the danger of blowing up the ship, but tanker owners say the safety of the vessel isn't so important once the crew is evacuated. The ship is less valuable than the cost of a billion-dollar cleanup. Environmentalists say burning oil produces air pollution, but Fingas claims it is no more smoky than the output of a forest fire. Even so, some oil is always left behind, since once the stuff burns down to the thickness of ten sheets of paper (one millimeter), the fire will go out.

Every method of spill control has its trade-offs. The use of chemicals is especially tricky. Dispersants, sprayed from the air, change the molecular structure of oil so it is no longer cohesive. The slick breaks into small droplets that sink or become diluted in the waves. When that happens, the oil is neatly out of sight, but far from gone. Dispersants change the threat from a coating on the surface to a series of small globs dispersed in the water column. What doesn't stain the beaches or choke the birds may still do immeasurable harm to marine life on the bottom of the bay. Their use is still debated.

Other chemicals are more exotic, like the elasticizer that turns oil into a solid sheet of sticky goo, a coagulant that turns it into a solid clump, and a product known as a sorbent that absorbs oil the same way sawdust does on a garage floor. Unfortunately these methods are considered marginally useful because they have one drawback or another (the elasticized oil, for instance, clings to everything).

One of the more promising methods for cleaning a beach relies on tiny creatures who feed on oil. Some ninety species of microorganism eat crude for lunch . . . and dinner. Trouble is, they linger over their food. In some cases, it takes two or three years to "bio-remediate" a shoreline. Even at that rate, though, it is twice as fast as the time it takes nature to scrub the beach.

Nature has a role in the cleanup process, too. At the start, evaporation will take care of 20 to 60 percent of a spill, depending on the type of oil and the weather. That leaves behind some pretty persistent tars, of course, but over time the waves will slowly lift the leftovers from the rocks and dilute them in the ocean. Most spills are gone within a year or two, or at least they are no longer visible. Even so, scientists examining shorelines closely have found leftover signs of a spill as much as a decade afterwards.

Here in Port Angeles harbor there is no outward sign of the damage this ship caused six years ago. Local officials say Arco did a pretty good job in the end. The pollution du jour is a hefty plume of smoke coming from a pulp mill. The cloud is visible through the porthole as a crewman steps into the captain's office to alert me that a launch is about to depart for town. Move quickly, I'm told, because the next one won't leave for another hour. As I head out the door, Carroll asks me to pick up a couple of cooking magazines for him. I chuckle to myself. Here I am a sailor about to hit port and I am looking for a copy of *Gourmet*.

17

The Beach

*(Port Angeles Harbor,
January 29, 5 P.M.)*

The rope ladder—Jacob's ladder, as they call it—hangs over the side of the ship motionless in the calm water. Last in line to go ashore, I ease my way down the black side of the hull, reassured by the grip of the bristly fiber and relieved that my feet can easily locate the rungs. Trying to act like a veteran, I leap the last two feet to the rear deck of the motor launch, but when I wave my arms clumsily to catch my balance, the novice in me is exposed. Chuckling with my audience, I choose a bench seat next to engineman Neal Curtis and look around at my fellow passengers, familiar people now in unfamiliar surroundings. The pale first engineer, Bob Rich, slumps a little under the weight of his illness. He is relieved to be free of his quarters and on his way to the hospital. Afterward, he'll head home by plane. He doesn't say much—a brief hello, a comment that he expects to be okay—and then stares out the back of the launch as the *Arco Anchorage* shrinks in the distance. Willie the cook-baker is animated, although he too has an appointment at the hospital. He is reciting an inventory of the sleazy joints he plans to visit in town. To Willie, the fact that Port Angeles is a town of loggers and fishermen is a good omen.

Pat Rogers, the steward, is a little down on his luck. He thought this was his final voyage before vacation, but at the last moment he received an ROB notice—"remain on board"—which means he must return tonight for another round trip because his replacement is unavailable. As for Curtis, he just wants to get away for a few hours. Maybe he'll suck a beer someplace far from the sound of boiler fires and spinning turbines. He has an emergency stash of money stuffed in a hole he cut along the top edge of his trousers, just in case the thugs try to rob him. By his own account, Curtis has been mugged in Portland, New York, and Pittsburgh, and even in this small town, Arco crewmen have been attacked. "It's the fate of a seaman. Seamen have money." Curtis has seen guys stripped of their clothing and jewelry, so he wears old jeans and a T-shirt with no embellishments. "I don't go to shore and make myself a mark. I like to pretend I'm someone else. I won't tell them I'm off a tanker. I'm a salesman."

When the launch reaches the dock, the salesman and I step ashore together and I feel again the sensations of solid earth. I've driven through Port Angeles dozens of times on my way to the beach, but arriving here from the deck of an oil tanker is a different experience altogether. Even though I have been at sea only a little over a week, the ground feels odd to my oceangoing feet. Dirt and concrete are foreign substances, and even the air seems warmer. I have to adjust my eyes to a different sort of daylight, like stepping out of a movie theater into the afternoon sunshine. I don't know why, but the others from the boat appear to be doing the same thing. And I don't know what's wrong with this town, but it seems to be rocking a good five degrees from side to side. We climb into a van provided by the motor launch company for a quick trip to a hotel parking lot near the main street. When we get there, we go our separate ways almost by design. Guys who have spent weeks aboard a ship together look forward to a few hours in the company of strangers.

The surroundings remind me of other times and I understand how keenly these guys must miss their wives, girlfriends, or families. Being on dry land links me to my wife in a way that was unimaginable on the ship, since I could hop a Greyhound bus from the station up the street and be home tonight. I know the sailors feel the same way, because they tell me that the beach beckons with a special siren song. Reality has it that the majority must ignore this feeling and get back on board the tanker tonight. They may not see a sidewalk again for weeks. Families are a voice on the telephone.

As Curtis climbs a steep hill to the first commercial street, he could be a college student or a tourist since he has no duffel bag or uniform to signify his profession. But his feet and heart belong to a sailor, and like any beached mariner, even the simple sensation of walking up hill is something to savor, something he doesn't experience on the ship.

They say a town's tallest structures denote the most important institution, and in Port Angeles those are the pulp mill smokestacks. Yet this is a border town between civilization and the wild. On either side of the skirmish line you quickly see the contrast: the ugliness of the main street, with its grim shop windows, and the staggering beauty of the Olympic Mountains that always stand taller than the chimneys of commerce. Today thousands of cars rumbled through this town on Highway 101, but only a cannon shot away is a roadless backcountry paved by winter snows. Just a short time ago, a man shot a mountain lion in his front yard. As if to emphasize the stubborn dominance of the mountains, the town tilts on a hillside so steep you could imagine an earthquake shoving it back into the sea from whence the settlers once came. The population of seventeen thousand people has varied little over the last ten years, a result of economic woes and the area's isolation from the more populated regions to the east across Puget Sound. The Olympic Peninsula's timber industry, the town's biggest employer, has taken a nosedive because of depleted forests and an argument over endangered species like the spotted owl. Too proud to die, the town is trying for alternatives such as a pulp mill recycling paper and residents exploiting newfound tourism.

Curtis turns right onto a street above the waterfront, and if he is mistaken for a tourist it is probably for the better. The town has an uneasy relationship with tankers. People aren't too bothered by ships like the *Arco Anchorage,* even though it is the only one that has ever spilled oil here. They are more concerned that some bigger tankers might be heading here in the future. A company has proposed building a tanker dock 18 miles west of Port Angeles and a 150-mile crude-oil pipeline to connect to the existing refineries at Cherry Point, Ferndale, and Anacortes. What scares local residents is that the new oil port would be conveniently located just outside the line that, under federal law, bars ships larger than 125,000 deadweight tons from sailing east of here. That means the port could accommodate vessels many times the size of the *Arco Anchorage*. Even though Port Angeles citizens could probably use the income such a place would generate, many here fought hard against a similar plan more than a decade ago and are doing so again. By all indications, the pipeline project is doomed because it is too expensive and the oil companies aren't anxious to invest the money in uncertain times. But as long as the idea percolates, it gets plenty of attention in town. Oddly enough, while people worry about a proposed tanker dock west of town, Port Angeles already ranks high as a major tanker port—a significant fueling stop for tankers sailing the West Coast as well as a parking lot for ships like the *Arco Anchorage* waiting to dock at the refineries.

Curtis is simply looking for a beer, though, not for an argument over pipelines, and he finds one pretty quickly. The nautical decor on the outside gives the tavern a salty facade, but on the inside the clientele of loggers and mill workers turns the flavor to sawdust. The hard-core out-of-work timbermen have sprouted like mushrooms from their permanent bar stools, like the guy with the tree-bark face who wears a hat that says he eats spotted owls for lunch. Curtis won't catch any flak here for the fact that his ship once despoiled the harbor, but he won't strike up any philosophical discussions either. He settles onto a stool at one corner of the U-shaped bar and tosses a pack of cigarettes onto the counter. He orders a schooner and stares straight ahead, guarding his flanks. The jukebox plays a lonely country song and in the background he can hear the clack of a pool game in progress. The voices next to him are slurred with the effects of afternoon beers; he won't initiate chitchat with them in this waterfront saloon. The guy next to him could be friendly, or he could ask for a loan and punch him in the face. Curtis says crewmen have gotten in fights in this town simply because they have a job and the locals don't. The sailor could probably make better use of his precious time ashore, but the tourists and the kids at the local community college have more options than a sailor on foot ever does. Bars like this thrive on their ability to filter mariners off the streets before they reach other activities. Sometimes when he is in town, Curtis takes a cab to one of the local shopping malls (where a couple of the guys have gone today). He strikes me as a man of imagination, not some jerk who hugs a bar whenever he can. He's a man of many interests who once sold a short story to a magazine about a guy being harassed by oil companies for inventing a gasoline-free car. But this happens to be one of those rare opportunities when a tanker sailor can enjoy some suds. The ship won't leave for another twenty-four hours, and as long as he doesn't get toasted drunk, Curtis isn't violating any rules.

I still must find a cooking magazine for Captain Carroll, so I excuse myself from the seedy bar and head up the hill toward the main street. At the bookstore, I'm amazed to see how many cookbooks and cooking magazines line the shelves. The challenge is not finding one, but deciding which one to buy. While I'm leafing through one recipe magazine, I strike up a conversation with a professorial fellow named Alan Bentsen, who turns out to be a fifty-three-year-old stockbroker and longtime resident. When I explain who I am, and what I am doing on a tanker, Bentsen, like others in town, turns out to have plenty of opinions about oil ships and petroleum. "The problem, of course, is that we use oil," he says, marking his place in a book with his index finger. "My solution is not so much how we get it in safely, but how we can use less of it. There's all kinds of things we can do, like use more efficient cars and lighting."

The bookstore manager joins in the conversation. If they have concerns, it is the proposed oil port and pipeline, not the *Arco Anchorage* or the spill in 1985, which is now a distant memory. No one thinks the spill had any long-term effects.

As the conversation continues, I glance at the bookshelves and my eyes are drawn to a history of steamships and a nonfiction account of the *Exxon Valdez* spill. The books here, and those in any library, will tell you a lot about shipwrecks and even some about oil spills. But it is remarkable how little literature there is available anywhere to describe the long-term effects of oil spills. We know the immediate effects. Birds die and the beaches are blackened. But what happens years afterward? Whether you are talking about Prince William Sound or Port Angeles Harbor, it is a debatable issue. In 1985, the National Academy of Sciences took a stab at compiling the available research on the long-term effects of spills. The six-hundred-page summary wandered all over the subject without coming to a more concise conclusion than this one: "The authors of this report conclude, based upon the evidence available, that there has been no evident irrevocable damage to marine resources on a broad oceanic scale, by either chronic inputs or occasional major oil spills. However, specific information that would enable unequivocal assessment of the impact of oil on the environment does not yet exist, particularly, with regard to certain specific environments and conditions. We, therefore, recommend further research in a number of areas . . ."

In other words, they don't know.

The subject is as large and murky as the ocean itself. Any scientist studying the long-term effects of oil must consider a number of variables.

Both oil and ocean water are chemical soups that never contain the same ingredients from place to place. With petroleum you have the decayed leftovers from plants and animals crushed for millions of years between rocks, a mixture as diverse as nature itself. With oceans, you have changing temperatures, depths, currents, and locations, plus a wide variety of marine life. Kuwaiti crude makes an entirely different splash in the Persian Gulf than Alaskan crude does in the Strait of Juan de Fuca. Even a scientist assigned to study a single spill must consider the impact on a multitude of species, each one with its own reaction to oil. When we ask a question about the long-term effects of oil, just whose skin are we talking about?

There is also the question of chronic versus occasional spills. There are places on the earth's crust where oil seeps daily into the ocean from cracks. And then there are the big tanker spills that put a whole gob in one place at one time.

The best way to study the effects of a sudden spill would be to dump the stuff into a body of water where oceanographers have documented the wildlife ahead of time. One place ideal for such a study is Buzzards Bay, a deep harbor that nearly divides Cape Cod from the

Massachusetts mainland. Since the place is home to Woods Hole Oceanographic Institute, the creatures have been better observed and counted there than in most places. On September 16, 1969, an unexpected experiment began when a barge drifted ashore at Fassett's Point, north of the institute, dumping some 180,000 gallons of No. 2 New England heating fuel into the water. Senior scientist Howard Sanders recalls how institute employees learned of the spill by catching the scent as it drifted on the wind to their homes above the water. They rushed to the scene carrying bottles of alcohol with which they could store samples of dead fish. Sanders couldn't believe what he saw as he stood on the muddy shore. "Literally millions of small animals were bubbling to the surface, some critters that we had never seen before." He was witnessing something that is often missed after a spill, the death of tiny invertebrates who are killed by the first waves of oil. They usually rot in short order and are not counted in the inventory of the dead. As months went by, Woods Hole scientists took advantage of the opportune spill. They observed the recovery of various species, for inhabitants such as the blue mussel a slow process. Yet a tiny worm known as the capitella, immune to the toxins in oil, thrived. As the others died, the capitella moved in and the bottom became home to as many as 225,000 worms per square yard. It was a city of worms with not much else left alive. The spill was a godsend, if you were a fan of the capitella worm.

Much of the wildlife returned—and the capitella diminished—in a couple of seasons. But eight years after the spill it was still possible to see oil pool up in footprints at low tide. Two decades after the spill, at the time of the *Exxon Valdez* cleanup, scientists returned to the site and could still detect remnants of oil.

In October 1974, another barge dumped No. 2 fuel oil, so the Woods Hole scientists had a chance to do a second study north of the previous site. This time the researchers looked at the plants and found that eighteen of forty-five species were missing from the area the next season.

But even in a well-studied and controlled area like Buzzards Bay, the scientists got only snapshots of a couple of spills. It would take researchers years and thousands of spills—not to mention billions of dollars—before they could speak with full authority about the effects on the oceans in general.

And the conclusions of science become as murky as the oiled oceans when different researchers make different assumptions depending on who pays their bill. When eighty oil and oil-related companies financed their own two-year investigation into the effects of oil on marine life in Louisiana, the conclusions were very different from those drawn by the Woods Hole scientists. In that case, the researchers said there were no signs of damage and that nature actually thrives near oil production facilities.

Whatever information does get published, there is often a counter-attack. When the Woods Hole scientists reported their findings at Buzzards Bay, they were roundly criticized by John Mackin, an emeritus professor of biology at Texas A & M University. The Mackin paper—distributed by Exxon—made a blanket condemnation of the Woods Hole work, saying the papers purporting to show long-term environmental damage from the Buzzards Bay spills were faulty. Among other things, Mackin claimed that some of the initial kill in Buzzards Bay was due to wind and waves, not oil. Mackin's judgment may have been colored by his own work history. Over the years, the late professor served as a consultant to Texaco, Gulf Oil, California Oil, Shell Oil, and Humble Oil. But his paper tossed an alternative view into the debate.

If Mackin's research was captive, however, it wouldn't be the first time. When the editors of the magazine *New Engineer* sought to find an expert to review Mackin's paper, the result was telling:

"Unfortunately, although we tried for nearly a year, we could not find a single scientist willing to take on the task. The reasons were never clearly stated, but the unspoken implication was that a reviewer who criticized Mackin might have difficulty securing research money from the two largest sources—oil companies and the federal government."

After the *Exxon Valdez* spill, scientists and researchers were once again arguing over the long-term effects of oil. For years after the spill, scientists were gagged by lawyers because most researchers were in the employ of either the governmental agencies or the companies who were preparing for pending lawsuits. Then at a meeting in Anchorage, Alaska—after some of the major suits had settled—government scientists and others presented what seemed like a balanced assessment of the condition of Prince William Sound. Killer whales and bald eagles were killed but had made a recovery a couple of years after the spill. As many as half the sea otters in Prince William Sound may have died, and some may still be in danger. As many as 645,000 birds died because of the spill and a sea bird known as the common murre, which was hardest hit, may take a long time to recover. But the evidence regarding the pink salmon was confusing. One salmon run following the spill was a record breaker and then there was a drop-off in 1992 and a collapse in 1993. Which do you blame on the spill— the bumper crop or the losses? More and more evidence points to the losses.

Exxon scientists refused to attend the Anchorage meeting or participate in the discussion. Then a couple of months later it was shades of Professor Mackin over again as Exxon scientists blasted the government research in statements to the press. They said the government scientists had bungled their data and misrepresented the facts. What irked the company most was a claim that Prince William Sound was clean before the spill and that remnants of oil persisted afterward. They disputed the findings, asserting that the researchers failed to differentiate between oil from the *Exxon Valdez* and oil from other sources.

Despite the wealth of data released following the spill, scientists remain nearly as uncertain as they were in 1985 when the National Research Council recommended further studies. Even one hundred million dollars spent on *Exxon Valdez* research barely dents the mystery. And with money and conflict creating a sideshow, while objectivity suffers, the public has little hope of getting solid answers soon.

Alan Turner, the Port Angeles bookstore manager, says he knows a tanker sailor when he sees one. "They come in with their duffel bags. That's how you know where they are from." He says the tankermen never talk business, or spills, but they will comment on the food they get aboard the ship. The food is very important.

Nathan Matlock, a teenager who has stopped in for a magazine, says the tanker sailors usually have other things on their mind besides the long-term effects of oil. "Sometimes they say to me, 'Don't you guys have any bars in this town?' " says young Matlock. " 'Hell,' I tell them, 'all we have is bars.' "

I wander back to the hotel and the van that will take us back to the motor launch. Along the way, I grab some film in a drugstore and a cream puff at a bakery. Down the hill I see the Black Ball ferry loading cars for its seventeen-mile journey across the Strait of Juan de Fuca to the city of Victoria, British Columbia. But when I notice a dark cloud gathering in the sky, the kind that dumps rain by the bucket, my wandering becomes more quickly paced.

At the hotel, a bunch of crewmen are sitting around a bar table sipping at short glasses. They hide the booze in mock surprise when I walk in. "Uh-oh, here's the reporter." No problem, I tell them, I know who's on watch tonight. In any case, there's no guard and no Breathalzyer test in Port Angeles. As I pull up a chair next to the chief steward, I feel as though I have become a familiar visitor to these guys, a man with a personality and a first name. I don't deceive myself into believing that once I leave I will linger long in their memories because it is the way of sailors to shrug off life's constantly shifting enrollment. But while I am here, a sailor might absentmindedly hand me a wrench, and one said I might make an okay deckhand with a lot of training. To me, meanwhile, the crew members have risen from a faceless roster to become well-defined characters, each with an individual texture. Promises are made that will probably not be called in, but are nevertheless the mark of friendly acquaintance. I will ski someday with the third mate, find a poster for an engineman, or give a tour of the newspaper to anyone who shows up.

As I settle into a cocktail-lounge chair, the conversation continues about mundane stuff like cars and gadgets. The only generality I can glean from the talk is that no one has returned from town with a story to tell. Even Willie is unfulfilled, it seems. The medical checkup consumed nearly all his time and the nurse was too wholesome to contort into a self-serving fantasy.

Within a half hour, everyone is assembled and resigned to another tour of duty. A collection of empty glasses are the remnants of shore leave as we toss a few dollars on the table. I watch closely, but no one staggers or speaks with slurred consonants. Apparently, the visit to a tavern and a bar were conveniences dictated by a shortage of time. Sailors make enough money these days that they are better golfers and real estate investors than they are barhoppers.

The launch seems to travel faster on our return trip to the ship. The tanker is stretched across the bay in front of us. In the dark I can still read the ten-foot-tall letters that spell the word ARCO. The letters are white against a hull that is otherwise black from stem to stern. A single porthole on the house is uncovered, a lonely light that reminds me for some reason of a one-eyed buccaneer lurking in ambush. Elsewhere in the harbor are a small Navy tanker carrying JP-4 jet fuel, a log ship, and a freighter. They look so innocent and small next to a loaded crude carrier.

18

The Final Passage

"Beginning to heave, Cap."
As we pull up the hook, the anchor chain clatters through the hawsepipe and chugs its way into a storage hold that's located below the foc's'le deck. Third mate Dean Davis reports our progress to the bridge over a walkie-talkie. The rusty necklace we are retrieving from the bottom weighs as much as a convoy of trucks, but the old winch handles the load easily. As for the ship, it is indifferent to the action, for it is nine thousand times bigger than its anchor.

I am hypnotized by the industrial muscle of the whole process and overwhelmed by the noise. Then I notice a hitchhiking starfish, as wide as a garbage can lid, coming out of the water, riding on the chain. It somehow eludes the powerful water cannon that cleans mud off the links just before the chain tops the deck. Crossing the threshold, the beast flops to our feet and lies there, soft and red against the cold gray steel. We are unfamiliar with each other, this bottom dweller and I, yet we are brought together by an oil tanker on a wintry evening. I'm an air breather with grease on my hands so I fit in this human place, but this poor creature lies there in the grips of death, as likely to survive on Mars as it would be to flourish on the bow of an oil-carrying ship. A seaman tosses the visitor into an empty bucket and casually sets him aside. We are not a haven for nature, we are a tanker on a mission. The anchor is snugged into place, and we are ready to sail.

A beam of the light from Ediz Hook strobes across the house and flickers against the windows of the bridge. The tide has turned in our favor, which makes us all that more anxious to leave, for we have been sitting in this harbor now for a full night and day. After we returned from Port Angeles last night, the ship was like a 7-Eleven store, never sleeping. As the eleven o'clock news faded into TV talk shows, a crew of workmen labored earnestly on the bow, fixing the injuries caused by our winter voyage. In the dark and the cold rain, the contractors from shore disassembled the tortured winches up on the fo'c'sle house and looked for the gremlins that had rendered them useless. The half-dozen men in blue coveralls, faces coated in grease, were still frantically probing the guts of the cantankerous machines when the morning talk shows made their debut. They appreciated the warm coffee in the crew's mess hall, but the sunrise was an unwelcome sight with so much work still to be done. Time marches impatiently when an oil tanker is sitting at port. This expensive ship is not earning a dime when it sits idle in harbor, so once we get word that the dock at the Cherry Point refinery is going to be free, all work on the winches must stop. We must weigh anchor and what remains broken must be fixed at the next opportunity, which in this case will be Cherry Point.

Besides working on winches, the crew also obtained a load of bunker fuel during our layover yesterday. A tugboat started the fueling process by shoving a two-hundred-foot-long barge against the hull of the *Arco Anchorage*. Bunkering, as it is called, is always a risky business. There is a great possibility of spills any time two vessels transfer petroleum, which occurs in a variety of ways. Two big tankers often sidle up to each other in ports like this to transfer whole cargoes of crude oil, a bumpered operation known as lightering that has its own dangers. Strict rules govern bunkering and lightering, but they are always an accident waiting to happen.

As soon as the barge was secured to the ship, two barge men readied a crane to lift the fueling hose to the ship. On the main deck of the *Arco Anchorage,* bosun Scotty Nehrenz lowered a milk carton over the rail and the barge man dropped in a clipboard containing the receipt for our fuel. As the bosun retrieved the paperwork and checked it over, he gestured impatiently to a seaman who was preparing the ship's manifold to receive the fueling hose. He also sent young Jimmy Doyle on a quick walk around the main deck's perimeter to see that all the drains, known as scuppers, were closed. If fuel spills on the deck, the closed scuppers will keep it from going overboard. "No sheens," is what the captain says. The company view is that even a quart of oil overboard will fire the public's ire.

As Doyle checked the scuppers, chief engineer Jim Vives walked onto the deck and started hollering about how pissed he was that it was taking so long to get this operation started. "Christ almighty, ten minutes to eleven and I'm opening the valves." Then he noticed that one of the men working on the barge had once been a third engineer in his engine room. Vives allowed that things must be pretty rough in the tanker business when a former ship's officer has to go to work on a barge. "What do you think a barge man makes a year?" Truth is, business is booming for barge jockeys, especially in the Pacific Northwest. Although it is a job that subjects a worker to plenty of fumes and long hours, they haven't lacked for business ever since the prices of bunker fuel rose in California and more ships began stopping in Washington to take on cheaper petrol. One weary barge worker said he had worked two hundred hours of overtime this month.

The command to heave anchor is a morale builder for the crew because we are anxious to bid this place good-bye. Our new pilot, Don Soriono, directs the helmsman to steer the ship past Ediz Hook and out into the Strait of Juan de Fuca. With the screw turning, and the engines rumbling, the old tanker feels like a ship again. The bridge is alive with navigation as we nose our way toward open water. The reddish orange radar screens display the passing scenery with electronic indifference while the compass indicators on the wall point the direction we are traveling. Our path home, in a pitch black world, is dictated by the pilot who barks out a series of compass headings he knows by heart. The helmsman repeats the pilot's commands with military precision, and everything seems so orderly. Then the radio on the back wall crackles with the voice of Seattle Traffic talking to a foreign tanker. The alien ship is reporting the fact that one of its radars is on the fritz. The unloaded foreigner wants permission from the Coast Guard to enter Rosario Strait with only one eye working. We're curious to see if the Coast Guard will let these guys get away with it.

Captain Carroll's face is illuminated by the Ediz Hook light as the beacon sweeps over the ship. He's got that Hinchinbrook look on his face—wondering about the weather—since rain squalls are in the forecast, and the winds are kicking up. I poke at his thoughts, asking whether he worries about Rosario Strait. He laughs. Tanker captains don't worry about such things, you silly boy. Carroll has been through these waters many times before. There is nothing to worry about. What could go wrong? "We've got the pilot with us, we've got good radar fixes, we've got escorts, we've been here before. It's not like—'Oh God, here's Rosario Strait.'"

We sail a dozen miles north and east out of Port Angeles before the tug escort appears a half mile ahead of us, and slightly to the left, just a dot of light in the darkness. We are nearing the entrance to Rosario Strait and this tugboat is our waltzing partner for the night. The name of our escort is the *Hunter,* not a tractor tug with their superior tanker-handling belly props but a stoutly powered favorite of Arco captains that Carroll is happy to have with us. Arco will soon announce its intention to hire nothing but tractor tugs in these waters, but for now we are content to dance with the *Hunter*.

The captain looks confident as the pilot guides the *Arco Anchorage* through the night. Carroll has a job to do, and the last thing he is probably pondering are the political battles fought over these waters that have resulted in tougher rules and practices than those found in other U.S. waterways, excluding Prince William Sound. Some tanker people don't like the regulations, but local environmentalists feel they are proof of the value of activism. You can tell whether the locals care about their waters by checking out the rules that govern ship traffic, says marine biologist and environmental campaigner Fred Felleman. "You go to the Gulf of Mexico ports and they will lie down for the oil industry—'Anything you want, sir.' " In the patchwork world of maritime regulation, the state of Washington gets more protection than most.

Not every battle was won, however, and more could be done. Back in the early 1970s, a now-defunct organization known as the state oceanographic commission proposed a series of unprecedented reforms aimed at protecting places like Rosario Strait from tanker mishaps. The commission, appointed by the governor, wanted all tankers entering these waters to have double hulls, twin propellers, and an engine with at least one horsepower for every two and a half deadweight tons. The idea was pretty progressive, and it showed how much people care, but the commission had no punch and nothing was ever done to make it law. Despite the organization's good intentions, only the federal government and the United Nations have the right to dictate ship construction standards. So tonight, as the *Arco Anchorage* sails into Rosario Strait, it sports a single hull, a single propeller, and an engine with only one horsepower for every four and a half deadweight tons. So much for those local efforts.

There was one area, however, where state government tried to exert some local authority and got some measure of success. While the legislature couldn't mandate rules for tanker construction, it tried to skirt the issue by making this region the only one in the country with a tanker weight restriction. They didn't use science to arrive at the 125,000-deadweight-ton size limit it imposed on loaded tankers sailing east of Port Angeles. Proponents simply started with a proposed 65,000-ton limit and raised it until, at 125,000 tons, they had enough votes to pass it.

Yet it was a stunning move, because no state had ever tried to impose a size limit on tankers entering its waters. Arco immediately sued the state of Washington and won when a federal judge ruled that only the federal government has the power to impose such limits on tanker construction. But no sooner had the judge tossed the idea overboard than the state's senior senator, Warren G. Magnuson, stepped into the fray. The old-style New Dealer (who owned property overlooking Puget Sound) was chairman of a committee that shaped the Coast Guard's budget. When Magnuson introduced a congressional amendment in 1977 and told the Coast Guard he wanted the 125,000-ton size limit, the once-reluctant regulators fell in love with the idea. By 1982 the size restriction was a permanent federal regulation, and Arco was forced to swallow it. Arco fleet president Jerry Aspland still bristles about it, and argues that it should be changed. It makes no sense, he says, since Arco's 190,000-ton tankers have double bottoms while smaller ships like the *Arco Anchorage* don't. And the bigger ships would make fewer trips to deliver the same amount of oil as the smaller ones. On the other hand, people like Felleman would like to make the "Magnuson line" more restrictive by moving it farther east to the entrance of the Strait of Juan de Fuca to protect more marine life. As it is now, the rule shelters human populated areas farther inland but not the richest marine habitats. "The Magnuson line has more to do with the abundance of people than it has to do with the abundance of resources," said Felleman.

But the line remains and everyone would agree it has taught Arco and other tanker companies a lesson—if you don't set your own standards in these waters, someone may set them for you. Aspland acknowledged as much after the *Exxon Valdez* spill when he suggested that tanker owners obey a voluntary speed limit in Rosario Strait of eleven nautical miles per hour. The owners accepted the "speed limit," but because it is voluntary it's like saying everybody on the highway will drive fifty-five miles an hour on the honor system. And even if the tanker owners obey the advisory, critics question whether the speed limit is slow enough. Aspland and others admit that tankers traveling slower than eleven knots might still overwhelm a tug and get in trouble. Tractor tugs will make a difference, but even they are no guarantee.

When the Davidson Rock beacon appears on the left beam of the *Arco Anchorage,* the pilot tells the mate to start slowing the ship. We are entering Rosario Strait, a one-way road where no other tanker is supposed to venture while we are sailing through (of course, exceptions are made). The tanker's bow is pointing north as we split the difference between Lopez Island on our left and Fidalgo Island on our right. It is pitch black, and the land masses fade into the gloom. As we sail onward, I'm having trouble distinguishing the lights on shore from those on the water. It's disconcerting not to know which luminary marks a navigation beacon and which one is someone's reading lamp in their living room. The mate tells me that a seaman's eye gets accustomed to the subtleties so he can tell the difference between a buoy and a house light.

We are still making fourteen nautical miles per hour but the propeller is slowing down and with it the ship. As I peer into the night I try to discern the outline of Lopez Island. I am a frequent visitor to the San Juan Islands, but this is quite another view from the bridge of an oil tanker. Islands that are usually playgrounds now seem like obstacles in the dark.

The San Juan Islands are a rocky archipelago arranged on a southeast-to-northwest diagonal between the Washington state mainland and Canada's Vancouver Island, hundreds of wafers of land providing a rural sanctuary to the farmers, entrepreneurs, trust-account recipients, and artisans who have the money or talent to live here. Only the biggest islands—Lopez, Shaw, Orcas, and San Juan—are served by government-owned ferries. Others are reachable by private ferry, private boat, or airplanes that land on private strips carved into the forest. For the wealthy, this is Cape Cod west, a monastery for folks on the run. Farms with long rustic fences occupy the lowlands and a few bridges remain that were built for the Model T. And one doesn't have to go too far to find the landmarks of local lore, like the British and American army camps, reminders of a war that was nearly fought a hundred years ago over the fatal shooting of a farmer's pig.

The pig war never amounted to much, but the cargo in the belly of the *Arco Anchorage* could surely destroy the tourism and flourishing wildlife of this place. The area around the San Juan Islands supports the highest concentration of wintering bald eagles in the Lower 48 states. The marine thoroughfares around the islands are used by the second-largest sockeye salmon run in the world. The rocky shorelines house one of the greatest collections of invertebrate marine creatures on earth, a living museum of sea slugs and mussels, anemones and octopuses.

It is a diver's dream, a kayaker's heaven, and for conservationists like Felleman, a place of special magic. Felleman's introduction to the San Juans was as a fisheries student at the University of Washington in 1983. A transplant from New York, Felleman chose to do his master's thesis on the voracious dining habits of the killer whale, a creature more revered than any other in these parts. To study them, he traveled for months in a small boat around the San Juans, where the whales are such a tourist attraction that there is a small park set aside for viewing them. Ranging in size from three to seven tons, with some as long as thirty feet, the killer whales in this area, numbering a little over one hundred, have been photographed as individuals and given names, making them all the more a royal treasure.

Yet with all their power, they would be helpless in the face of an oil spill since they breathe and travel on the water's surface. When the *Exxon Valdez* spill hit Prince William Sound, it quietly snuffed out more than a dozen killer whales, and mysteriously their bodies were never found. The Prince William Sound whales had been photographed and monitored the way they are down here, and when researchers checked on them days after the spill there were vacancies in the pack.

So how would it play if the *Arco Anchorage* hit the rocks tonight and we slaughtered the resident killer whale population? Many people would probably say it was an assassination and demand that Jack Carroll be thrown in jail. What the whale provides, for environmentalists, is a political lightning rod, a visible creature whose intelligence and playfulness inspires the musing of bipeds. To Felleman, though, the whale is merely an indicator of a greater resource lying below the water's surface. The way Felleman sees it, tanker owners and others who scoff at the danger are ignoring the real value of the ocean. "All they need is a fluid that is buoyant to conduct business, they don't need it to be vital."

No loaded tanker has ever spilled a major amount of its cargo in these waters. We passed a spot a while back where the unloaded tanker *Bunker Hill* exploded some thirty years ago, killing five crewmen and sending the flaming ship to the bottom. Investigators initially thought the ship hit an old practice bomb or a mine, something that is occasionally, although rarely, found in waterways such as these. But it was another tank-cleaning accident—some rusty metal fell into a tank and sparked the explosion.

At a little past nine o'clock, the evening sky is as black as crude oil and our ship is passing Bird Rocks as it sails deeper into Rosario Strait. A dot on the radar screen indicates the position of Bird Rocks, but I can't see them with my eyes. They are five times closer than Bligh Reef was when we sailed through Prince William Sound, but they are not the closest obstacle we will slip past tonight. The choke point of Rosario Strait is dead ahead.

I feel a bit of excitement as the *Arco Anchorage* closes on the narrowest portion of the strait, a channel between Peapod Rocks and Buckeye Shoals. The jagged reefs are about a mile apart, a crack compared to the twelve-mile-wide waters in which the *Exxon Valdez* went aground on Bligh Reef. Peapod Rocks and Buckeye Shoals are rimmed by submerged crags too deep to be visible but shallow enough to rip six feet of steel off the bottom of our ship. When the *Arco Anchorage* goes through, its hull will be less than three boat-lengths from danger.

As I study the scene on the radar screen, a Coast Guard voice comes over the radio, talking once again with the foreign tanker that has only one radar in working order. Seattle Traffic is giving the guy permission to enter Rosario Strait despite his problem. A chuckle breaks the silence somewhere near the wheel. "That's what you are going to get if they rescind the Jones Act. Foreign tankers with one radar."

"That's discrimination," says the chief mate. "We have to have two."

Our dual radars agree that Orcas Island, my favorite island in the chain, is the dominant feature now on the left of the ship. I stroll to the bridge wing to see it shrouded in the darkness. Orcas is the crown jewel of the San Juans, a treasure that reaches twenty-five hundred feet to the top of Mount Constitution and is draped with a dense forest of evergreen trees. Only an occasional light tells me the natives are awake, and if anyone were watching us from shore it would take a well-trained eye to know that we are the *Arco Anchorage,* slipping by in the dark, making a fully loaded passage to Cherry Point. From their perspective, we are an eventide ghost, invisible on the water except for our tiny lights. The beach dweller whose porch light I see is probably enjoying a fireside book, little aware of the trouble we are carrying in our tanks. If we were to hit the shoals ahead of us, the islander might kiss his shoreline good-bye. There is a swift current tonight that would carry the stuff in his direction. But spills are not what folks think about on a windy and rainy January evening, unless they happen to be on the bridge of an oil tanker, heading through the eye of a needle.

With around two miles to go until we reach the narrows, the pilot orders the helmsman to execute a dogleg turn to the right. Carroll is a silhouette standing near the front window of the wheelhouse, and as I sidle up to the handrail, the shadow speaks. "It might be pretty windy at Cherry Point. I'll check when we get closer. I've got to make sure it's not blowing too hard off the dock. If it is, I'll anchor off Sandy Point." Carroll is considering his options for docking, not the rocks that lie ahead. He'll let the pilot handle the narrows. The lights of Peapod Rocks and Buckeye Shoals are now a little more than a mile ahead, lurking on either side of the ship.

Meanwhile, down in the depths of the engine room, Bill Harrison smells smoke. The third engineer can't see where it is coming from, but he can taste the acrid mist and feel it in the back of his throat.

He checks the machinery nearest him and scans the control panel for advice. There are no obvious signs of trouble. "Shit." This is all he needs. Nothing is more dangerous than a fire in the engine room, which could disable the ship in seconds, leaving it unable to steer or stop. Or worse still the whole damn thing could explode.

The narrow gap between Peapod Rocks and Buckeye Shoals is now seven-eighths of a mile away, and up on the bridge the pilot is unaware of any problem below.

Harrison is not sure whether he has a serious problem, or whether it is something very simple. If there is real trouble, he must remember that the steam-powered fire-fighting pump has been diverted to do the work of the malfunctioning scrubber pump (which provides seawater to clean and cool the inert gas). Harrison can use a smaller electric pump to fight a fire, and he could quickly reconvert the big steam-driven one if he had a big blaze, but this is the type of thing you read about in accident reports: "The engine room crew was unable to start the fire-fighting process because . . ."

"Okay," Harrison says to himself, "what are the possibilities?" He remembers that the tug escort comes close to the ship in these waters. The tug's exhaust fumes are sometimes sucked into a gooseneck ventilator shaft up on the house and are drawn right down into the engine room. Figuring that is what he is smelling, Harrison calls the bridge and asks the mate to tell the tug to change its position. But the smoke only gets thicker. An accident report would say the third engineer made his first mistake when he mistook the smoke for tug exhaust.

Peapod Rocks and Buckeye Shoals are now five-eighths of a mile away, and those on the bridge have no idea that smoke is rising in the engine room.

Harrison sees no reason to sound an alarm yet, since he doesn't know whether he has a serious problem. It is ten o'clock and time for engineman Neal Curtis to make his rounds. He, too, has smelled the smoke, so he hurries his work. Whether there is trouble or not, Curtis usually conducts an hourly inspection, an extra precaution you don't get in unmanned, automated engine rooms. He starts at the bottom of the engine room and works his way up, examining each piece of equipment. As he does so, Curtis glances up seven stories to the ceiling and notices for the first time how much smoke is wafting through the place. It is light in color and still pretty thin, but the fact that he can see any at all is not a good sign. Engine room problems are the number one cause of ship fires, so like Harrison, Curtis starts to worry. He can't tell yet where the smoke is coming from, but it seems to be concentrated around the high-pressure turbine. He climbs a steep set of steel stairs and heads in that direction. The accident report would note how the engineman found the source of smoke during his routine rounds.

Peapod Rocks and Buckeye Shoals are now less than a half mile away, and Carroll is unaware of any trouble in the engine room.

Curtis summons Harrison and shows him the source of the smoke. A small "sight glass" on the surface of the high-pressure turbine is leaking lubricating oil. The "sight glass" is a viewing port, maybe two inches in diameter, where an engineer can see the caramel-colored lubricating oil flowing to the machinery. The oil that is leaking is soaking onto a fireproof insulation blanket that surrounds the turbine. The oil-soaked blanket is smoldering and giving off ever-thickening smoke. The third engineer doesn't call the bridge because he assumes he can fix the problem quickly. The turbine is nine hundred degrees Fahrenheit inside, and the steel on the outside is nearly as hot. If the sight glass were to break, hot oil would come bubbling out under ten pounds of pressure per square inch. The accident report would describe how the oil caught fire the moment it hit the hot steel, and how the engine room filled with smoke so thick the two men couldn't see.

Peapod Rocks and Buckeye Shoals are now a quarter of a mile away, and the mate is taking a reading off the radar screen, checking the ship's position as it enters the narrows.

Fortunately, the glass hasn't broken. Harrison pulls on a pair of fireproof gloves and checks his shirtsleeves to be sure the cuffs are buttoned. He doesn't want any skin exposed as he climbs onto the turbine to rip off the smoldering, oil-soaked shroud. What he is doing is worse than walking on hot coals, but he has no choice. He positions his feet very carefully on whatever brackets and pipes he can find that are not as hot as the turbine itself. The composite soles of his steel-toed boots absorb the hellfire just inches below him. The soles are thick and they give him some time, but he can't stay there for long. Like a cowboy hog-tying a steer, he stands spread-eagled and bent over the nine hundred-degree turbine, elbows flying and gloved fingers tearing away at pieces of smoking insulation. The smoke stings his eyes and irritates his skin. As he works, he keeps glancing at his right foot, which is just inches away from the glass window of a thermometer attached to the turbine. Caramel-colored oil is flowing through the thermometer, too. "The only thing I'm worried about is breaking the thermometer glass. If I break it, we would have hot oil coming out onto the hot turbine at a very high pressure." The accident report would describe how Harrison was burned in the flash fire that followed, and how the blaze spread to the rest of the machinery.

Peapod Rocks and Buckeye Shoals are now a few hundred yards ahead of the ship.

Harrison rips off the last pieces of insulation and hops off the turbine without breaking any glass or burning his feet. The soles of his boots are smoking as he pulls out a nearby garden hose that's used for deck cleaning and douses the smoldering blanket of insulation. The fire is out. Nobody on the bridge is any wiser because Harrison didn't have time to report the problem and now there isn't one. He hops back on the turbine and stops the oil leak by screwing down a nipple underneath the sight glass that had vibrated loose.

The scene in the aftermath is hardly anything to get excited about: a black garden hose lying atop a pile of blackened insulation. But Harrison is pretty irritated because it is more serious than it looks. He says if the oil had caught fire he would have been forced to shut down the turbine, to stop the flow of oil, before he could really fight the blaze. "That's five minutes later. In other words, you are basically fucked."

The accident report would have dwelled on the fact that Harrison and the other engineers had been working six hours on and six hours off during their journey south. It would have raised the question of why the chief engineer and other crew members were not summoned to the scene. As it is, Harrison has saved the day and there will be no accident report. It is not a reportable incident, just one of those things.

Harrison will need a good shower when his shift is done in a couple of hours. "My eyes are burning, plus my skin is all itchy." He probably owes Curtis a beer. "Neal Curtis is a good man. I'm glad he spotted this. I'm lucky to have him."

The incident was surely a close call, what some experts would call a "near miss." Consider what could have happened. The wind is now blowing at more than thirty-five miles an hour and the current is moving fast. With the engine room on fire, or smothered in a blanket of fire-fighting foam, the ship would have lost all ability to stop or maneuver. If the tug had been unable to control the ship, it would have drifted in the direction of Peapod Rocks just off the Doe Bay side of Orcas Island. It is debatable whether a grounding or an explosion would have broken the ship apart first, but there is no question that the San Juan Islands and hundreds of miles of shoreline north and east of here would have been devastated.

As it is, it is just another day at the office. Back up on the bridge,

Captain Carroll is talking by radio to an old friend, the captain of the *Arco Prudhoe Bay,* which is the ship that was taking up our place at the Cherry Point dock while we waited in Port Angeles. The voice is none other than John Piotrowski, Carroll's old mentor, the guy who taught him to be a skipper. Piotrowski says the winds were kicking up in the bay around Cherry Point and although they've now calmed down a bit they are likely to gust again, probably about the time Carroll arrives. "See you in Valdez."

"Yeah, the winds will come up just as we're docking, just as we are a ship's length away," Carroll says to me. "It always happens that way."

As we sail past Lummi Island and catch the lights of the British Petroleum dock at Ferndale, the whistling air picks up velocity. A rain is falling sideways, and it stings the face.

Out on the bridge wing, bosun Nehrenz is staring straight ahead, blinking away the heavy drops of rain that add to the misery of his lookout duties. I can see the lights of the Arco refinery in the distance, a busy place, hungry for our cargo. It looks like the city of Oz, with lights strung up the sides of the tall cracker towers and a gas fire belching out the top. Nehrenz is anxious to see his wife, for she is somewhere in the vicinity of the lights. Whenever the ship docks at Cherry Point she comes to see him. If he can get some time off, they check into a nearby motel and spend a little time together. "It's great to have a good wife." I know how he feels. My wife is somewhere out there, too.

Two other oil tankers are pulling away from the docks at the Arco and BP refineries. One, of course, is the *Arco Prudhoe Bay* and the other is the *Prince William Sound.* Yes, the latter is the same tanker we so soundly beat in the race from Hinchinbrook when it took a left turn into a storm and we turned right over the hundred-fathom curve. Now we find that it has slipped ahead of us as we slept in Port Angeles, and it has already off-loaded its cargo. The turtle wins the race, after all.

As tanker operations go, this one is a traffic jam. The *Prudhoe Bay* passes less than three-quarters of a mile on our port side. "See you, John," the skipper says over the radio. "See you, Jack," comes the reply.

At the same time, the *Prince William Sound* is a close string of lights passing us on the right. And, of course, there is always that foreign ship somewhere behind us, sailing up the strait with one radar.

Dean Davis stands at the throttle, casually adjusting the ship's speed at the pilot's request. In the dead of night and the middle of a blistering rainstorm, Davis looks as sharp and as scrubbed as a schoolboy. I wonder if he'll skipper a ship into Cherry Point someday, and whether he will talk over the radio with his mentor Jack Carroll.

Down on the main deck, Jean Holmes is walking toward the fo'c'sle where she will oversee the handling of the lines. She is a bundle of yellow Gortex pitched forward against the wind and horizontal rain. Will she keep going against the trials of sea duty and make captain herself someday? I hope so, but it is a hard road.

In heaving gusts of wind we are maneuvering into a flood tide, just as Carroll expected.

Newman has his gnarled hands around the steering wheel now, looking as crusty as the ship itself. The *Arco Anchorage* may outlast the cynical seaman, or maybe he will stay on the job despite his feelings. The ship has six years left before its thin hull will be illegal and Newman has Lord knows how many trips left in him before his patience wears too thin. It will take a lot of something inside this sailor to keep him going that long. "Got to hook up the tugs, put the lines out, and tie this bitch down," he is saying in the darkness. "Got to do it again, and again, and again, and again, and again."

Carroll looks tired. He is already days past the time when this tour should end, but Robert Lawlor, his relief, is attending radio school. As a result, Carroll must do a few more trips in this worst winter in fifteen years.

"The *Arco Anchorage* is what some call the worst ship in the fleet, maintenance-wise. You've got some engineers who don't get along. You've got the weather sometimes. It just drains me. I'm looking forward to a vacation."

The tugs push the big ship into place against the Cherry Point dock. The guys on shore are getting the gangplank ready. Soon we will experience the firm sensation of solid ground. The cargo will gush ashore and be processed to feed the engines of commerce and pleasure. My own car is idling on a tank of regular unleaded gasoline right now, somewhere in the darkness, keeping my waiting spouse warm.

As soon as the gangplank hits the dock the action I saw in Valdez will repeat itself and there won't be much time for socializing. In the peace of these closing moments, the captain and I bid each other farewell. I wish him a following wind and trouble-free career. Being from Texas, he allows as how he hates the rain, but he figures I, the Seattleite, must love the stuff. We laugh, knowing it is probably true.

The ship looks haggard and worn in this drenching winter rain. As I gaze at the gaggle of pipes on the main deck, I can't predict whether this long hull will go quietly into oblivion on June 1, 1998, the last day it is allowed to operate with a single skin, or whether it will hit some rocks beforehand and attain a dubious place in history. I wonder the same thing whenever I see an oil ship these days. Most owners say their tankers are safe, and they cite reasons why. But with the year that just ended being the worst for spills, worldwide, it is no surprise that the year we are entering is destined to be the second worst. Tonight, a tanker named the *Aegean Sea* is sailing into Egypt, almost identical in size and age to this one, but equipped with a double hull, it seems invulnerable. At the same time, cruising toward Rotterdam in the Atlantic Ocean is a smaller tanker named the *Braer* which, at 90,000 deadweight tons, is not the kind of super tanker people associate with trouble. And if the *Maersk Navigator* seems awfully big and dangerous carrying 254,000 deadweight tons south of Japan tonight, it is reassuring to know it is only three years old and part of a Danish fleet known for very safe operations. These three ships are not the type you would worry about, no more than you would lose sleep over the *Arco Anchorage* docking quietly at a refinery north of Bellingham in a sheet of rain shortly after midnight.

But exactly ten months from now, the *Aegean Sea* will go aground in a storm off Spain and the double hull will rupture. One month later, the fully loaded *Braer* will lose power in a hurricane-force storm off the Shetland Islands and will be pounded to oblivion on the rocks. Two weeks later, the fully loaded *Maersk Navigator* will slam into a smaller tanker in the Strait of Malacca, causing the second major spill in that waterway in four months. In total, nearly fifty-three million gallons of petroleum will be spilled by three ships in less than six weeks.

Individual tanker accidents are random and unpredictable events. You might not see one in a particular area for years, and then you will get two of them in a matter of weeks. Coast Guard statisticians made a computer run and could discover no time of day, season, or place where we should especially gird ourselves. The one thing the accident reports tell us with certainty is that the accidents usually begin with a cascade of events and errors much like the one we experienced tonight.

If the world is to prevent these spills, the regulators must require the reporting of near-miss incidents, and study them along with accident reports to find the weak points in the system and patch them. Some organization must take charge of the maritime safety system with enough authority to tell shipowners around the globe what to do. And it should not take decades to require fundamental safety systems such as inert gas and double hulls, or to force shipyards to build tankers with sufficient steel to withstand the tremors of the ocean. Prevention is the only answer when ships are hauling a dangerous substance that cannot be stuffed back into the container.

In a few years, the crew of this vessel will have new faces and more double-hulled tankers will be parting the waves. There may be a better vessel-traffic system in these waters, and there could be tougher rules and even better inspectors.

But it is just as likely—given the pattern of history—that people will have forgotten the lessons of the *Exxon Valdez*. Double hulls will not solve the problem if ships carry the maximum amount of oil with the minimum amount of steel and people; if vessel-traffic systems exist in only a few waterways of the world; if standards for crew training do not change; if the regulators are fragmented and weak; and if the profit margin squeezes out safety. History shows that things return quickly to business as usual in this tanker trade.

The gangplank is now married to the main deck and my shoreside mate awaits me somewhere over the rise in the nasty weather. Soon I will rejoin the petroleum users on the freeway and the tanker will have another bout with the Gulf of Alaska. On the company books, voyage number CF-396 is over. Leave it to Newman to have the last words.

Maybe he is pessimistic, or maybe he is wise, but with the engines shut off, and the old ship at idle, the veteran seaman has some parting advice for my notebook. He says it doesn't matter much whether you build ships with double hulls, put in more steel, stick on double propellers, and install "all kinds of other good stuff." It doesn't matter whether the sun is shining or the wind is blowing. The difference between an uneventful trip and a disaster is attitude.

"Our real enemy isn't the elements or anything like that. It's complacency, indifference, and arrogance."

Bibliography

For the reader's convenience, reports on specific vessels are grouped together under the name of the ship.

Abrams, Alan. "Environmentalists Press for Further Tanker Changes." *Journal of Commerce,* 7 October 1992.

———. "Final Test Results Cast Doubts on Mid-Deck Tanker Design." *Journal of Commerce,* 6 February 1992.

———. "NTSB Blames Inspection Miscue for Fatal Persian Gulf Tanker Blast." *Journal of Commerce,* 7 April 1992.

———. "Ship Inspection Firm Sued over Sinking That Killed 2." *Journal of Commerce,* 29 July 1992.

———. "Tanker Industry Reluctantly Gears for Vapor Rules." *Journal of Commerce,* 13 January 1992.

———. "Tanker Inspections Are Questioned by Oil Executives." *Journal of Commerce,* 3 June 1992.

"ABS Mess," editorial. *Journal of Commerce,* 13 April 1992.

ABS 2000, Approaching the Goals. Paramus, New Jersey: American Bureau of Shipping, 1991.

Alvarez, A. "Sinking Fast." *New York Times Magazine,* 17 May 1992.

Bibliography

"Alyeska Pipeline Service Company Covert Operation." Draft Report of the Committee on Interior and Insular Affairs of the U.S. House of Representatives. Washington, D.C., July 1992.

American Bureau of Shipping 125th Anniversary. Paramus, N.J.: American Bureau of Shipping, 1987.

American Waterways Operators, 1991 Annual Report. Arlington, Va., 1991.

Anderson, David. *Report to the Premier on Oil Transportation and Oil Spills.* Victoria, B.C.: Queens Printer for British Columbia, 1989.

Andrews, Paul. "Maggie Maneuvers Around." *Seattle Times,* 6 October 1977.

———. "Supertanker Ban Overturned." *Seattle Times,* 24 September 1976.

Arco Anchorage. Deposition of George Kirk Greiner, Jr. (investigator). Lacey, Washington, Pollution Control Hearings Board, 14 August 1987.

Arco Anchorage. Deposition of Raymond L. Leson. Seattle: Pollution Control Hearings Board, 5 August 1987.

Arco Anchorage. Findings, *Raymond Leson* vs. *State of Washington,* Pollution Control Hearings Board, April 1988.

Arco Anchorage. Grounding, December 21, 1985. Seattle: U.S. Coast Guard, 28 May 1986.

Arco Anchorage. On-Scene Coordinator's Report, T/V Arco Anchorage Major Oil Spill. Seattle: U.S. Coast Guard, 14 February 1986.

Arco Anchorage. Transcript of Proceedings, Pollution Control Hearings Board, *Raymond Leson* vs. *State of Washington,* September–November 1987.

An Assessment of Tanker Transportation Systems in Cook Inlet and Prince William Sound. Report to the Alaska Oil Spill Commission by Engineering Computer Optecnomics, Inc. Annapolis, Md., 8 December 1989.

Bangsberg, P. T. "Ship Crash Rekindles Malacca Concern." *Journal of Commerce,* 22 September 1992.

Beedel, Capt. R. "An Introduction to MARS, The International Marine Accident Reporting Scheme." *Seaways* (London), July 1992.

Behr, Peter. "Supertankers Face Extinction." *Washington Post,* 5 January 1986.

Bernstein, Peter J. "The Sea Itself May Die." *The Nation,* 16 September 1978.

Bjorkman, M. *Coulumbi Egg Oil Tanker.* Design construction and certification handbook. Monaco, August 1991.

Blumenthal, Ralph. "Ship Inspectors' Costs Paid Directly." *New York Times,* 30 November 1989.

Bovet, David. *Preliminary Analysis of Tanker Collisions and Groundings.* Washington, D.C.: U.S. Coast Guard, January 1973.

Briefing Package for Commander, 13th Coast Guard District, Marine Safety Office, Puget Sound. Seattle: U.S. Coast Guard, 13 July 1992.

Broom, Jack. "Crack Down on Shoddy Ship Pilotage, Says Bottiger." *Seattle Times,* 16 January 1986.

Broom, Jack, and Ross Anderson. "Could It Happen Here?" *Seattle Times,* 2 April 1989.

Brown, Tom. "Lifeline to Alaska." *Seattle Times,* 23 August 1992.

Budget in Brief. Washington, D.C.: U.S. Coast Guard, 1990 and 1993.

Bulls Tankrederi A/S, Annual Report, Jorgen Jahre Shipping. Oslo, 1991.

Calicchio, Domenic A. Variety of reports reviewing pilotage, 1991 and 1992.

Cameron, Juan. "Cracking the Tanker Safety Problem." *Fortune,* April 1977.

Campbell, William H., Jr. *Single Boiler Reliability Experience on U.S. Flag Ships.* Washington, D.C.: U.S. Coast Guard, 1977.

Card, James C. "Effectiveness of Double Bottoms in Preventing Oil Outflow from Tanker Bottom Damage Incidents." *Marine Technology,* January 1975.

Chadbourne, Scott H., and Thomas M. Leschine. 1988 Petroleum Transportation Estimates for Puget Sound and the Strait of Juan de Fuca. December 1989.

"The Chedabucto Bay Spill—Arrow, 1970." Oceanus (Woods Hole, Mass.: Woods Hole Oceanographic Institution), Fall 1977.

Chen, Y. A., and A. K. Thayamballi. *Consideration of Global Climatology and Loading Characteristics in Fatigue Damage Assessment of Ship Structures.* Jersey City, N.J.: The Society of Naval Architects and Marine Engineers, n.d.

"A Close Look at Marine Surveying." *Boating,* September 1978.

Coast Alert, Scientists Speak Out. San Francisco: Coast Alliance/Friends of the Earth, 1981.

Coast Guard, Limited Resources Curtail Ability to Meet Responsibilities. Report by the Comptroller General to the Chairman, Committee on Commerce, Science and Transportation. U.S. Senate, 3 April 1980.

Code of Federal Regulations, Title 33, Parts 1–199, Navigation and Navigable Waters. Washington, D.C.: U.S. Government Printing Office, 1988.

Bibliography

Code of Federal Regulations, Title 46, Parts 41–69, Shipping. Washington, D.C.: U.S. Government Printing Office, 1988 and 1989.

Cohen, Lucille. "$75 Million Refinery Fulfills Dreams of Anacortes Founders, Shell Oil's Decision to Speed Growth of the New York of the West." *Seattle Post-Intelligencer,* 15 July 1953.

Coordination and Planning for National Oil Spill Response. Washington, D.C.: General Accounting Office, September 1991.

Coping with an Oiled Sea: An Analysis of Oil Spill Response Technologies—Background Paper. Washington, D.C.: Office of Technology Assessment, 1990.

Coughlin, William P. "Exxon Curbing Overtime on Ships in Bid to Justify Smaller Crews." *Boston Globe,* 30 April 1989.

Coulter, Henry W., and Ralph R. Migliaccio. "Effects of the Earthquake of March 27, 1964, at Valdez, Alaska." U.S. Geological Survey Professional Paper 542-C. Washington, D.C.: National Academy of Sciences, 1971.

Crane, C. Lincoln, Jr. "Maneuvering Safety of Large Tankers: Stopping, Turning, and Speed Selection." *Maritime Reporter/Engineering News,* 1 January 1974.

A Crew Exposure Study; Phase II, Volume II; at Sea. U.S. Department of Transportation, U.S. Coast Guard, 1985.

Crew Size and Maritime Safety. Report of the Marine Board, National Research Council. Washington, D.C.: National Academy Press, 1990.

Crude Oil and Product Movements in Washington State—1986. Western Oil and Gas Association.

Curtis, Clifton. Statement on Behalf of the Oceanic Society and Friends of the Earth before House Committee on Merchant Marine and Fisheries, 11 May 1989.

"Custom Oil Spill Data, Oil Spill Intelligence Report." Cutter Information Corp. Special report on tanker and barge spills compiled for the author, July 1, 1992.

Dane, Abe. "America's Oil Tanker Mess." *Popular Mechanics,* November 1989.

Davidson, Art. *In the Wake of the Exxon Valdez.* San Francisco: Sierra Club Books, 1990.

Davies, John. "Depressed Charter Rates Raise Maintenance Concern." *Journal of Commerce,* 26 October 1992.

————. "Ex-NY Port Official Defends Vessel Traffic System." *Journal of Commerce,* 18 June 1992.

Decision and Report, loss of the VLCC *Albahaa B* off the East Coast of Africa on 3 April 1980. Monrovia, Liberia: Bureau of Maritime Affairs, August 1982.

Decision and Report, explosion, VLCC *Atlas Titan,* at berth, Setubal, Portugal, 27 May 1979. Monrovia, Liberia: Bureau of Maritime Affairs, August 1979.

Decision and Report, breaking and sinking of MT *Aviles* in the Indian Ocean on 28 June 1979. Monrovia, Liberia: Bureau of Maritime Affairs, May 1984.

Decision and Report, major hull fracture of *Energy Concentration* in Europoort. Rotterdam, The Netherlands. Monrovia, Liberia: Bureau of Maritime Affairs, November 1981.

Decision and Report, fire and loss of the ULCC *Energy Determination* in the Strait of Hormuz, 1979. Monrovia, Liberia: Bureau of Maritime Affairs, June 1983.

Decision and Report, fire and explosion in the engine room, MT *Haralabos,* at Ras Gharib, Egypt, 26 November 1992. Monrovia, Liberia: Bureau of Maritime Affairs, August 1983.

Decision and Report, structural failure and loss, *Hawaiian Patriot,* in Pacific Ocean, 24 February 1977. Monrovia, Liberia: Bureau of Maritime Affairs, April 1979.

Decision and Report, steering failure, MT *Hellespont Courage,* Northwest Coast of Ireland, 9 February 1988. Monrovia, Liberia: Bureau of Maritime Affairs, n.d.

Decision and Report, sinking of ST *Irenes Challenge* near Midway Island, 17 January 1977. Monrovia, Liberia: Bureau of Maritime Affairs, February 1980.

Decision and Report, collision, M/S *Mimosa* and M/T *Burmah Agate,* 1 November 1979. Monrovia, Liberia: Bureau of Maritime Affairs, July 1981.

Decision and Report, explosion, breaking in two, and sinking of VLCC *Mycene,* 3 April 1980. Monrovia, Liberia: Bureau of Maritime Affairs, March 1982.

Decision and Report, S.S. *Pacocean.* Monrovia, Liberia: Bureau of Maritime Affairs, February 1970.

Decision and Report, explosion/fire, VLCC *Pegasus,* off Sirri Island, 16 December 1988. Monrovia, Liberia: Bureau of Maritime Affairs, February 1991.

Decision and Report, collision, MT *Phillips Oklahoma* and *Fiona,* North Sea, East Coast of Ireland, 17 September 1989. Monrovia, Liberia: Bureau of Maritime Affairs, January 1991.

Decision and Report, sinking of *San Nicolas,* Gulf of Mexico, 5 March 1972. Monrovia, Liberia: Bureau of Maritime Affairs, n.d.

Decision and Report, explosion/fire, *Seatiger,* Neches River, Texas, 19 April 1979. Monrovia, Liberia: Bureau of Maritime Affairs, February 1980.

Decision and Report, collision of *Stolt Sheaf* and *Altair* in the Pacific near Panama, 20 June 1988. Monrovia, Liberia: Bureau of Maritime Affairs, January 1990.

Bibliography

Decision and Report, explosion/fire, S.T. *Universe Defiance,* Atlantic Ocean, 15 April 1977. Monrovia, Liberia: Bureau of Maritime Affairs, March 1981.

DeFries, C. E., president of National Marine Engineers' Beneficial Association. Statement to House Subcommittee on Merchant Marine, 10 May 1989.

Development and Assessment of Measures to Reduce Accidental Oil Outflow from Tank Ships. U.S. Coast Guard, May 1989.

DiBenedetto, William. "Navy Tests Tanker Designs, Grapples With Indoor Oil Spills." *Journal of Commerce,* 7 January 1992.

Dietrich, Bill. "Oil Beginning to Wash Ashore on Mainland." *Seattle Times,* 28 July 1991.

———. "Oil Spill: One Week of Frenzy." *Seattle Times,* 31 March 1989.

Dike, Tom M. "Close Aboard Situation between Tanker *Overseas Alaska* and Freighter *Pacbaron."* U.S. Coast Guard internal memo, 23 April 1992.

"Double Bottom Rule Shunned for Tankers." *Journal of Commerce,* 1 August 1974.

Doyle, Jack. *Crude Awakening, The Oil Mess in America: Wasting Energy, Jobs and the Environment.* Washington, D.C.: Friends of the Earth, 1993.

Drydock Examination Book. U.S. Coast Guard, n.d.

Dunn, Laurence. "Tanker Development." *Tanker Register,* 1970.

Effective Manning of the U.S. Merchant Fleet. Committee on Effective Manning, Marine Board. Washington, D.C.: National Research Council, 1984.

Embiricos, Philip A. *The Quest for the Environmental Ship.* An Intertanko Discussion Paper, May 1991.

"Ensuring Ship Safety," editorial. *Journal of Commerce,* 3 May 1993.

"Escort Vessels for Certain Oil Tankers." Proposed Rule, U.S. Department of Transportation, Coast Guard. *Federal Register,* 7 July 1992.

Evans, Mary. *Research Report, Effects of U.S. Coast Guard Enforcement Performance on Oil Tanker Safety, for State of Alaska Oil Spill Commission.* 4 December 1989.

"Evans Signs Bill Banning Oil Supertankers on Sound." *Seattle Times,* 31 May 1975.

The Expert 5, issues 1 and 2. Ridgefield, Conn.: Maritime and Environmental Consultants, 1989.

Explosion and Fire aboard the U.S. Tankship Jupiter, Bay City, Michigan, 16 September 1990. Marine Accident Report. Washington, D.C.: National Transportation Safety Board, 1991.

Exxon New Orleans, Marine Casualty Narrative Supplement, Injury to deckhand Paahana, 18 March 1992.

Exxon Philadelphia, Report of Marine Accident, Injury or Death, loss of power 10 miles west of entrance to Strait of Juan de Fuca, 26 April 1989.

Exxon Philadelphia, Report of Marine Accident, Injury or Death, loss of power, Latitude 45.32 N and Longitude 129.26 W, 14 January 1988.

Exxon Philadelphia, Special Inspection, loss of power off Cape Flattery, 17 February 1988.

Exxon San Francisco, U.S. Coast Guard report on loss of power near Port Angeles on September 15, 1989.

Exxon Seamen's Union. Various newsletters and reports.

Exxon Shipping Company. Various memoranda regarding automation and de-manning on *Exxon Baton Rouge, Exxon San Francisco,* and *Exxon Philadelphia.*

Exxon Valdez, chronology of spill, National Transportation Safety Board files.

Exxon Valdez, General Accounting Office Report, 30 October 1989.

Exxon Valdez, grounding of, Bligh Reef, Prince William Sound, March 24, 1989. Washington, D.C.: National Transportation Safety Board, 31 July 1990.

Exxon Valdez, grounding of, complete National Transportation Safety Board investigation files.

Exxon Valdez, Oil Spill Restoration, Volumes I–IV, Prepared by *Exxon Valdez* Oil Spill Trustees, April 1992.

Exxon Valdez, Proposed Findings of Fact, Conclusions and Recommendations. Exxon Corporation, 17 July 1989.

Exxon Valdez, Proposed Probable Cause, Findings and Recommendations, Robert LeResche, Oil Spill Coordinator, State of Alaska, 17 July 1989.

Exxon Valdez, The *Exxon Valdez* Oil Spill, A Report to the President, from Samuel K. Skinner and William K. Reilly, May 1989.

Fararo, Kim. "Scientist Warns Valdez of Benzene in the Air." *Anchorage Daily News,* 21 March 1992.

———. "Study Absolving Alyeska Flawed, Air Experts Say." *Anchorage Daily News,* 27 August 1992.

Farnsworth, B.A., and Larry C. Young. *Nautical Rules of the Road, The International and Inland Rules.* 3d ed. Centreville, Md.: Cornell Maritime Press, 1990.

Bibliography

Farrington, John W. "The Biogeochemistry of Oil in the Ocean." *Oceanus* (Woods Hole, Mass.: Woods Hole Oceanographic Institution), Fall 1977.

Federal On-Scene Coordinator Report, Major Oil Spill, M/V Glacier Bay, Cook Inlet, Alaska, July 2 to August 3, 1987. Anchorage: U.S. Coast Guard Marine Safety Office, 24 March 1988.

Final Report of the States/British Columbia Oil Spill Task Force. October 1990.

First Report of the Washington State Marine Oversight Board. Report Card on the Status of Safety of Oil Transportation in Washington's Waters. Seattle, March 1993.

Focus on IMO. Various issues. London: International Maritime Organization.

Ford, Royal, and William Coughlin. "Studies Show Tankers Crack and Spill Oil Because They Are So Big." *Boston Globe,* 6 July 1989.

"Freeing the Tiller," editorial. *Journal of Commerce,* 15 April 1992.

Frontline, Highlights of the Year. Annual report of Frontline AB. Stockholm, Sweden, 1991.

Galyean, Dr. Paul H. "Differential GPS—A Vital Player in Future Vessel Traffic Systems." *Sea Technology,* March 1992.

Geselbracht, Laura L. *Washington's Compensation Recovery Mechanisms for Aquatic Resource Damages from Pollutant Spills: A Review and Appraisal.* Seattle: University of Washington, Institute for Marine Studies, February 1989.

Golob's Oil Pollution Bulletin. Various editions. Cambridge, Mass.: World Information Systems.

Gordon, Huntley. "Big New Cherry Point Refinery Weathers Storms and Protests." *Seattle Times,* 21 March 1971.

Grandolfo, Jane. "Troubled Waters." *Houston Post,* 12 August 1990.

Gray, William O. "Prevention of Pollution." Speech for Conference on Oil Pollution Claims, Liability and Environmental Concerns, London, November 4, 1992.

Greiner, Capt. Kirk, USCG-Ret. Letter regarding pilots, 16 December 1989.

———. "Steering Gear Failures—Have We Done Enough." Undated paper.

Grounding of the S.S. Hillyer Brown at Cold Bay, Ak., March 7, 1973. U.S. Coast Guard report prepared for National Transportation Safety Board, 15 January 1975.

Grounding Probability Studies. Prepared by George G. Sharp., Inc. New York: U.S. Maritime Administration, 7 January 1977.

Grove, Noel. "Giants That Move the World's Oil, Superships." *National Geographic,* July 1978.

Gugliotta, Guy. "Billionaire Slices Civilization from Brazilian Jungle." *Seattle Post-Intelligencer,* 9 July 1978.

Gutierrez-Fraile, Rafael. "The European E-3 Tanker." Paper presented to Tanker Legislation Symposium 1991, Washington, D.C., 24–25 September 1991.

Gwinn, Mary Ann. "A Deathly Call of the Wild—Mournful Cry of a Loon Echoes through a Land Devastated by Oil Spill," *Seattle Times,* 4 April 1989.

Hamel, Charles. *Hamel Environmental Accountability Project.* Various issues. Self-published. Alexandria, Va.

Hanksworth, Thomas W. Letter regarding Northern Tier Pipeline, 14 November 1989.

Hill, Christopher, Bill Robertson, and Steven J. Hazelwood. *An Introduction to P & I.* London: Lloyd's of London Press Ltd., 1988.

Hooke, Norman. *Modern Shipping Disasters 1963–1987.* London: Lloyd's of London Press Ltd., 1989.

Horne, George. "Giant U.S. Tanker Named in Boston, 106,500-ton *Manhattan* is Biggest Built in Country." *New York Times,* 11 January 1962.

———. "Sinclair to Build Push-Button Ship, 51,000-Ton Tanker to Use Half of Normal Crew." *New York Times,* 29 October 1961.

Horne, Janet. "Environment Will Bounce Back, Says Dr. Ray." *Seattle Times,* 26 January 1977.

Howard, Craig. "Human Fallibility Cited as Key Ship Loss Factor." *Journal of Commerce,* 27 October 1971.

———. "Tanker Advisory Center Finds—Double Bottoms Cut Oil Pollution." *Journal of Commerce,* 22 July 1977.

———. "Vessel Losses in 1970 Highest in 50 Years." *Journal of Commerce,* 1 October 1971.

How Effective Is the Coast Guard in Carrying Out Its Commercial Vessel Safety Responsibilities? Comptroller General Report to the Congress of the United States, 25 May 1979.

"How the Oil Spilled and Spread: Delay and Confusion Off Alaska." *New York Times,* 16 April 1989.

Hoye, Paul F. "Tankers: A Special Issue." *Aramco World,* July–August 1966.

Bibliography

Human Performance Factual Report, Accident, Exxon Valdez. Washington, D.C.: National Transportation Safety Board, Bureau of Technology, 16 February 1990.

Hurn, Jeff. *GPS, A Guide to the Next Utility.* Sunnyvale, Calif.: Trumbull Navigation Ltd., 1989.

Iarossi, Frank J., Exxon Shipping Company president. "Surrendering the Memories," June 1988.

Inquiry Report, explosion and fire on board S/T *Spryos,* 12 October 1978, Jurong Shipyard, Singapore, January 1979.

Inspection Program Improvements Are Underway to Help Detect Unsafe Tankers. GAO Report. Washington, D.C., October 1991.

Instructions, Engineering Piping Systems, Single-Screw Tanker, Sparrows Point Hulls. Bethlehem Steel Corporation, Sparrows Point, Maryland.

International Conference on Marine Pollution 1973. London: Inter-Governmental Maritime Consultative Organization, 1973.

"International Conference on Tanker Safety and Pollution Prevention." Draft Environmental Impact Statement. U.S. Coast Guard, February 1978.

International Convention on Standards of Training, Certification and Watchkeeping for Seafarers, with Annex. London, 7 July 1978.

International Maritime Organization. Various reports and summaries of treaties.

International Oil Pollution R&D Abstract Database. Tysons Corner, Va.: Interagency Coordinating Committee on Oil Pollution Research, June 1992.

International Safety Guide for Oil Tankers and Terminals. 2d ed. London: Witherby & Co., Ltd., 1984.

Interpretation of Various Issues Regarding Pilots and the Pilotage Regulations. Navigation and Vessel Inspection Circular No. 3-91. Washington, D.C.: U.S. Coast Guard, 21 February 1991.

Jahre Viking. "Keppel Restores the World's Largest Tanker." *Keppel Now,* First Quarter 1992.

Jahre Viking. "Lloyd's Maritime Seadata." Speech. November 1992.

Jones, Stan. "Empty Promises." *Anchorage Daily News,* 15 October 1989.

Keith, Virgil. "The *Exxon Valdez* and *American Trader* Oil Spills: What Can Be Done to Prevent Future Spills?" Report to 1991 International Oil Spill Conference, San Diego, Calif., 4–7 March 1991.

————. "Tank Vessel Design and Arrangement; Double Hull and Double Bottom Considerations." Paper delivered at a conference. 1990.

Keith, Virgil, Joseph D. Porricelli, Jan P. Hooft, Paul J. Paymans, and Franz G. Witt. "Real-Time Simulation of Tanker Operations for the Trans-Alaska Pipeline System." Reprinted from *Society of Naval Architects and Marine Engineers* 85 (1977).

Kimon, Peter M., Ronald K. Kiss, and Joseph D. Porricelli. "Segregated Ballast VLCCs." *Marine Reporter/Engineering News,* 1 April 1973.

Kolstad, James L., acting chairman, National Transportation Safety Board. Letter to U.S. Rep. Walter B. Jones, chairman, House Committee on Merchant Marine and Fisheries, regarding pilot licensing, 7 November 1989.

Lagerberg, Brian, and Mark Anderson. *Washington State Petroleum Markets Data Book.* Olympia, Wash.: Washington State Energy Office, 1992.

"Large Oil Tanker Structural Survey Experience." A position paper by Exxon Corporation, 1 June 1982.

Lawn, Daniel J. "Alyeska Prince William Sound Tanker Spill Prevention and Response Plan, Prince William Sound District Office." Draft. Valdez, Ak: Alaska Department of Environmental Conservation, 21 May 1990.

————. *Analysis of Ballast Water Tanker Practices.* Valdez, Ak.: Alaska Department of Environmental Conservation, 1991.

Ledbetter, B. Glenn. "That's the Way Things Are." *Pacific Maritime,* July 1985.

Leis, R. D. *Double Hull Effectiveness Analysis.* Washington, D.C.: U.S. Coast Guard, 1976.

Levine, Sydney. "Has Tanker Resale Mart Bottomed Out? Maybe, But Don't Bet the Boat on It." *Journal of Commerce,* 26 October 1992.

"Licensing of Pilots; Manning of Vessels-Pilots." Department of Transportation, Coast Guard, Washington, D.C.: *Federal Register,* 6 June 1988.

"Licensing of Pilots; Manning of Vessels-Pilots." Rule and Proposed Rule, Department of Transportation, Coast Guard. Washington, D.C.: *Federal Register,* 24 June 1985.

"Licensing of Pilots." Proposed Rules, Department of Transportation, Coast Guard. Washington, D.C.: *Federal Register,* 28 November 1980.

Lloyd's List International, 1991—A Year of Major Losses. A Lloyd's List Archive Publication. Colchester: Lloyd's List, 1992.

Bibliography

Lloyd's World Shipowning Groups. Colchester: Lloyd's of London Press, Ltd., 1992.

Ludwig, Daniel K. The Associated Press Biographical Service, 8 May 1980.

———. *Current Biography,* 1979.

MacDonald, Comdr. James L., USCG-Ret. Letter to L. A. Colucciello, National Transportation Safety Board, regarding *VTS Valdez,* 26 April 1989.

Machinery Inspection Book, U.S. Coast Guard, n.d.

Mackin, John G. Biographical data, résumé provided by spouse.

Maersk, A.P. Moller. Various reports and pamphlets, Copenhagen.

Maersk Neptune, ramming of *Mont Fort,* 15 February 1988, Upper New York Bay. Washington, D.C.: National Transportation Safety Board, November 1988.

Magnier, Mark. "Philippines Takes Steps to Ensure Honesty in Seafarer Licensing." *Journal of Commerce,* 16 October 1992.

———. "Precautions Fail to Deter Pirates Off Singapore." *Journal of Commerce,* 5 May 1992.

———. "Shortage of Skilled Ship Officers Sparks Call for Shipowner Initiative." *Journal of Commerce,* 16 October 1992.

———. "Singapore Ship Braves the Waters to New Vietnam, Piracy Looms as a Risk, Graft as a Certainty." *Journal of Commerce,* 10 June 1992.

Magnuson, Sen. Warren G. Testimony to the Senate Committee on Commerce, Science and Transportation, regarding the Puget Sound Tanker Safety Act of 1989, 7 May 1989.

Maider, Ian. "Otters are Back, Trade Follows." *Anchorage Daily News* (Associated Press), 13 June 1993.

Malseed, William A., Shell Oil Company. Statement to Washington State Senate Transportation and Utilities Committee on cleanup capabilities, 2 April 1975.

Management Improvement Could Enhance Enforcement of Coast Guard Marine Safety Programs. GAO Report. Washington, D.C., 15 August 1985.

Mandan, Collision of the Hong Kong–Registered Motor Tank Ship *Mandan* with the U.S. Army Corps of Engineers' Barge Flotilla. Marine Accident Report. Washington, D.C.: National Transportation Safety Board, March 1992.

Marian, Lt. Tom. "The Art of Managing Space in Puget Sound." *48 Degrees North, The Sailing Magazine,* 12 July 1992.

Marine Accident Reports, National Transportation Safety Board, issues 1–7.

Marine Digest. Various editions (Seattle).

Marine Electric, U.S. Bulk Carrier, capsizing and sinking, 12 February 1983. Marine Accident Report. Washington D.C.: National Transportation Safety Board, March 1984.

Marine Exchange of Puget Sound. Various vessel arrival and departure reports, and a report on lightering.

Marine Pilots, Statutes and Regulations. Alaska Department of Commerce and Economic Development, Anchorage, Ak: February 1992.

MARS Report No. 1, International Marine Accident Reporting Scheme. London: *Seaways,* October 1992.

Matsukaze, grounding at Crescent Bay in the Strait of Juan de Fuca on 28 April 1988. U.S. Coast Guard investigation report and various attachments, plus correspondence with Central Marine Company Ltd. of Japan.

McCoy, Charles. "Alyeska Record Shows How Big Oil Neglected Alaskan Environment." *Wall Street Journal,* 6 July 1989.

McKenzie, Arthur. *Guide for the Selection of Tankers.* New York: Tanker Advisory Center, Inc., 1989, 1990, 1991, 1992.

———. "Petroleum Tankers Should Be Built to a Higher Standard." Presented to Committee on Tank Vessel Design, Marine Board, National Research Council, Washington, D.C., 6 November 1989.

———. *Petroleum Tankship Operations.* New York: Tanker Advisory Center, Inc., 1990, 1991, 1992.

———. *The World Tanker Fleet: Trends in Quality Standards.* New York: Tanker Advisory Center, 1991.

McKenzie, Douglas. *Model Test Results of Oil Loss from a Mid-Deck Tanker During High-Energy Groundings.* Self-published report. January 1992.

McPhee, John. *Looking for a Ship.* New York: Farrar Straus Giroux, 1990.

Mega Borg. Report from the Working Group Appointet [sic] to Investigate the *Mega Borg* disaster. Norwegian Maritime Directorate, 1990.

The Memorandum of Understanding on Port State Control. Annual Reports. Rotterdam, The Netherlands, 1989–92.

Merchant Fleets of the World. Washington, D.C.: U.S. Department of Transportation, Maritime Administration, April 1989.

Metula, Report of the VLCC *Metula* Grounding, Pollution and Refloating in the Strait of Magellan in 1974, U.S. Coast Guard.

Bibliography

Mielke, James E. "Oil in the Ocean: The Short- and Long-Term Impacts of a Spill." Congressional Research Service Report to Congress, 24 July 1990.

Mobiloil, grounding of U.S. tankship S.S. *Mobiloil* in the Columbia River near Saint Helens, Oregon, 19 March 1984. Washington, D.C.: National Transportation Safety Board, November 1984.

Mongelluzzo, Bill. "Ship Bureau Chief, Board In Bitter Battle." *Journal of Commerce,* 12 March 1992.

Morison, Robert F. "U.S. Softens Its Stand on Double Bottoms, Will Consider Segregated Systems." *Journal of Commerce,* 18 January 1978.

Morrow, Edward A. "U.S. Court Stuns Tanker Owners; Decision Permits Unlimited Damage Suits if Vessels Are Not Gas-Freed." *New York Times,* 19 December 1959.

"Mortality among United States Coast Guard Marine Inspectors." Washington, D.C.: *Archives of Environmental Health,* May/June 1989.

Mostert, Noel. *Supership.* New York: Alfred A. Knopf, 1974.

Nalder, Eric. "Case for Double Bottoms: Oil Spill Called Avoidable." *Seattle Times,* 22 April 1990.

———. "Tankers Full of Trouble." Six-part series. *Seattle Times,* 12–17 November 1989.

Navigation Safety and Bridge Management Manual. Long Beach, Calif.: Marine Transportation, Atlantic Richfield Company, n.d.

Newsletter of the International Tanker Owners Pollution Federal Ltd. London: various issues.

1991 Puget Sound Water Quality Management Plan. Puget Sound Water Quality Authority, June 1991.

North Puget Sound Tanker Escort & Tug Assistance Study. Prepared by Glosten Associates Inc. for Arco Marine, Inc., and Foss Maritime Company, September 1991.

Ocean Wizard, loss of starboard and port boilers and emergency generators in the Pacific Ocean in July 1989. U.S. Coast Guard Report, 20 October 1989.

Oil and Hazardous Substances Pollution and Contingency Plan, Puget Sound Zone. Seattle: U.S. Coast Guard Marine Safety Office, 7 February 1990.

Oil in the Sea: Inputs, Fates and Effects. Washington, D.C.: National Academy Press, 1985.

"The Oil Industry in the Pacific Northwest." *Pacific Northwest Executive,* January 1988.

Oil Pollution Research and Technology Plan. Washington, D.C.: Interagency Coordinating Committee on Oil Pollution Research, 24 April 1992.

Oil Spill Intelligence Report. Arlington, Mass.: Cutter Information Corp., various editions.

Oil Spill Prevention Act. Summary. Washington State Department of Ecology, August 1991.

Oil Spills Continue Despite Waterfront Facility Inspection Program. GAO Report. Washington, D.C., June 1991.

Oil Transfer Manual, Arco Anchorage.

Oil Transportation by Tankers: An Analysis of Marine Pollution and Safety Measures. Washington, D.C.: U.S. Congress Office of Technology Assessment, July 1975.

100 Spills, 1,000 Excuses. A Report by the Wilderness Society, Washington D.C., March 1990.

Overseas Shipholding Group, Annual Report 1991. Report to Stockholders, 11 June 1992.

Oversight Report of the Committee on Merchant Marine and Fisheries together with additional views. U.S. House of Representatives. Washington, D.C.: U.S. Government Printing Office, 1981.

Pacbaroness, On-Scene Coordinator's report, major pollution incident, 21 September 1987. Los Angeles–Long Beach: U.S. Coast Guard Marine Safety Office.

Pace, Eric. "Daniel Ludwig, Billionaire Businessman, Dies at 95." *New York Times,* 29 August 1992.

Parker, Walter B. "Alaska & Oil, The Next 20 Years." Anchorage, Ak. 20 April 1993.

———. "Oil Spills in the 90's: A Global Challenge." Delivered to the Alaska World Affairs Council, Anchorage, Ak. 6 April 1990.

———. "Our State Land Heritage." An address to the 1988 Alaska State Land Use Symposium, Anchorage, Ak.

———. "Tanker Bill Keeps Old, Small Ships Sailing Too Long." *Anchorage Daily News,* 17 April 1990.

Parker, Walter B., and Virgil Keith. "Transportation Options in the Chukchi and Beaufort Seas: On Site Oil Tanker Loadings." Delivered to the International Society for Offshore and Polar Engineering, San Francisco, 1992.

Bibliography

Petition for Reconsideration, Radio Officers Union and American Radio Association, in the matter of requests of 22 large oceangoing cargo ships for exemption from radiotelegraph requirements. Federal Communications Commission, 5 August 1988.

Piernes, Guillermo. "The Catastrophic Clearing of the Vast Amazon River Basin." *Seattle Times,* 25 February 1979.

Pilotage in the Coastal Towing Industry. Arlington, Va.: American Waterways Operators, 1992.

Poet, Report on the disappearance of the U.S. Flag Freighter *Poet* in October 1980, Committee on Merchant Marine and Fisheries, 16 September 1982.

Policy Regarding Marine Inspection and Port Safety Activities When the Potential for Exposure to Benzene Exists. Washington, D.C.: U.S. Coast Guard, 1988.

"P&O Subsidiary Introduces Black Box Recorder for Ships." *Journal of Commerce,* 30 March 1992.

Porricelli, Joseph D., and Virgil F. Keith. "A Systematic Process for Evaluating Measures Which Minimize Oil Tanker Outflows." Paper presented at the annual meeting of the Society of Naval Architects and Marine Engineers, La Jolla, Calif., 1 April 1978.

Porricelli, Joseph D., Virgil F. Keith, and Richard L. Storch. "Tankers and the Ecology." Paper presented at the annual Meeting of the Society of Naval Architects and Marine Engineers, 11–12 November 1971.

Porter, Janet. "Charterers Willing to Pay Higher Rates for Modern Ships." *Journal of Commerce,* 14 July 1992.

———. "EC Considers Stricter Laws On Tanker Safety." *Journal of Commerce,* 20 July 1992.

———. "Experts Fear Pirate Attacks Could Result in a Disaster." *Journal of Commerce,* 30 March 1992.

———. "Global Salvors Need Saving Fast, Classifier Warns." *Journal of Commerce,* 5 May 1992.

———. "High-Risk Ships Flunk Insurers' Inspections." *Journal of Commerce,* 3 June 1992.

———. "Insurance Rates Soar for Run-Down Ships." *Journal of Commerce,* 27 May 1992.

———. "More Scrapping Urged to Help Tanker Market." *Journal of Commerce,* 25 August 1992.

———. "New Tankers, Low Scrapping Level to Keep Rates Soft, Analysts Say." *Journal of Commerce,* 6 February 1992.

———. "Pollution Act Standards Test Tanker Industry." *Journal of Commerce,* 9 April 1992.

———. "Shell Toughens Tanker Inspection Procedures." *Journal of Commerce,* 11 February 1992.

———. "Shipowners, Insurers Hit Impasse Over Need for More Ship Inspections." *Journal of Commerce,* 7 July 1992.

———. "Shipowners Urged to Fund Training of 3rd World Seamen." *Journal of Commerce,* 9 June 1992.

———. "Ship Safety Agency Looks to Crack Down on Irresponsible Flags." *Journal of Commerce,* 13 October 1992.

———. "Soaring Bulk Ship Casualty Rate Sparks Call for Study of Cargoes." *Journal of Commerce,* 6 February 1992.

———. "Swedish Shipowners Call for Crackdown on Inspection Groups." *Journal of Commerce,* 10 July 1992.

———. "Warnings Sounded On Uninsured Ships." *Journal of Commerce,* 20 October 1992.

Potential Pacific Coast Oil Ports: A Comparative Environmental Risk Analysis. Vols. 1 and 2. Vancouver: Fisheries and Environment Canada, February 1978.

Proceedings: Workshop on Reducing Tankbarge Pollution. Maritime Transportation Research Board, 1980.

"Progress in Flags of Convenience." Special report. *UN Chronicle,* June 1982.

Progress toward Improvements in Marine Steering Reliability. Washington, D.C.: National Transportation Safety Board, 25 January 1979.

Protocol of 1978 Relating to the International Convention for the Prevention of Pollution from Ships, 1973. London: Inter-Governmental Maritime Consultative Organization.

Protocol of 1978 Relating to the International Convention for the Safety of Life at Sea, 1974, London: Inter-Governmental Maritime Consultative Organization.

Provincial Marine Oil Spill Preparedness and Response Strategy. Environmental Emergency Services, Victoria, B.C., n.d.

Pryne, Eric, and Lyle Burt. "Ray Won't Fight Oil-Port Ban." *Seattle Times,* 6 October 1977.

Bibliography

Puerto Rican, Explosion and Fire on Board U.S. Chemical Tankship *Puerto Rican* in the Pacific Ocean near San Francisco, 31 October 1984. Washington, D.C.: National Transportation Safety Board, April 1986.

Purtell, Comdr. T. W., and Lt. Comdr. J. P. Brusseau Mielka. *Marine Structural Casualty Study.* Report to the Marine Inspection Program Casualty Review Council, Washington, D.C.: U.S. Coast Guard, 27 April 1988.

Qualifications for Pilot Applicants, Washington Administrative Code, 296-11-075.

Quam, Whickham J. "Oil Barges, Tankers and Toxic Fumes." *Monitor,* April–June 1988.

Ratcliffe, Mike. *Liquid Gold Ships.* London: Lloyd's of London Press, 1985.

Reduced Manning/Automation, Exxon Valdez. Exhibit No. 10G. Washington D.C.: National Transportation Safety Board, 1989.

Reducing Tanker Accidents. Exxon Background Series, September 1973.

Regulation for Tank Vessels Engaged in the Carriage of Oil in Domestic Trade. Environmental Impact Statement. U.S. Coast Guard, August 1975.

"Regulation Requiring Double Bottoms on New Tankers and Segregated Ballast on New and Existing Tankers." Draft Environmental Impact Statement. U.S. Coast Guard, May 1977.

Regulations to Implement the Results of the International Conference on Tanker Safety and Pollution Prevention. Regulatory Analysis and Environmental Impact Statement. U.S. Coast Guard, February 1979.

Reinhard, George F. Letters on various tanker issues, 1971 through 1992, testimony to Congress, and clipping file.

Rempel, William C. "Alaska Oil Ships in Sea of Troubles." *Los Angeles Times,* 15 May 1989.

Report of Board of Investigation, stranding of the SS *Torrey Canyon,* March 18, 1967. Monrovia, Liberia: Bureau of Maritime Affairs, May 1967.

Report of Hearing by U.S. Coast Guard, in the matter of mariner's document issued to Charles Beaudette. Seattle, 14 March 1989.

Report of Hearing by U.S. Coast Guard in the matter of mariner's document issued to Mark Hawker. Seattle, 28 December 1988.

Report of Hearing by U.S. Coast Guard in the matter of mariner's license issued to Andrew C. Subcleff. Anchorage, April 1988.

Report of Pilotage Study Group. Washington, D.C.: U.S. Coast Guard, September 1989.

Report of preliminary investigation, steering failure of MT *Hellespont Courage,* off Ireland, 9 February 1988. Monrovia, Liberia: Bureau of Maritime Affairs.

Report of the Tanker Safety Study Group. Washington, D.C.: U.S. Coast Guard, 6 October 1989.

Report of Violation, Puget Sound Vessel Traffic Service. Various documents.

Report on the Marine Safety Training and Qualification Program. Washington, D.C.: U.S. Coast Guard, Office of Marine Safety, Security and Environmental Protection, 16 December 1988.

Report on the Tanker Design for Prevention and Mitigation of Oil Spills. Japan: Ministry of Transport, 1990.

Report on the Trans-Alaska Pipeline Service (TAPS) Tanker Structural Failure Study, Office of Marine Safety, Security and Environmental Protection. Washington, D.C.: U.S. Coast Guard, 25 June 1990.

"Risk Analysis of the Oil Transportation System." *Pacific Northwest Sea* (Seattle), Oceanographic Institute of Washington, 1972.

Roberts, Allen S. "Mozambique Plans Charges against Captain of Sunken Tanker." *Journal of Commerce,* 18 June 1992.

Rockwell, Keith M., and Alan Abrams. "Safety Agency Backs Mid-Deck Tanker Design." *Journal of Commerce,* 10 March 1992.

"RTCM Recommended Standards for Electronic Chart Display and Information Systems." Sixth Draft Report, Radio Technical. Washington, D.C.: Commission for Maritime Services, 25 March 1989.

Rubin, Jonathan. *Description and Analysis of Alaska's Formula to Assess Civil Penalties and Applications of this Formula to the Port Angeles and Anacortes Oil Spills.* Seattle: University of Washington, Institute for Marine Studies, 19 March 1989.

————. *Petroleum Toxicity and Fate in the Marine Environment with Implications for Development of a Compensation Schedule for Spilled Oil.* Seattle: University of Washington, Institute for Marine Studies, March 1989.

Safer Tankers and Cleaner Seas. Exxon Background Series, November 1992.

The Salvage Association (London). *The Association's Operations, 1988–89.*

Salvage Manual. Arco Marine Inc.

Sanders, Howard L., J. Frederick Grassle, George R. Hampston, Linda S. Morse, Susan Garner-Price, and Carol C. Jones. "Anatomy of an Oil Spill: Long-term Effects from the Grounding of the Barge *Florida* off West Falmouth, Massachusetts." *Journal of Marine Research,* 1980.

Sanders, Howard L. "The West Falmouth Oil Saga." *New Engineer,* May 1974.

―――. "The West Falmouth Spill—[involving the barge] *Florida,* 1969." *Oceanus* (Woods Hole, Mass.: Woods Hole Oceanographic Institution), Fall 1977.

Sansinena, Marine Casualty Report, S.S. *Sansinena* explosion and fire in Los Angeles Harbor, Calif., on December 17, 1976. Washington, D.C.: U.S. Coast Guard, 25 November 1977.

Sansorb, Sorby Alaska Inc. Anchorage, Ak., 5 April 1991.

Scates, Shelby. "Ray Fights Back, Calls Magnuson a Dictator." *Seattle Post-Intelligencer,* 8 October 1977.

Segregated Ballast Tanker Study, Ship Configuration. Study Group Report. 18 April 1975.

Shipboard Productivity Methods. Maritime Administration, Office of Advanced Ship Operations. Washington, D.C.: U.S. Department of Transportation, February 1987.

Ship Construction Report. Shipbuilders Council of America, July 1991.

Shorrock, Tim. "Union, Environmentalists Push Radio Officer Law." *Journal of Commerce,* 27 December 1991.

Sinking of the F/V Jack Jr. Findings of Fact, Alameda, Calif.: U.S. Coast Guard, 1987.

Sipes, Radm. J. D., USCG. *Trans-Alaska Pipeline Service (TAPS) Tanker Structural Failure Study.* Washington, D.C.: U.S. Coast Guard, 25 June 1990.

Sloyan, Patrick. "Huge Tankers Worry Navy; Stopping Ability Causes Concern." *Seattle Post-Intelligencer,* 7 October 1970.

Smith, J. P., P. Daniels, B. Paramore, and J. Porricelli. *Tank Analysis Report Relative to Vessel Collisions, Rammings and Groundings.* Vol. 1. Washington, D.C.: U.S. Coast Guard, 11 December 1976.

Sohio Intrepid, Report of Vessel Casualty or Accident, loss of power near Sinclair Island on 8 December 1983, U.S. Coast Guard.

Solomon, Caleb, and Daniel Machalabe. "Troubled Waters: Oil Tankers' Safety is Assailed as Mishaps Average Four a Week." *Wall Street Journal,* 20 June 1990.

"Sound Tanker Design . . . And Much More," editorial. *Journal of Commerce,* 22 February 1992.

Spaeth, M. G., and S. C. Berkman. "The Tsunami of March 28, 1964, as Recorded at Tide Stations." Coast and Geodetic Survey Technical Bulletin (Rockville, Md.) 33 (July 1967).

Spill Prevention. Olympia, Wash.: Puget Sound Water Quality Authority, September 1989.

Spill, The Wreck of the Exxon Valdez. Final Report, with appendixes. Anchorage, Ak.: Alaska Oil Spill Commission, February 1990.

Star Connecticut, ground of, near Barbers Point, Hawaii, 6 November 1990. Washington, D.C.: National Transportation Safety Board, March 1992.

State of Alaska vs. *Joseph Hazelwood.* District Court for the State of Alaska, Valdez, 31 March 1989.

Statistical Study of Outflow from Oil and Chemical Tanker Casualties. Washington, D.C.: American Petroleum Institute, Lloyd's Register, May 1990.

Status and Management of Puget Sound's Biological Resources. PTI Environmental Services, for U.S. Environmental Protection Agency, January 1990.

Steiner, Rick. "Lessons of Exxon Valdez Spill Lost on Greedy World." *Seattle Times,* 24 March 1992.

Stuyvesant, fracture of no. 5 port cargo tank bottom plating and heavy weather damage, Gulf of Alaska, 7, 8, and 9 January 1987. U.S. Coast Guard, 23 June 1989.

Stuyvesant, fracture of no. 5 starboard cargo tank sideshell plating and heavy weather damage, Gulf of Alaska, 4 October 1987. U.S. Coast Guard, 26 June 1989.

Stuyvesant, Report, Inspection & Investigation of Major Bottom Shell Fracture, Bay Tankers, Inc.. New York, 9 June 1987.

Stuyvesant, Technical Report No. 7650, Bottom Plate Fracture, Bay Tankers, Inc., 22 May 1987.

Surf City, explosion and fire, Persian Gulf, 22 February 1990. Washington, D.C.: National Transportation Safety Board, 31 March 1992.

Summit Venture, ramming of Sunshine Skyway Bridge, Tampa Bay, Fla., 9 May 1980. Washington, D.C.: National Transportation Safety Board, 10 April 1981.

Sunde, Scott. "Poor Visibility Makes It Hard to Track Oil." *Seattle Post-Intelligencer,* 29 July 1991.

Survey of U.S. Coastal States Oil Pollution Statutes. New York: Hill, Betts & Nash, August 1991.

Tank Vessel Operations: Puget Sound. Department of Transportation, U.S. Coast Guard. Washington, D.C.: *Federal Register,* 26 April 1982.

Bibliography

"Tanker Captain Sent Home after Failing Sobriety Tests." Associated Press, 6 March 1992.

Tanker Double Bottoms, Yes or No? Washington D.C.: American Institute of Merchant Shipping, 1989.

Tanker Legislation 91, Living with OPA and State-Level Tanker Laws. Conference sponsored by Marine Log in Washington, D.C. Various papers.

The Tanker Register. Clarkson Research Studies Limited, 12 Camomile Street, London EC3A 7BP, England 1986.

Tankers in the World Fleet. Washington, D.C.: U.S. Department of Transportation, Maritime Administration, January 1988.

Tanker Spills: Prevention by Design. Marine Board, National Research Council. Washington, D.C.: National Academy Press, 1991.

Tankship Hull Inspection Book, U.S. Coast Guard, n.d.

"Thar's Gold in Them Hulls, Tax-Propelled Tanker Deals Are Loaded with Profits." *Fortune,* August 1952.

Third Report of the Commission on Merchant Marine and Defense. 30 September 1988.

Thompson Pass. Report of Structural Failure. U.S. Coast Guard, 30 January 1989.

Thorne, Charles. *How Can the People of the State of Washington Coexist with the Oil Industry?* Self-published report to the Oceanographic Institute of Washington, 1 December 1970.

———. Testimony to House Government Operations Subcommittee on Conservation and Natural Resources, December 1971.

Title 46, Code of Federal Regulations. Coast Guard, Department of Transportation.

Townsend, Richard. *Shipping Safety and America's Coasts.* Washington, D.C.: Center for Marine Conservation, 1990.

Trans-Alaska Pipeline Service (TAPS), Tanker Structural Failure Study—Follow-up Report. Office of Marine Safety, Security and Environmental Protection. Washington, D.C.: U.S. Coast Guard, May 1991.

Transporting U.S. Oil Imports: The Impact of Oil Spill Legislation on the Tanker Market. New York: Petroleum Industry Research Foundation, Inc., prepared for the U.S. Department of Energy, June 1992.

Turner, Norma. "The Case against a Supertanker Oil Port." *Seattle Times,* 4 October 1991.

"27 Crew Lost After Oil Tanker Cracks Up in the Atlantic." Reuters, 10 November 1988.

Ulman, Neil. "Uneasy Passage, Tanker Skirts Danger in the English Channel, Battles Tedium at Sea." *Wall Street Journal,* 21 October 1971.

Unsworth, Edwin, Chris Dupin, and Jon Jacobs. "Safety at Sea." *Journal of Commerce,* March 1989.

United States Coast Guard vs. *Raymond L. Leson.* Decision and Order, 1986.

Update, Oil Pollution Act of 1990. Various editions. U.S. Coast Guard.

The U.S. Oceangoing Tank Barge Industry. Arlington, Va.: The American Waterways Operators, 1990.

Vessel Organization Manual, Exxon Valdez. Exhibit No. 40. Washington, D.C.: National Transportation Safety Board, 1989.

Vessel Traffic Systems, Analysis of Port Needs. Department of Transportation, U.S. Coast Guard, August 1973.

Vessel Traffic Systems. Department of Transportation, U.S. Coast Guard. Washington, D.C.: *Federal Register,* 10 July 1974.

Vessel Traffic Systems, Users Manual. Department of Transportation, U.S. Coast Guard, April 1987.

"Voyage into Oblivion." *Los Angeles Times,* 27 January 1986.

Washington Coast Sensitive Areas Mapping Project. Various booklets, prepared by the Department of Landscape Architecture, University of Washington, for the Washington State Department of Ecology, March 1992.

Washington State Energy Use Profile. Olympia: Washington State Energy Office, 1988.

Wastler, Allen R. "Marine Pilot Selection Process Comes Under Fire," *Journal of Commerce,* 4 February 1992.

Wenk, Edward, Jr. Letter to Department of Ecology Director Christine Gregoire, 10 July 1990.

———. *The Wreck of the* Exxon Valdez, *Lessons for Prevention.* Self-published report. 7 November 1989.

Wenk, Edward, Jr., Richard Storch, Thomas Laetz, Eric Lichty, and Charles Black. *Improving Maritime Traffic Safety on Puget Sound Waterways.* Report. Seattle: University of Washington, 15 December 1982.

Bibliography

Wenk, Edward, Jr., Juris Vagners, James Crutchfield, and Steven Flajser. *Comments on the Final Environmental Impact Statement for the Proposed Trans-Alaska Pipeline*. Self-published report. 1 May 1972.

Whitely, Peyton. Series on Pilots. *Seattle Times,* 13–18 February 1977.

Whitney, David. "Oil-Spill Seminar One-Sided." *Anchorage Daily News,* 15 May 1990.

Wills, Jonathan. *A Place in the Sun.* St. John's, Newfoundland: The Institute of Social and Economic Research, Memorial University of Newfoundland, 1991.

Wills, Jonathan, and Karen Warner. *Innocent Passage: The Wreck of the Tanker Braer.* Edinburgh: Mainstream Publishing Company, 1993.

Wilson, John Arthur. "Candidates Differ on Oil-Tanker Ruling." *Seattle Times,* 25 September 1976.

Wohlforth, Charles. "Rare Loon May Be Hardest Hit by Spill." *Anchorage Daily News,* 17 May 1990.

Wolferstan, W. H. *Oil Tanker Traffic: Assessing the Risks for the Southern Coast of British Columbia.* Victoria, B.C.: APD Bulletin & Ministry of Environment 1981.

Wooton, Sharon. *"Tenyo Maru* Spill: Taking Stock, Wake-up Call." *The Herald* (Everett, Wash.), 4 August 1991.

World Prodigy, grounding of, off the coast of Rhode Island, 23 June 1989. Washington, D.C.: National Transportation Safety Board, March 1991.

———. "World's Largest Tanker Completed in Japan." *Jiji Press,* 13 December 1980.

———. "World's Largest Tanker Hit by Iraqi Planes." *Journal of Commerce,* 17 May 1988.

Yamanaka, Keiko, and Michael Gaffney. *Effective Manning in the Orient, a Review of Asian Developments.* Washington, D.C.: American President Lines, for Maritime Administration and Office of Technology Assessment, March 1988.

Yergin, Daniel. *The Prize: The Epic Quest for Oil, Money & Power.* New York: Touchstone, Simon & Schuster, 1992.

Index

Index

Index

Index

Index

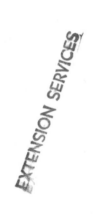

INSPIRED AMATEURS

INSPIRED AMATEURS

BY
KEVIN GUINAGH

Essay Index Reprint Series

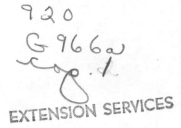

EXTENSION SERVICES

BOOKS FOR LIBRARIES PRESS, INC.

FREEPORT, NEW YORK

BOOKMOBILE

LIBRARY OF CONGRESS CATALOG CARD NUMBER:

67-26746

PRINTED IN THE UNITED STATES OF AMERICA

CONTENTS

ACKNOWLEDGMENTS

THE author's sincere thanks are due:

To Messrs. Dodd, Mead and Company for permission to quote passages from *The Life of Jean Henri Fabre*, by Augustin Fabre, from *The Life of the Scorpion*, by Jean Henri Fabre, and from *The Mason Bees*, by Jean Henri Fabre.

To Messrs. Harcourt, Brace and Company for permission to quote passages from *Antony van Leeuwenhoek and His "Little Animals,"* by Clifford Dobell.

To Messrs. Little, Brown and Company for permission to quote a passage from *Schliemann*, by Emil Ludwig.

PREFACE

BY ARTHUR E. MORGAN

Chairman of the T.V.A.

THERE would be some consolation in having nine lives, like a cat, if one could live them simultaneously. Yet it would be incomplete consolation at that, for the lives I want to live run into the scores or the hundreds, and nine would be only tantalizing. Whenever some person lives one of the lives I have wanted to live, or does one of the things I have wanted to do, I feel a twinge of jealousy, almost of resentment, that an intriguing and virgin field has been occupied by another. To establish a claim to spiritual respectability I should add that this primitive reaction of envy is more or less counteracted by a feeling of satisfaction that an alluring field is not neglected, but is giving interest and zest to some one.

When Mr. Guinagh informed me that he was writing this book, I had a feeling of envy that so supremely alluring a subject should be preëmpted. Yet this is one of the many fields I am destined to pass by without entering to explore, and so it is a pleasure to stand at the entrance and draw attention to its absorbing interest.

A book which interested and greatly encouraged me as a boy was entitled *Illustrious Shoemakers*. It consisted of short biographies of men who had dared to lay down the shoemaker's last in order to lead the world in some field. It appears that the mending of shoes does not demand the full attention of an active mind,

and so the old-time shoemaker had time to think. I
have almost completely forgotten the contents of that
book, but I can still recall the sense of freedom and of
added courage it gave me. It is not always true, I
found, that the shoemaker should stick to his last, and
even so humble a calling might be the doorway to significant accomplishment.

Mankind has always paid its highest allegiance to the
amateur. The name which has been held in reverence
by more men than any other since the birth of the race
is that of a carpenter who became an amateur teacher,
sociologist, and guide to a way of life. A great body
of professionals has grown up who presume to explain
and mediate this amateur to the world. But how often
has their professionalism cut men off from the great
amateur spirit whose name they bear?

Could there be a more perfect example of this professional interference than the contrast between the amateur and the professional spirit toward prayer? The
Great Amateur said, "Use not vain repetitions, as the
heathen do. . . After this manner therefore pray ye";
and he gave them in the "Lord's Prayer" an example
of a spontaneous expression of the spirit. Whereupon
the professionals for nearly two thousand years, forgetting the admonition, "use not vain repetitions," have
taught the *Paternoster*, and have furnished strings of
beads for counting the repetitions.

Not even the creative amateur brings his works into
being from nothing. He catches the spirit of what
went before, and gives it larger meaning. The Great
Amateur was in this sense the fulfillment of the Hebrew
prophets, and the greatest and most creative of them
were not the professional mumblers of formulas, but

were also amateurs. The prophet Amos is typical. When the professionals, fearing his radical ideas, urged that he go back to his home and earn his bread by the trade of prophecy, he disdained their advice, saying, "I was no prophet, neither was I a prophet's son; but I was an herdsman, and a gatherer of sycamore fruit: And the Lord took me as I followed the flock, and the Lord said unto me, 'Go, prophesy unto my people Israel.'" Amos was a true amateur.

Andrew Carnegie had an idea that throughout America there might be genius burning itself out without opportunity for expression. Perhaps his school reader had contained the lines:

"Full many a gem of purest ray serene
The dark unfathom'd caves of ocean bear;
Full many a flower is born to blush unseen
And waste its sweetness on the desert air."

So he created the Carnegie Institution of Washington to be a clearing house for those ideas which had not found opportunity for expression. I recall, from memory, from the final report of the first president of the institution, a statement to the effect that no such desert flowers or ocean gems had been forthcoming, no "mute inglorious Milton" had been discovered. He stated, if I remember correctly, that no worth-while idea had been presented to the institution which was not the product of long and vigorously disciplined preparation on the part of the person who had achieved it.

I have sometimes wondered whether Mr. Carnegie did not make the mistake of selecting a professional to search for amateurs. Yet there is truth in this retiring president's statement. To be an amateur does not mean to be unprepared. Get behind the appearance of any great idea or of any great accomplishment, no matter how suddenly it may seem to have arrived, and nearly always we shall find a substantial background of growth and preparation. Often a large part of the preparation of a lifetime is crowded into a few years of very intensive effort.

In other cases there is gradual and steady achievement over a long period; but wherever there is any achievement worth while, either in thought or in action, that accomplishment nearly always is the product of a great total of effort. This is no less true for the amateur than for the professional. In thirty years of varied engineering experience I have not recognized half a dozen new and worth-while engineering suggestions made by persons who lacked substantial training in that field.

Schliemann as a boy dreamed of his excavations. His profession was but an interlude to the expression of his dominant life interests. In my own case, interest in education, as the fundamental process for improving the cultural fabric of society, had an earlier origin and a deeper root than my professional interest in engineering. As Mr. Guinagh so well observes, it sometimes is necessary to be an amateur in order to be free.

Sometimes, as in the case of Henry Ford, or that of Edward Bellamy, the author of *Looking Backward* and of *Equality*, achievement comes from straight thinking about the realities of life rather than from the reading of books or from work in the laboratory. Had Henry Ford been "properly" trained in the axioms of economics, he might never have acted upon those common-sense conclusions on fundamental economics which by

his action have so profoundly changed economic thinking in the last two or three decades. Occasionally what
is most needed is not great knowledge, or even keener
thinking, but a fresh outlook and freedom from indoctrination. In political life, for instance, the Machiavel-
lian philosophy of shrewd, worldly wise duplicity
sometimes appeals strongly, even to very intelligent
persons, who enjoy the zest of using mental shrewdness,
and have confidence in their superior acumen. The
ultimate futility of that philosophy may be clearest to
the simple-minded but straight-minded amateur.

Sometimes I dread the results of universal education,
especially higher education. We become so indoctrinated with traditional ideas which may not be true, and
we become so humble before the imposing prestige of
accepted professional opinion, that we lose the power
of independent creative thinking. We need a "Society
for the Preservation of Ignorance," so that occasionally
someone of great mental vitality and directness may
look at the world anew and tell us what he sees. But
I would have honorable membership in that society confined to men of creative drive and insight.

The impracticability of this suggestion illustrates a
profound fact. This great fact is that in administering
the affairs of life our choices are not between right ways
and wrong ways, but between ways all of which are
at least partly wrong. If a man becomes thoroughly
familiar with a subject before making his own contribution, he thereby commonly becomes so indoctrinated
with accepted ideas that he may lose his own creative
originality. The great Leonardo da Vinci, but for his
unconscious acceptance of current religious cosmology,
might have become the first evolutionary geologist.

That conventional indoctrination blocked the free action of his mind in the presence of suggestive facts.

On the other hand, lack of mastery of what men have thought and achieved leaves one mentally in the childhood of the race, with small chance of summing up all preceding human experience in any field, and then of surpassing it. Years ago while waiting for the railroad train in a southwestern Minnesota town, I spent my spare time in exploring the personalities of the village. Among my discoveries was that of the village printer who was also an inventor. He became very confidential and took me to see a perpetual motion machine he had made. On looking it over I remarked, "Oh, that is an Archimedes screw." Whereupon the inventor replied indignantly, "No, it isn't. I never met that gentleman. This is my own invention."

We forever face this dilemma of either losing our creative originality through being indoctrinated with what other men believe, or of remaining primitive children in our minds because we have not equipped ourselves with the accumulated knowledge of the race. The professional man as a rule must travel the conventional and accepted road of preparation and must submit himself to indoctrination in order to gain professional recognition. The amateur can strive to achieve a new balance of preparation and of freedom from indoctrination. The professionals will bring about the gradual perfection of present methods and, by the use of the scientific method, will sometimes follow the necessary sequence of ideas into new and unexpected worlds. The amateur, free from the necessity of achieving professional standing, will occasionally follow his nose into new and original points of view, and will be one of the chief sources of new creation and of readjusted emphasis; but he may waste his life over false issues. We need both the amateur and the professional.

One of the most powerful forces for molding our intellectual theories is self-interest. The physicians of America are generally opposed to public medicine. The amateur, who views the situation without self-interest, may have a sounder view. Just at present the foremost presidents of our endowed universities are decrying increased taxation of large fortunes. Unconsciously they speak from professional self-interest. With fewer great fortunes there will be less endowment. Were they living in a world of caterpillars they would deplore that apparent disorganization and loss of effectiveness which accompanies transformation from the caterpillar stage through the chrysalis stage to the mature insect form. Like children who resent giving up present interests at bedtime, men cling to those occupational interest patterns which have given meaning and stability to their lives. Sometimes the amateur is necessary to create a new pattern.

Mr. Guinagh could not, in the course of any single volume, exhaust his subject. He can only open the doors to a most alluring field and bid us explore further for ourselves. Just to indicate how far the subject is from exhaustion, Mr. Guinagh does not mention that prince of amateurs, Leonardo da Vinci. Painter, sculptor, architect, mechanical inventor, unconsciously responsible for the cotton spinning industry, military engineer, geologist, greatest anatomist of his day, psychologist and philosopher, he found the world intriguing at many points.

Nor does Mr. Guinagh more than mention the first

of all American amateurs, Benjamin Franklin. He was printer, writer, diplomat, business man; it was purely as an amateur that he discovered the identity of lightning and electricity. Observing a seed in a whisk broom in a friend's house, he planted the seed and started the broom corn industry of America. Seeing a sprout on a piece of willow furniture which had been dropped in Dock Creek, in Philadelphia, he planted this sprout and started the willow furniture industry on this side of the water. He founded the University of Pennsylvania and the American Philosophical Society. These are by no means all of his undertakings. He did not shrink from action out of deference to the superior ability of the professional.

The elaborations of science have not closed the door to the amateur. Rather they have opened many new doors. For years, a Mr. Harrison, a shopkeeper on the Kentish coast east of London, collected curious flints along the chalk cliff and made a careful study of them. Since he had neither social status nor professional standing, he was scorned by professional anthropologists. The British Museum would not list his collections. Finally, however, this amateur triumphed. His curious flints are now recognized as man-made implements, and because of his work the recognized age of man in Britain has been extended half a million years.

The real distinction, however, is not between amateurs and professionals, but between minds and personalities that are creative and those that are not. The creative mind takes the wisdom of the past as food to be digested, assimilated and made over into its own living being; the non-creative mind takes the accepted cultural inheritance as ready-made clothing to be worn according

to the authentic style.   The ideal man would be he who
could take all the past has to offer, using it as the source
of material for his own creative activities, without being
indoctrinated or mastered or warped, while being enlarged and taught.   We sometimes see men with the
driving vigor and stubborn critical discrimination which
enables them to be informed but not indoctrinated.
Wherever that quality appears the distinction between
amateur and professional begins to fade.

The routine administration of our world, and a large
proportion of the most brilliant and creative contributions to human progress, will be the work of professionals.   Yet creative minds are not made to order and
do not result from training, and so professionals are
forever getting into deep ruts and losing the broader
view.   It will continue to be the work of the amateur,
wherever he may unexpectedly emerge, to see life fresh
and new, to refuse to deaden creative power by conformity, and to make those profound readjustments of
emphasis and attention which men must achieve if they
are to keep on the main highway of survival and progress, and are to escape the blind paths of provincialism
and over-specialization which have diverted so many
peoples and so many species, and led them to extinction.
The amateur must help save our civilization from being
only the digging ground for future archeologists, and
he can have a good time in fulfilling that function.
Mr. Guinagh has done a service in introducing us to
him.

I

THE SHOEMAKER AND HIS LAST

I

THE SHOEMAKER AND HIS LAST

WE often hear the cautious advice that the shoemaker should stick to his last. Those who like to have their doctrines fortified by ancient authority should glory in this proverb, for the Greek painter Apelles is credited with being its author. The origin of the proverb is told by the Elder Pliny. The painter Apelles, in his unusual desire to hear honest criticism, hid himself behind one of his pictures. A shoemaker who chanced to pass that way observed that the shoes he had painted had one latch less than the approved style; the artist quickly corrected the error. When the shoemaker later noted that his suggestions had been heeded, he began to criticise the leg that wore the shoe. It was then that the artist's head appeared from behind the picture to remind the shoemaker that he should give no opinion beyond the shoe. This advice, originally spoken to a shoemaker, has now a general application and may be directed by mere artisans to artists.

Despite the age of this proverb — let the shoemaker stick to his last — I am for letting the shoemaker look up from his last if he chooses. The fact that this proverb has been quoted for centuries need not disturb us. Antiquity is the most fruitful mother of error, wrote Arnobius, a Christian writer of the third century. Let the shoemaker be heard if he has a message. Perhaps in his mind are germinal ideas that may blossom into inspiration, if allowed the sun and air. He may become an inspired amateur in some art or science, and

3

the world may beat a path to his door, as in the case of the man of mouse-trap fame. Although I tell the shoemaker that he may look up from his last, I do not go the whole way with Herr Emil Ludwig in maintaining that the inspired amateur beats the professional every time. His statement is not without rhetorical exaggeration.

If the matter were debated, the discussion would turn upon the definition of inspiration. Those who have read something of the disputes on the inspiration of the Bible will remember that men speak of the inspiration of Shakespeare and the inspiration of the Holy Ghost. Herr Ludwig might cogently contend, if challenged, that not every amateur is inspired, but that those who are inspired of the Holy Spirit, as it were, often reach above and beyond men who have spent their whole lives over these same problems.

Our grandfathers never missed the opportunity of showing the Latin derivation of a word whenever it had any bearing on a subject under discussion. Today one offers such information with considerable reluctance, for readers often class such observations under the heading of pedantry. But everybody who has begun the study of Latin knows that the word *amateur* is derived from *amator,* meaning a lover. An amateur in the sense in which I shall use the word is one who pursues some interest because he loves it. His zeal is not inspired by his lust for money. His daily bread does not depend on the success or the orthodoxy of his work. Money may come to him in the pursuit of his interest. This, if he be human, he will hardly refuse, but he places his rewards in the satisfaction of his curiosity, the joy of possession, the sense of achievement.

That man will be regarded as an amateur who becomes absorbed in some subject in which he has never been professionally trained, but who develops an interest alien to his education and occupation.

We are not concerned with that distinction between the amateur and professional which exists in athletic circles whereby a man becomes professional when he has received payment for even a part of a single game. By this Midas-touch of gold the man who may be a tyro of tyros is suddenly by some strange alchemy transmuted into a professional.

Nor are we concerned with those amateurs who are uninspired. The world is full to overflowing with such men. These are the dilettanti, the devotees of hobbies, who pursue a subject intermittently. It is not my purpose to rail at such interests. You may be one of that vast host which finds recreation in collecting stamps, first editions, or butterflies. Far be it from me to ridicule the interest that makes your life worth living, that refreshes your mind for the battle of the ensuing day. As the machine lessens the hours of employment, educators are constantly emphasizing the importance of finding some absorbing activity to aid men in spending their leisure with profit and pleasure. You may be taking lessons on the violin; you need no man to spring to your defence, though you may later be thankful for a little fatherly advice. It is in defence of you that G. K. Chesterton wrote, in his usual paradoxical manner, about the importance of doing things badly.

These pages are not written in justification of the rights of the amateur who is uninspired. He needs no apologist. I am interested in certain amateurs who rose out of the class of dilettanti to a height where they overshadowed many professionals. I have no interest in proving that these inspired amateurs beat the professionals every time; in fact, I have no definite thesis to prove. I am simply interested in sketching, because they are interesting, the lives of men who distinguished themselves in a field in which they were not specifically trained.

The inspired amateur approaches a subject with certain advantages. In the first place he is not controlled by the groove of the past called tradition. There is a healthy attitude toward tradition, but there is also a deadening technique resulting from the adoration of one's predecessors which finds expression in the smug exposition beginning: "This is the way we have always done it."

Often the amateur knows nothing about the history of the subject which he is assaulting and for this reason he may not realize in his hardihood that he is rushing into a situation where angels fear to tread. The kingdom of ideas suffers violence sometimes, and the violent bear it away. If the beginner knew at the outset all the volumes written on the subject before he began to interest himself in it, he would be discouraged at the mountain of reading that lay in his path and probably would retreat. For those who finally succeed it may be said that their blissful ignorance was an asset.

In this connection it is interesting to recall a conversation that once took place between the two great French scientists, Fabre, "The Insects' Homer," and Pasteur, the chemist. The latter, although the subject was entirely out of his field, was appointed by the French government to rehabilitate the silkworm industry. He knew nothing about the work and did not conceal his

ignorance when given the appointment. Whereupon,
the official who commissioned him said that he would
therefore be in a better position to conquer the disease,
since he would have no ideas on the subject except those
that would come as the result of his own observations.
Pasteur came to consult Fabre. The latter has left us
an account of this interview, which was a spur to his
own researches, although he did not like Pasteur's
haughtiness toward him :

A few words were exchanged concerning the prevailing
evil ; then, without further preamble :
"I wanted to see some cocoons," said my visitor ; "I have
never seen any ; I know them only by name. Could you
get me some ?"
"Nothing simpler. My landlord is himself a dealer in
cocoons, and he lives across the road. If you'll be good
enough to wait a moment, I will bring you what you want."
A few long strides and I had reached my neighbor's
house, where I stuffed my pockets with cocoons. On my
return I offered them to the scientist. He took one, turned
it over and over in his fingers ; curiously he examined it,
as we should some singular object which had come from
the other end of the world. He shook it against his ear.
"It rattles !" he said, quite surprised. "There is some-
thing inside !"
"Why, yes !"
"But what ?"
"The chrysalis."
"What's that, the chrysalis ?"
"I mean the sort of mummy into which the caterpillar
turns before it becomes a moth."
"And in every cocoon there is one of those things ?"
"Of course ; it's to protect the chrysalis that the cater-
pillar spins."
"Ah !"
And without more ado, the cocoons went into the pocket

of the scientist, who was to inform himself at leisure concerning this great novelty, the chrysalis. . . The ancient gymnasts presented themselves naked for the contest. This ingenious thinker, who was to fight the plague of the silkworm nurseries, had also hastened to battle wholly naked: that is, devoid of the simplest notions of the insect he was to save from danger. I was astounded; more I was filled with wonder.

A second advantage of the inspired amateur is that he has no obligation to be sound. He may make the most exasperating statements, suggest the most radical solutions, and the world will not even take time out to correct him. But those who aspire to being authorities in a field must exercise caution in their statements, for the word may be passed around that the professor is unsound. This cry "unsound, unsound" will go up from the ranks of his colleagues and will produce as much isolation for the radical as the shout of "unclean, unclean" did for the leper of medieval days. Novel ideas in a professional mind may mean the loss of prestige and bread. The ambitious young professional has a tendency to learn the methods invoked by other members of his profession, adopt a safe style, and avoid a figure of speech as if it were poison.

Another advantage of the inspired amateur lies in the fact that, pursuing a subject solely for itself and for the interest he has in it, he often expends more energy on it than the man who makes his living thereby. Many men are not interested in the work at which they earn their bread. They suffer it but do not love it. The inspired amateur, on the contrary, does not keep one eye on the clock to determine how long he must stay at his office, desk, or laboratory before he is free. The amateur, the lover, never feels that time passes slowly. The hours this wooer spends with his love speed far too quickly for him. His private study is his recreation. This intense interest brings with it that concentration without which few men have ever written their names in bronze.

It must not be inferred that professional men as a class are not interested in their work, nor that there are not many professional men who are inspired. The outstanding work in any major field of study has been effected by men who were regularly disciplined by formal instruction and who pursued a routine of labor from day to day. At the same time it cannot be denied that there are some members in every profession who are uninspired.

If anyone discerns anything derogatory to the professional in these pages, it must be remembered that these gibes are intended for the uninspired professional. Such a man often possesses the form but not the content, the shadow but not the substance. It is he who sets about with solemn air to expound the obvious. When he finds a detail has been incorrectly stated, he may dilate on the discovery out of all proportion to its significance. It cannot be denied that trifles make perfection, but to overemphasize a trifling flaw betrays a lack of that prime quality of a balanced mind, a sense of perspective.

Your uninspired professional is often selfish. He is interested in maintaining the security of his position and to this end he will make appeals to narrow loyalties, will insist on the letter of the law, and demand those little courtesies which seem to come most frequently when they are unsought. Instead of considering a statement in itself, he is prone to inquire for the credentials of the man who made it. If he learns that the idea comes from an amateur, he may observe that the newcomer has injected himself into a controversy that has been traditionally regarded as delicate. To him it is a personal insult if an amateur ventures to question the theories that have received the blessing of the leaders in the field. If he is hotly pursued, he rushes inside the stockade of authority.

One of his sharpest weapons is the query: "How long have you been at this subject?" He likes to talk of how long he has studied or practised, wishing at the same time to have it inferred that the years spent at a study infallibly make men wise. Perhaps he has been doing the same thing over and over for years, without the least effort at improvement. With all his service, he may never have risen superior to the performance of his fifth year. An uninspired professional, then, may resemble the blind horse walking the treadmill, vainly believing that he is covering vast sweeps of territory when, in reality, he has never left the spot where he began.

But again let it be made clear that these faults belong to the uninspired professional. Whoever thinks he reads between the lines of these pages a covert attack on professionals in general will probably be forced to admit, if closely questioned, that he has been reading too many detective stories. When one praises an amateur he does not by the very fact belittle the professional. These sketches are written in the hope that they may entertain a little and instruct a little, but certainly not with the intention of supporting any theory maintaining the unqualified superiority of the amateur over the professional.

II
PREACHER CHEMIST
JOSEPH PRIESTLEY

II

PREACHER CHEMIST

JOSEPH PRIESTLEY

To be a sickly boy in the eighteenth century was not always a disadvantage in life. Strong sons were early put to some hard work while their weaker brother was often forced to find a way of making his living with his brain. The frail lad knew that the only way he could win the respect of physically strong men was by showing the world what he could do in the realm of ideas.

Little Joseph Priestley, sitting in a far corner of the living-room in his aunt's home at Leeds, was just such a boy. He was doing his best to read, but who could keep his mind on a book when those ministers over there in front of the fire were discussing, as usual, the torments of the damned? Always they kept at those terrifying themes, hell, its eternity, the pains awaiting those predestined to punishment even before they were born. The boy was tired. He wanted to go to bed, but who could sleep with those frightful pictures before his mind? Besides, his aunt had told him that one of the ministers was going to speak to him a little later. When the questions of theology were finished, his aunt began:

"I wanted to talk to you, doctor, about Joseph's education. His mother, poor thing, died in the hard winter of '39 after giving birth to her sixth child in six years. My brother is having a hard time with the other children. I suppose he will be marrying soon again. Joseph is twelve now and a good boy. He has never given me cause to rebuke him. He reads all day long,

13

and it is my firm belief, doctor, that he is destined to be a minister."

The doctor turned to the boy in the corner of the room and asked him if he desired to serve God.

Young Priestley tried to express satisfaction at such a prospect, but when he began to talk he stuttered uncontrollably. "I — I — It would p — p — p-lease me very much."

The aunt and the doctor quietly discussed the boy. Joseph knew what they were saying in spite of the minister's attempt to lower his voice. "The boy is sickly . . . he stutters . . . either of these is an obstacle to a successful career in the ministry."

In spite of his handicaps, he was given the opportunity to study. By the time he was sixteen, he had a fair knowledge of the learned languages, and without a master had assaulted French, Italian, and German. His ambition to be a minister seemed foiled by illness when his health suddenly improved. After studying in a seminary supported by the Dissenters, he found himself in his twenty-second year a minister earnestly preaching the word of God. The parish he was given was not a rich one. His salary was only thirty pounds a year, a mere pittance to be sure, but what could a stuttering minister expect? Priestley held on in his lonely parish. He was hardly popular. He was too troubled with questions of belief to be bowing and smiling and chatting, the approved technique of winning lay approval. As a consolation in his trouble, he had taken up the study of the scriptures. While toiling over ancient texts, the conviction grew within him that he could not honestly subscribe in his soul to some of the doctrines he was supposed to profess and expound in the pulpit.

Disturbed by his biblical studies, he glutted an appetite for facts on science. For the education of the public and the benefit of his purse he offered a series of twelve lectures on *The Use of a New and Correct Globe of the Earth*. His talks were scarcely appreciated—there were only ten listeners at the last session—and when he counted the collection, he had just enough to pay for the materials he had bought to illustrate the lectures. He shrugged his shoulders, realizing that at least he had added to his scientific equipment. Unhappy preacher, he dreamed quite pardonably of a richer benefice, but his next call was to a still smaller parish.

There was a great advantage in this smaller charge. Here he could open a school. He now became a most exacting schoolmaster, teaching thirty boys and half a dozen young ladies from seven in the morning to four in the afternoon. How he resisted any suggestion they made in favor of an occasional extra holiday! Didn't he himself instruct private students even after four o'clock? People soon began to say that he was a better schoolman than a minister. His work was so successful in the classroom that it opened for him an appointment as tutor of languages in Warrington Academy.

While he was at the academy, he always managed to spend a month of each year in London. It was on one such vacation that he met the philosopher from Philadelphia who had performed that notable experiment with the kite and key. Franklin immediately recognized a strain of genius in the young man and suggested that he write a history of electricity. The American was willing to furnish the books for the necessary research. With these spurs to his ambition—the praise and encouragement of a great man almost twice his age

— he rushed to the task. Within a year he had finished the volume, which brought him election to the Royal Society.

With such honors in his thirties he should have been happy. But he had taken on new responsibilities. He had married. The cry of the financially embarrassed pedagogue has been heard in every age, and Priestley raised his voice to swell the chorus. How could he rear a rapidly increasing family on his salary? He had scientific fame, but did that butter bread? Now he remembered that his duty in life was to preach the word of God, a calling that would pay much better. When he received an invitation to a congregation of liberal views at Leeds, he accepted. Here he threw himself into the writing of controversial pamphlets by which he soon offended many within and without his church.

Even the clerical mind must relax. Priestley sought rest from the ardors of doing God's work by performing those experiments which have made his name immortal in the annals of pneumatic chemistry. His preparation was limited to a few lectures given by a Doctor Turner of Liverpool, the author of that beautiful bit of rationalization pointing out that, although England had lost the American colonies, she had been compensated for her loss by the planet Uranus, then recently discovered by Herschel. But these lectures were of little help to Priestley. He did not know the "approved" methods of his day. And we are glad that he didn't. As he himself pointed out:

I have often thought that upon the whole, this circumstance was no disadvantage to me; as in this situation I was led to devise an apparatus, and processes of my own, adapted to my peculiar views. Whereas, if I had been previously accustomed to the usual chemical processes, I should not have so easily thought of any other; and without new modes of operation I should hardly have discovered anything materially new.

The pious parishioners in Leeds began to gossip when they saw their new minister entering the brewery near his house. What in the world could he be doing there? Rumor had it that his interest was not in the beer but in the gas that bubbled to the top of the liquid in the fermenting vats. A likely story! But wasn't it just a bit undignified for a minister to be found so frequently in a brewery? If they had followed him they would have seen a sight that was already causing employees of the brewery to fear for his sanity. They watched him as he bent hour after hour over the fermenting vats of beer. In one hand he held a lighted candle, in the other chips of wood which he lighted from time to time and placed near the surface of the liquid. The flame was always extinguished by the bubbles of gas.

"What strange air is this!" he thought. "If we had enough of this we might extinguish great fires. . . How marvelous are the ways of the Creator!"

When he moved to a new neighborhood he found it inconvenient to be returning constantly to the brewery. It was then that he invented the pneumatic trough — for which alone he would be known — by which he collected quantities of this gas. He mixed some of this new gas with water and agitated it. What a pleasant drink it made! In fact it was as pleasant to taste as expensive seltzer water. Thus was carbon dioxide discovered, without which the soda fountain would be a very flat institution indeed.

"The father of soda water" received a great deal of

fame from his experiment. Men rushed to do him honor. The Copley medal was conferred on him by the Royal Society. The College of Physicians viewed the experiment. That learned body recommended that the navy use it to combat the horrors of the scurvy, from which sailors suffered in those days. But this was just another in the long list of incorrect prescriptions for the scurvy that doctors had given. A seaman was later to show the physicians how to prevent the sea scurvy.

Patrons have a way of stepping forward to offer aid when the days of need are past. The minister's fame attracted Lord Shelburne, who urged Priestley to be his secretary. The salary was splendid — over eight times what he had received in his first parish — and there was a house to boot. Priestley, however, was not fascinated by the arrangement. His lordship had a nasty way of ending friendships, but in this case there was to be a generous allowance if they separated. The offer was too good to be passed by.

Once established as his lordship's secretary, he had an abundance of time, and he spent much of it in writing religious tracts. Whenever he needed recreation he went to his crude laboratory.

A burning-glass furnished him as much amusement as it does a small boy. He directed the sun's rays on many different substances and collected the resulting "air." When he focused the rays of the sun upon a red powder, the oxide of mercury, it gave off a new kind of air with which he was not acquainted. By chance a lighted candle was at hand. He put it into the gas. It flared up. He inserted a wire, previously brought to a red heat; it took on an added brightness.

If this were ordinary air he knew that the candle would have been quickly suffocated, the wire would not have appeared to come to life.

His theory about this new air was quickly formed. He would learnedly call it dephlogisticated air, that is, air minus phlogiston. And what was phlogiston? It was a chemical myth that had been handed down to Priestley's era. By it men attempted to explain the mystery of fire. It was that mysterious, invisible substance that escaped in combustion. When coal was burned, the advocates of this theory explained, little of the weight of it remained in the ashes, and this was caused by the fact that coal contained so much phlogiston. Opponents pointed out that metals when heated increased in weight. But the chemist, who was bound to save his theory, was not stopped by any such objection. He explained that in such cases there existed negative phlogiston. Priestley liked this old theory, and he held on to it to his dying day. He could deny that there was a spiritual principle in man, he could assert that man was nothing but matter, but throw over phlogiston, never!

For months he thought about this new air. Then one day he wondered if it might not be better than common air. That could be determined quickly if a mouse were put into a vessel containing some of it. When he appeared in the kitchen with a trap his wife asked:

"Why, Joseph, whatever are you about now? I thought you were at work on your *Harmony of the Gospels*. Really I think it is more in keeping with the dignity of your calling than wasting your time with mouse traps."

"I'll do no more on the Harmony today. I need some mice. A little experiment, my dear."

Returning with his captive mice to his laboratory, he put the mouth of a vessel containing this new air upside down in water. Then he passed a mouse through the water into the vessel, carefully placing it on a little deck so that it would not drown.

"When I have imprisoned full-sized mice in ordinary air," he reasoned, "they have died in about fifteen minutes. This may be better than ordinary air. At any rate I'll observe carefully and play the flute meanwhile. . . The flute is an admirable instrument, the solace of many an hour that would otherwise be very dull. Moreover, it is easy to play. I think I must speak a word for it some day in one of my papers."

Fifteen minutes passed. Other mice in ordinary air had been unconscious in that length of time. This one was still active. The flute was put aside. In a half hour the mouse became sluggish. In any case, it lived twice as long in this new air as others did in common air. But when he removed the wet mouse from his prison and placed it over near the grate, it quickly revived.

"If this air is better than common air," he mused, "it will do me no harm to breathe in a little of it myself." He inhaled some of the gas through a tube. Not only was his new gas colorless and odorless, but it was tasteless as well. The effect upon his lungs was exhilarating. "Perhaps my air may be of help to those suffering from lung trouble," he thought.

Priestley would hardly be surprised, if he returned from his grave today, to find thousands of people who attribute their recovery from pneumonia to the use of the oxygen tent.   This experiment was made on March 8, 1775, a red letter day in the history of science, for on that day this preacher-chemist saw something of the practical value of the oxygen that he had discovered some seven months before.

While Doctor Priestley remained with his patron, he made many other noteworthy chemical discoveries. Meanwhile, he continued to make contributions to religious speculation.   During these years he became convinced of a doctrine — most startling for a minister — that man is entirely material and that his only hope of immortality is in the resurrection.   This from a minister who could believe in the myth of phlogiston!   The press heaped violent criticism upon his head, terming him little more than an atheist.   Soon ill luck, which had forgotten to plague him for a time, returned.   He and his patron quarrelled.   Shelburne had recently remarried and might be supposed to have less need of a companion.

When he sought to find a place for Priestley in Ireland, the doctor reminded his lordship of the contract by which he was to receive an annuity, in case his services would no longer be desired.   Just at this time, a liberal congregation called him to Birmingham.   Though for a period of ten years he gave an example of honest thinking and decent living, still he was the devil incarnate to many.   He was happy in his seventh year of his sojourn in Birmingham.   It was then that he wrote his autobiography, the story of a happy man whose bliss was in his breast.   Indeed, he seems to have forgotten his troubles when he wrote:

I esteem it a singular happiness to have lived in an age and country, in which I have been at full liberty both to investigate, and by preaching and writing to·propagate, religious truth; that though the freedom I have used for this purpose was for some time disadvantageous to me, it was not long so, and that my present situation is such that I can with the greatest openness urge whatever appears to me to be the truth of the gospel, not only without giving the least offense, but with the entire approbation of those with whom I am particularly connected.

Little did he realize when he wrote these words that his greatest trials lay before him. He had applauded the success of the French Revolution and had been made a citizen of the French Republic, in appreciation of the propaganda he had spread in England in behalf of civil liberty. This served to increase his unpopularity with the rank and file of the English people. Not only had he deserted God but he was dishonoring his king as well.

Priestley was friendly with a small group of Birmingham liberals, who planned to hold a dinner and drink a temperate toast on the second anniversary of the fall of that hated prison, the Bastille. The city was seething with rage. A handbill had suggested that the wholesale activity of the guillotine in France would soon be witnessed in England. About the hour set for the banquet, an angry crowd began to collect. It was plain that there would be trouble.

Someone suggested that they burn down the church where Priestley assisted on Sundays. They did—for God and king. The mob, "of many hands but no head," was mad by this time. The cry went up, "Burn Priestley's house." The doctor had not gone to the banquet. He had spent the evening at home, playing backgammon with his wife. Into the room rushed a breathless man who cried, "Flee for your life : the mob has burned the old and the new meeting-houses. They are headed this way! They will surely kill you, doctor ! You have only a moment."

"God have mercy on us !" cried his wife. "Here's your cloak, Joseph."

"This is a false alarm. It can't be true. Impossible !"

Once in the street, he knew that his informer was right. The sound of tumult was close at hand. "One can never be sure in this life," he said to his wife as they rode away from their home. "These poor people are doing a great wrong and some day they will be sorry. I had thought the cause of liberty was making some progress. I only hope that they will not destroy my papers and philosophical instruments. . . Father, forgive them — they know not what they do."

The leaders of the crowd cursed on finding that their prey had escaped. A few gave chase but to no purpose. To satisfy their fury, they dumped his scientific instruments and his library into the street. Then they wrecked the house. Since there was no Priestley to burn, they burned his effigy instead. Little did they know that he was close enough to hear the rioters demolishing his home.

For three days and three nights the mob raged. The trials that followed were a sham, though three of the rioters were executed. Said King George in grandiose manner :

Though I cannot but feel better pleased that Priestley is the sufferer for the doctrines he and his party have instilled, and that the people see them in their true light, yet I cannot approve of their having employed such atrocious means of showing their discontent.

Escaping to London in disguise, he soon discovered that the members of the Royal Society, who respected his scientific work, were fair-weather friends. They avoided him now in his religious and political difficulties. It took courage to be identified with a man who had been denounced by Gibbon, the historian, and Burke, the statesman. Priestley knew there was no hope for him in his native land. He looked toward America, whither his sons had gone. America, a land of freedom, would welcome him.

Philadelphia, then the capital of the United States, received him with great enthusiasm because of his scientific and political reputation. But it was his desire to preach rational Christianity in the new world. This was the one thing that Americans were not interested in hearing, especially when the doctor's voice was weak and his teeth gone. Ministers looked askance at this new heretic who had created such a furore across the sea. He settled with his sons in Northumberland, one hundred and twenty-five miles from Philadelphia, a journey of five days in those times. Later an opportunity to teach at the University of Pennsylvania was open to him, but poor health, dogging his steps from youth, forced him to decline the offer. He lived on for about ten years, experimenting and prophesying the future of world events with the help of three-month old newspapers and the Bible.

Though Priestley was a great observer, he was weak in drawing conclusions from what he brought to light. Early in his scientific studies, he had adopted the theory of phlogiston, and through his life he expounded this idea with the fervor of a fanatic. When he was dying, he took his lance in hand to fight his last battle for this theory. He himself had unearthed the information that had destroyed this myth, for he had performed his experiment with the oxide of mercury for the French scientist Lavoisier, who used it to upset this theory of the difficult name. His last work was *The Theory of Phlogiston Established.* This, he hoped, would bolster up his scientific reputation, which, in turn, would interest men in his religious convictions and ultimately lead them to God. "If a scientist like Priestley can be a Christian believer, so can I," was the reasoning he expected. He wanted his work as a theologian to be recognized. "It is in this light chiefly," he wrote, "that I regard it. How insignificant are all subjects compared to those which relate to religion."

His life was a tragedy, as life has often been for men who advanced too far ahead of their times. A century after Priestley fled from Birmingham before the mob's rage, the grandchildren of his persecutors saw his monument unveiled and heard Thomas Huxley sound his praises. The city had repented of its blunder, but those who should have witnessed this triumph were beyond the reach of that humiliation, being long in their graves. Nor will the injustice done a man who should have been treated with respect in view of his honest purpose and spotless life give any modern fanatic pause. Bigots are always burning in the flesh or in effigy those who disagree with them. The pathetic irony of it all is that they will never know the scorn in which they are held when succeeding generations rise up to condemn their prejudices.

III

THE COUNT AND HIS BEGGARS

BENJAMIN THOMPSON

"He was strong, but untrained, and his language was not always such as a truly disciplined man of science would employ." — *John Tyndall.*

III

THE COUNT AND HIS BEGGARS

BENJAMIN THOMPSON

IN THE days when our republic was in its infancy, there were numerous inspired amateurs abroad in the United States. The opportunities of formal training were scanty, but in spite of this barrier men of native energy and intelligence made use of books, the common man's university, and often attained distinction in a field in which they were neither trained nor regularly employed. Many of the wealthy who could give their sons an education more thorough than any available in the states were sent across the sea to the mother country to acquire that polish which could not be obtained on this side of the water. But men of originality and force might be neither close enough to an institution of higher learning nor wealthy enough to attend its sessions if they were. When such men were intellectually curious, they often pursued a subject with an originality which their thinking might not have manifested, had they been trained in the tradition of the schools.

One immediately thinks in this connection of Benjamin Franklin, who distinguished himself in a variety of fields. With scanty formal training, ending when he was ten years old, he so improved his opportunities in private study that he was highly honored by his contemporaries and is even more so today. By profession a printer, he attained distinction in science, diplomacy and literature. In the field of electricity, he was an inspired amateur, fortunate in his notable experiment wherein he identified lightning and electricity. We have already seen in the case of Priestley that he was the inspiration of a history of electricity which brought its writer a name in science and membership in the Royal Society.

There is a contemporary of Benjamin Franklin whose career in many respects parallels his, though his fame does not approach Franklin's. That man was Benjamin Thompson, later Count Rumford. Both were born in the British Colony of Massachusetts, Franklin at Boston and Thompson at North Woburn, towns only twelve miles apart. In youth both were poor, ambitious and to a great extent self-educated, though Thompson went for a short period to the lectures of a professor of natural philosophy at Harvard. In spite of the fact that they had many friends in common, they never met, possibly because Franklin was so many years Thompson's senior.

Thompson was early apprenticed to an importer of merchandise. He seems not to have been overmuch interested in the work, but kept objects of mechanical interest handy to occupy his mind when business was slack. When increasing difficulties with England threatened the importing trade, he was forced to look for employment in another field. Like many another great man he taught school — but not for long. So unromantic an occupation could not hold a restless disposition like his for any extended time. The widow of Colonel Benjamin Rolfe fell in love with this handsome young teacher of nineteen and, if we may believe his own ungallant account of the matter, he suffered himself to be married to a woman fourteen years his senior. But the schoolmaster knew there were com-

pensations. The widow had means and a social position, and to a young man of his temper, believing
himself destined for great enterprises, considerations of
this nature were not to be scorned.

Although Benjamin Thompson was of humble origin,
he had that mysterious trait of personality which attracted people far above his station. He seems to have
won friends of influence easily; in consequence, he
made many enemies. When he was a young man of
twenty, Governor Wentworth of New Hampshire
caught sight of him on horseback and was so struck
with his appearance that he sought his acquaintance.
Thompson impressed the governor, and before long, in
spite of the young man's absolute ignorance of military
training and discipline, he was made a major over the
heads of many veteran officers in 1772.

Being close to the governor's ear, he suggested the
surveying of the White Mountains, and in this the
governor not only concurred but expressed himself as
desirous of taking part in the work personally. Meanwhile, experienced soldiers in His Majesty's service
uttered deep curses against this upstart, whose commanding figure on a charger was his sole title to the
rank of major. Opposition soon arose among American
patriots, too. Accused of being unsympathetic to the
cause of colonial liberty, he was brought before the
vigilantes, but nothing could be definitely proved against
him. Meanwhile, he stoutly maintained his innocence.
At the outbreak of the revolution when he was twenty-
two, he fled from persecution to England, leaving behind
his wife and infant daughter. With him he carried
despatches from General Gage to Lord Germain, Secretary of State.

Once in England, he was rewarded for his loyalty to the king. Later as a lieutenant colonel, he saw service in South Carolina and Long Island. When peace came, he desired to be sent to the West Indies, but instead, upon returning to England, he was discharged with a generous pension. At the time there was a rumor in military circles to the effect that the Turks and Austrians would soon be at war. A soldier of fortune, he decided to offer his services to the Austrians. While en route to Vienna, he took part in a military review at Strassburg. Once again his striking figure on horseback attracted attention. The duke made his acquaintance and gave him letters to his uncle, the Elector of Bavaria.

The elector liked this handsome foreigner. He understood so much about gunpowder and the making of cannons. Since Austria was not going to fight the Turk, would he not enter the elector's service and settle in Munich? Would he accept the dignity of Count of the Holy Roman Empire? Certainly. He would call himself Count Rumford—after the place where his wife's estate was located. Of course, King George's permission had to be obtained before Thompson could enter the elector's service, for he was a subject of His Majesty. The king not only approved but expressed his pleasure by knighting him.

Count Rumford was aware that his new position was not an empty title. Wherever he turned, shocking disorder was to be seen. The army was wretchedly clad, poorly fed, and therefore dissatisfied and undisciplined. But now he was Minister of War and it was his duty to improve the pay and comfort of the soldiers.

It was his feeling that a peace-time army must be kept

busy—even at projects that were non-military. Soon soldiers who had lately been loafers were employed in a public works program, making and repairing highways, draining marshes, repairing the banks of rivers. To encourage industry each soldier was given a small piece of land to cultivate. Excellent seeds were supplied. Rumford was especially interested in promoting the planting of potatoes. When the soldiers returned to their homes, they took with them this new interest in agriculture. The soldiers, their children and even peasants attended the barrack schools where supplies were free. With his characteristic economy he saw to it that the used paper was saved for the making of cartridges.

If the army's condition was pathetic when the count came, how much more so was the condition of the poor of Munich! On many a street corner a small child would hold out its hand to passers-by and say, "I am cold and hungry and afraid to go home. My mother told me to bring home twelve *kreutzers,* and I have only been able to beg five. My mother will certainly beat me if I don't carry home twelve *kreutzers."* And a *kreutzer* was only a half a cent!

Everywhere there were beggars. Some, like the child described, were truly pitiable. Some were kidnapped children, who had been purposely maimed or blinded to present a more touching sight. Not all the paupers, however, were crippled and weak. Some were strong. These plagued those who passed by until they gave them an alms to be rid of them. Sometimes in their begging they would enter houses and take whatever they saw. Munich had a population of sixty thousand, and its beggars ran into the thousands. To them begging was a profession. Regularly they appeared on certain beats which they regarded as their exclusive territory and from which they routed any newcomer attempting to cut in on their clientele. There were alliances by marriage within the caste and gang wars when lines were crossed.

The citizens of Munich hated the condition, but previous efforts to uproot it had proved unavailing. As Chief of Police, Count Rumford was given full scope to remedy the condition. Here the professional soldier became an amateur sociologist. He realized that to some it would "appear extraordinary that a military man should undertake a work so foreign to his profession as that of forming and executing a plan for providing for the poor." For this reason he felt it necessary to defend his interest in the poor.

Probably because he was an amateur, free from tradition, his method was entirely novel. Poverty, he said, was increased rather than lessened by the remedies commonly applied to remove it.

To make vicious and abandoned people happy, it has usually been supposed necessary, *first* to make them virtuous. But why not reverse this order! Why not make them first *happy*, and then virtuous! If happiness and virtue be inseparable, the end will be as certainly obtained by the one method as by the other; and it is most undoubtedly much easier to contribute to the happiness and comfort of persons in a state of poverty and misery than by admonitions and punishments to reform their morals.

First, he must make men happy. To do that, they must be made industrious. They must be given work. But these beggars could do nothing. All they knew was the art of begging. Clearly they must be taught how to do something that would bring them a wage and make them self-supporting. He answered the proposition that they should be given a dole, with this fundamental principle of his:

It is most certain that all sums of money or other assistance given to the poor in alms, which do not tend to make them industrious, never can fail to have a contrary tendency, and to operate as an encouragement to idleness and immorality.

He was a soldier but he had a heart. The poor must be helped, and the charitable and willing exertion of individuals must effect this aid. "No body of laws, however wisely framed, can in any country, effectually provide for the relief of the poor without the voluntary assistance of individuals." It was the demonstration of interest that he felt of supreme importance in this social work — not the levying of taxes. But again, the usual method of showing concern for the pauper was to give him an alms. This did no good at all because it did not tend to make the poor industrious, and it took power from any organized method of aiding them.

Clearly then his first task was to find some method of employing paupers. The elector gave some money toward his scheme, but how could there be much hope of success, when every plan to date had failed? A large, abandoned factory was bought and completely renovated. Master carpenters, smiths, turners, spinners, weavers, clothiers, dyers and saddlers were engaged to teach the poor the trades. The necessary raw materials and tools were stocked. Rumford's preparations were purposely completed by a New Year's day. This would be a splendid time for his manoeuvre, since on this fes-

tival people were a little more generous and the beggars
a little more audacious.

Rumford's plan was to take into custody all who were
found begging. He himself made the first arrest. Going into the street with some of his lieutenants, he was
immediately accosted by a beggar. Putting a hand on
his shoulder, the count said, "You are under arrest. Go
quietly with these officers to the station where your
case will be investigated. If you are worthy, you will
be taken care of."

Many soldiers were busy that day, and in the cleanup
twenty-six hundred were arrested. They were immediately released with instructions. Those who could
work were told to appear the next day at the factory,
The House of Industry, where they would be paid for
working and would receive a full meal free of charge.
But there was to be no more begging.

Now it was necessary to solicit private funds, especially for those who were genuinely in need of aid.
Rumford himself approached people for subscriptions.
The names of those who gave were made public, and
contributions of the smallest amount were accepted from
the poorest people, principally for the good it did them.
Likewise, the list of those who received the dole was
made public. They had been bothered by beggars and
now they knew that if the scheme were encouraged,
they would actually save money. Butchers and bakers,
who had previously been forced to give meat and bread,
were glad to make their donations directly to the House
of Industry.

The first attempts at teaching the poor were very
discouraging. In the first three months, the experiment
lost money. So many of these people had so little skill

that they ruined a great deal of raw material. In the beginning, the spinners were put to work on hemp which, if destroyed, would be less costly than wool and cotton. They were paid while learning and though their inferior products were not marketable, nevertheless he encouraged them. Soon there were evidences of developing skill. As the quality of the work improved, the House of Industry began to show a profit. Those who had gone hungry were now well fed. Those who formerly went almost naked in the cold of winter were not only earning clothes for themselves but clothing the army as well. The experiment was, moreover, changing these unfortunates into happy men and women.

Of course, there must be discipline, but he insisted that there be no harshness or force. He knew the value of rewards in shaping human conduct. Those who made exceptional progress were praised and pointed out to strangers, put in a position of prominence. When their work was worthy of notice, they were given a special uniform of which they were very proud. Mothers came to their work with their small children. They were put in chairs around the wall and received three *kreutzers* at the end of the day. As they grew to observe the constant industry around them, they cried to be given a chance to learn to spin. Child labor, of course, but an hour in the morning and an hour in the afternoon were set aside during which these children had to attend a school in the building.

Count Rumford did not organize his enterprise and then abandon it after it was started. Here was enough work for him—and glory too. As he walked through the House of Industry, he was not count, but a king. Mothers working at spinning wheels stopped at their work to wish him God's blessing. They were happy. Men who had formerly been able to use their hands for nothing but to reach for alms proudly displayed their work and were pleased when he praised their skill.

The people loved this count. He had not given them money to be rid of them. No, he had treated them as human beings. His personal interest — "the demonstration of concern," which he claimed necessary in dealing with the poor — was what won their affection. When he was ill on one occasion, the poor went in procession to the cathedral to offer public prayers for him, though he was a Protestant, and they Catholic. Their great benefactor was supposedly dying, a martyr, in his service to them. Later when he fell ill at Naples, they set apart an hour each evening, after they had finished their work, to pray for him.

"I dare venture to affirm," he later wrote, "that no proof could well be stronger than this that the measures adopted for making these poor people happy were really successful." One may judge of the esteem in which he was held when the people of Munich erected a monument to him while he still lived. It was dedicated to "him who eradicated the most scandalous of public evils, idleness and mendicity; who gave to the poor help, occupation, and morals, and to the youth of the Fatherland so many schools of culture." Beneath was the command, "Go, wanderer! try to emulate him in thought and deed, and us in gratitude."

RUMFORD's scientific interests fitted very well into his social program for the poor. Throughout his entire life he was interested in heat, particularly in its practical uses. He was constantly trying to produce more heat from less fuel, a study which benefited rich and poor alike. It was his belief that most grates did little more than heat the chimney. Often in those days the houses of the wealthy were full of smoke, because the architect did not understand the proper construction of grates and chimneys. He claimed to have rid about five hundred homes of this defect.

In his opinion much good food was wasted because of the improper construction of the stove. Food was scarce in the homes of the poor and should not be ruined in preparation. Nor should fuel be wasted. On a trip to Italy he observed how wasteful were the cooking fires in institutions for the poor. This was especially deplorable because fuel was scarce in Italy. He gave directions for the rebuilding of these fire-places, and when they were put into use, only one-eighth of the fuel formerly used was required.

The economic preparation of nutritious food was a study of greatest importance for the poor. In his essays he goes into details about the cost of food for the great numbers that took dinner each day at the House of Industry, often as many as fifteen hundred persons. Interesting, too, is another essay : *Of the Excellent Qualities of Coffee and the Art of Making it in the Highest Perfection*, which is accompanied with various illustrations of urns.

Later, when he took up residence in England, he founded the Royal Institution, enlisting by the power of his personality, the co-operation of the most notable people in England. But his associates disagreed with him over the purpose of the society. Rumford, like Franklin, was primarily interested in the practical side of life. It was his belief that the Royal Institution should be interested in the study of economical ovens and the proper construction of fire-places. Other officers felt that the institution should direct its efforts toward purely scientific research. Rumford was not much interested in this and so withdrew from the enterprise.

But it must not be imagined that Rumford had no interest in the theory of subjects dear to his heart. On the contrary, he made a well-known contribution concerning the nature of heat. In that day it was commonly held that heat was a substance, a kind of fluid. Rumford had spent a great deal of his time studying this phenomenon and always had his eyes open for anything that would help him solve a problem so vexing to the scientists of that time.

One day in Munich, while supervising the slow process of drilling a cannon, he stooped to pick up some of the metallic grindings that fell from the boring tool. What made these chips so hot? A few grains of metal did not produce all this heat. It was friction. He saw it all in a moment, but how was he to prove it to the learned men of the Royal Society?

He planned his experiments and carried them out while still in favor at Munich. Into a piece of discarded cannon, which had been partly bored, he inserted a dull drill. This was put into a container, holding about nineteen pounds of water. Then the horses furnishing power for the drill were started. After two and one-half hours, the water about the cylinder was boiling. All this heat did not come, he argued, from the bit of metal dust that was drilled out by the borer. The heat was not furnished by the metal, nor did it come from the air. Heat was not a material. If it were a material, its supply would be exhausted by friction, but this heat was inexhaustible and depended on the friction expended. Heat must therefore be a motion. When Humphry Davy, his protégé in the Royal Institution, demonstrated by rubbing two pieces of ice together that the friction would bring about liquefaction, Rumford's theory was further established.

Count Rumford spent eleven years of his life in Munich. Eventually opposition arose to a foreigner who possessed so much power. He went to England but was recalled, however, when Austrian and French armies threatened to capture Munich. He returned in time to prevent the occupation of the city. By way of appreciation his patron sent him as Ambassador to the court of the King of England. Upon his arrival he found that the king would not accept one of his own subjects in that capacity. Nettled at this, he decided to go to America where he would live as a German nobleman near Cambridge, Massachusetts.

What would the states, now free, say to that? President Adams was pleased and offered the count his choice of two military positions. While these negotiations were in progress, he became interested in organizing the Royal Institution and altered his plan of going to America. But after his differences as to the policy of the institution, he retired to France, where he moved in the most distinguished circles.

There he met the widow of Lavoisier. He was free to marry now, since his wife in America had died several years before he left Munich. What promised to be an ideal marriage turned out dismally. In less than four years they separated with the most hostile feelings toward each other. He had locked out her guests; she had retaliated by pouring boiling water on his flowers.

Rumford was essentially a courtier, pleasant — when he wanted to be — and ingratiating, a man who had the faculty of getting on in the world. Yet he had more than a pleasing personality. He possessed a mind rich in a variety of fields. Besides being a soldier, who was an inspired amateur in science and sociology, he was a skilful musician, a mathematician, an exact draughtsman, a linguist, a student of medicine and surgery, an author, and an inventor. In most of his work Count Rumford had service to others in view; the benefactions of this international man were so numerous and widespread that four nations mourned his passing.

IV

A MUSICIAN LOOKS AT THE STARS

WILLIAM HERSCHEL

"Music was long his pursuit, astronomy his
pastime; a fortunate event enabled him to make
astronomy his pursuit, while keeping music for a
pastime." — *Agnes M. Clerke.*

IV

A MUSICIAN LOOKS AT THE STARS

WILLIAM HERSCHEL

THE Seven Years' War was the World War of the eighteenth century. In this conflict a million men lost their lives on battle fields from India to America. Prussia and England united against France, Austria, Russia, Sweden and Saxony. Great Britain had sided with Frederick of Prussia because the English kings, the Georges, were from Hanover and they wanted to save their heritage from the rising power of Prussia's war lord, Frederick the Great. England was especially interested in overcoming the French forces. This she did, though there were battles in which the British were totally routed.

One of these battles was fought at Hastenbeck in Hanover, and one of the soldiers who took part in that conflict — at a safe distance — was William Herschel. As he lay in a ditch on the night after this battle, he told himself that this war was a stupid business. He had enlisted some four years before because he wanted to play in the band with his father and brother. That feature of the army he liked, but this wallowing about in a muddy ditch, especially when a man was sickly . . . Wasn't a person a fool to stay on helping men, mad with ambition, to build up empires? Well, he had ambitions of his own. One only lives once. Why not desert? He would go to England where his regiment had been quartered two years before.

Life was hard for the deserter the first few years, but

soon his musical talent brought him employment. Ten long years passed before he reached the enviable position of organist at fashionable Bath. Here he became a popular teacher. Why shouldn't he? He was handsome, affable, talented. With boundless energy he set about the task of giving lessons, conducting concerts and composing music.

But he could not keep at his music perpetually; there had to be some recreation. Years before, when in the Hanoverian Guard, he had given evidence of his serious interest by buying Locke's *Essay on Human Understanding*. Since that date he had constantly studied to supplement what he had been taught at the garrison school at home. To unbend his mind from the rigors of a day spent at teaching music, he gave his evenings over to the study of mathematics, optics and astronomy.

After becoming established at Bath, he went back to his home at Hanover to visit his family. He had made good and he was welcome. None was more anxious to see him than his sister Caroline. She had been brought up very strictly by her mother who, unable to write herself, felt that education for women was superfluous, that woman's place was in the kitchen. The father of the family was not so strict with Caroline. He early discovered that she, like her brothers, had musical ability, but when he wanted to give her lessons, Frau Herschel objected, and it was only when she was not at hand or in an exceptionally benevolent mood that the father could give Caroline any instructions. When the father died, Jacob, the oldest of the brothers, came into the dignity of head of the house and carried out the policies of his mother with reference to his sister Caroline.

"You don't look very happy, Lina," we can imagine

William saying when he came home. "Why are you so gloomy?"

"You don't know how lonesome I am here at home since father died, and you have gone so far away to England. I often wonder what will happen to me when the family breaks up."

"Well, you'll be getting married one of these days."

"No, I'm getting too old. Girls my age are married. I know I'm not beautiful, William, and you know it, too. I have never been allowed to do anything but work. There's nothing I can do that interests anybody. Even when I wanted to learn some dressmaking and millinery, brother Jacob stormed about it and only let me go if I'd make only useful things — no fancywork. Jacob doesn't know it, but I did learn to do some fancy stitches. Sometimes I have a chance to knit before the boys get up and want their breakfast."

"Now don't worry," said William sympathetically. "You practise your singing — you have good timbre in your voice — and then one of these days I'll come for you."

On a later visit William suggested that he take Caroline to England. The family vote was decidedly against the plan. Who would cook and scrub and polish if she went away? But finally she was permitted to go when William offered to pay the wages of a servant to take her place.

If Caroline was busy at Hanover, she was still more so at Bath, for life in her new surroundings was always at fever heat. But there was a world of difference between the day's work in Hanover and here in England. Now everything she did was new, interesting and educational. She took lessons in English, music and the business of becoming a lady. Her brother was so busy that they had little time together except at meals. It was then that he educated her. Her progress in singing pleased him so much that soon she was playing the leading roles in his oratorios and training the sopranos. In addition to this, she copied the music for the vocal parts and for an orchestra of over one hundred pieces.

The more routine work that he could pass over to Caroline, the more time William had for study. Night after night, when his sister felt he should have been sleeping, he was sitting up in bed reading books on astronomy by candlelight. Each night the subject so fascinated him that he read on for hours, forgetting the passing of time. Though thirty-five years of age, he had not yet peered through a telescope. He decided to satisfy his curiosity and rented a small reflector. What he saw only awakened a deeper interest instead of satisfying him. He must rent a larger reflector. But no larger instruments were made, though he was told that one could be manufactured for him, if he had the money.

But his budget could stand no such expense. If men made these telescopes, he told himself, he could do it, too. He bought tools from a Quaker who used to polish mirrors and went at the making of telescopes with the enthusiasm he showed in everything. Immediately the Herschel home began to look more like a factory than the residence of a popular young music master. Their mechanically minded brother Alexander had put in his appearance. He was given a lathe which was set up in one of the bedrooms. The furniture in the drawing-room was pushed to the wall to make room for a cabinet-maker's tools. "What would my good mother say,"

Caroline asked, "if she came into this house and saw everything in such disorder? I can even hear her scolding." But Caroline swallowed her indignation and before long she was absorbed in her brother's desire to build a telescope bigger and better than any previously built.

But this craft was not to be learned in a single day. It was a tedious and discouraging business, especially when they had nothing to instruct them except their own mistakes. Herschel never told the world how he made his telescope, but it is easy to imagine some of the difficulties he encountered. There was the problem of finding a metal that would take a high polish and retain it. Then they must learn to cast this molten metal. Of what substance would the mold be made? After many experiments he came to use loam mixed with sifted manure.

Time and time again his castings developed flaws. Once he succeeded in making a good casting, the long task of grinding the concave surface and polishing it by hand began. All this had to be very accurate, if true images of the stars were to be reflected. He tells us that after about two hundred mistakes he finally produced a satisfactory, five and one-half foot telescope. It had cost him much toil and study, but when he had finished it, he was out in the front rank of telescope makers.

Now that he had learned his art, he kept on improving his instruments so that he could see farther and farther into the depths of the heavens. This was now his passion — to make bigger and better telescopes. But the day was never long enough. So many hours had to be given over to music, and much of the night was spent in viewing the skies. Eight years of constant toil followed the day when he first looked through a telescope. Then one night while studying the constellation Gemini, his instrument reflected an unexpected light.

"This is no ordinary star, Lina. It has a disk. I think it is a comet."

Immediately Herschel wrote a letter to the Royal Society on the subject. But after he observed the star's course in the heavens, he was convinced that it was a planet — the first that was ever discovered by a telescope, the other five having been known from antiquity: Jupiter, Mercury, Saturn, Venus and Mars. Herschel had extended the boundary of our solar system, for this new planet was farther distant from the earth than Saturn and required over eighty years to complete its orbit. And the organist had done it all in his leisure with instruments he had made himself! The learned world was aghast.

George III was interested and wanted to see the star. Herschel was glad of the opportunity to visit court and brought his instruments into the royal presence. But before they would gaze at the stars, there was this matter of his desertion of the Hanover army to be considered. Solemnly the king handed him papers in which he was declared absolved of his disloyalty. His Majesty was pleased with Herschel and his discovery, a pleasure that was doubtless increased by the fact that the discoverer came from Hanover, whence the Georges came. To show his appreciation, he appointed Herschel to the post of Royal Astronomer with a pension of two hundred pounds a year. When William spoke up to say that his sister Caroline was indispensable, she was given a pension of fifty pounds a year.

Once Herschel was out of the kingly presence, he shouted for joy. Now he was free from that soul-sapping routine of giving lessons to every mother's daughter who could pay the fee. Now he would accomplish things. Immediately he wrote to Lina about the king's pleasure at seeing the new planet and the honors that had been heaped upon him. Even the small telescope he had brought with him was superior to those at the Royal Observatory. The praises people were showering on him only proved how little they knew. "I will make such telescopes and see such things —."

The king had honored Herschel; Herschel would honor the king. He wrote a pompous letter to the Royal Society in which he stated that there was no reason why the new body should be called after some god or goddess of antiquity. Why not call it *Georgium Sidus?* Was the discoverer not "a subject of the best of Kings, who is the liberal protector of every art and science . . . a native of the country from whence this illustrious family was called to the British throne . . . a member of that society which flourishes by the distinguished liberality of its royal patron; and, last of all . . . a person now more immediately under the protection of this excellent monarch and owing everything to his unlimited bounty?" But in spite of his flowery appeal the new planet was called Uranus.

When a man reaches eminence, he is often inclined to sit back and enjoy his new ease with dignity. But honors were not fatal to Herschel's advance; rest was the farthest thing from his mind. How could he rest when he wanted to see farther and farther into the heavens? To do this he would have to make a thirty-foot telescope or perhaps a forty-foot one. His ambition was checked when he remembered his income. It was difficult enough to keep Alex and Lina on two hundred pounds a year, without sinking money into a project so expensive as a forty-foot telescope. How to get sufficient money was his problem. Different governments would pay him handsomely if he would build some of his excellent instruments for them. He hated the idea of slaving to make telescopes that would pass into other hands, but he saw no other way out. Later he was to marry a wealthy widow, who would chase the wolf from the door. But now he needed funds.

Herschel began to manufacture telescopes, but the king, learning of his ambition, loosened the royal purse strings and gave him some two thousand pounds and a generous annual allowance for the maintenance of the instrument. In the midst of the work, he ran out of money. Unforeseen difficulties had arisen. The first reflecting mirror had been too thin. The second cracked in the cooling. But the king did not desert him. Another two thousand pounds came from the royal purse. His third mirror, weighing well over a ton, was not satisfactory until it had been worked on for ten months.

Meanwhile the whole enterprise had captured the public fancy. Sightseers came to walk through the tube. Among the number was King George, accompanied by the Archbishop of Canterbury. The king went ahead, and the archbishop stumbled along after him, unable to find a sure footing in the darkness. His Majesty turned to him and with royal humor said: "Come, my lord bishop, I will show you the way to heaven."

With the new telescope Herschel discovered the fifth

and sixth moons of Saturn. Yet he was not happy about this new instrument. The mirror was sensitive to changes of temperature, which caused inaccuracy. After a short time the reflector lost its luster and it was never repolished. Moreover it was too unwieldy for practical purposes, two men being required to operate it. He figured that if he were to make a review of the heavens with this instrument, it would take eight hundred years.

Modern attempts to make larger telescopes are in a direct line with the work of this amateur. How interested he would be in the present manufacture of the world's largest reflecting mirror, poured in Corning, New York, to be put in position on Palomar Mountain, California. We can imagine him among the throng of those who recently looked on when the cooled reflector, weighing twenty tons, was taken from the oven. How interested he would be in this new reflector, weighing sixteen times as much as the one in his forty-foot telescope and having a diameter of two hundred inches, four times his own.

In praising Herschel one must not forget that he accomplished so much because his sister devoted her whole life to his success. She was always at his side to help him. When he was sweeping the heavens with his instrument, she was ready to jot down what he observed, even though the weather was often so cold that the ink froze. Then during the day she would make calculations based on what they had observed the previous night. When he was busy polishing a mirror, and could not stop until it was completed, she would put food into his mouth or read aloud to him from the novels of Fielding and Sterne. At other times she helped at tasks so uninspiring as the sifting of the manure needed for the castings. But her work was not always menial. She, herself, learned to watch the skies and discovered two nebulae and five comets.

When her brother died at the age of eighty-four, she decided to go back to Hanover to die, but death does not always come when it is welcome. She lived on for twenty-five more years, reaching almost a hundred, always busy making catalogues of stars. She was not forgotten in her lonely retreat. Many illustrious savants came to visit her; many distinctions were conferred upon her in terms so flattering that the modest Caroline thought that those who wanted to do her honor were making sport of an old woman.

But sometimes as she sat propped up in her bed, her eyes would dim with tears as she dreamed of those days in England when her brother and she were so busy and so happy. Again she was singing and he was conducting, or she saw herself smiling as she read some amusing scene from *Don Quixote* while William was polishing a mirror. Then she remembered his marriage. It upset her at the time, but nobody would ever learn her thoughts; she had destroyed her diaries for those years. After all, who could be angry with him for marrying so kindly a widow? Certainly the son, John, born of that marriage, had fulfilled his father's dreams. But John had never had to fight his way up from poverty. It was William who was the superman.

V

SCIENCE IN A MONASTERY GARDEN
GREGOR MENDEL

"Biology was one of his numerous avocations, like playing chess, organizing fire brigades, running banks and fighting governmental taxes. He was really a physicist, and brought to one of the great problems of biology the attitude of mind and the quantitative method of attack which has been in use for some time by physicists and by astronomers, and which was just coming to be used more widely by chemists." — *Professor E. M. East.*

V

SCIENCE IN A MONASTERY GARDEN

GREGOR MENDEL

AN ambitious young man once wrote to Luther Burbank, the plant wizard, asking him what works of
Mendel he should read. Perhaps the youth was only
interested in adding another autograph to his album,
but it may be that he had heard of Mendel's famous
theory and, being a lonely scholar, honestly sought direction from the great plant-breeder. Burbank was
never slow to speak his mind. "My advice to you," he
wrote, "is to start Mendel by reading Darwin, and then
let Mendel go and read more Darwin." In other words,
there was nothing worth while in Mendel.

The practical doer is often inclined to ridicule the
man who tries to work out a rule or formula. Burbank's advice is typical of the practical man's lack of
sympathy with the theorist. He was a nurseryman who
gave up that work to become an amateur botanist. His
ability lay in the keenness of his senses. This enabled
him to pick out at a glance young plants possessing
those characteristics which he wished to perpetuate, but,
though he had a world of patience and industry, he had
not the scientific temper. He certainly did the youth
who sought his advice no service in prejudicing him
against Mendel's experiments. His dismissal of the monk
and his work with an airy gesture leaves the impression
that he was giving advice in a matter about which he
had no first hand acquaintance. Certainly he could
hardly have read the monk's brief paper.

But Burbank was not the first man to ignore Mendel's work. In fact nobody ever paid any attention to him during his life. He was born a generation before his time. He performed a brilliant experiment, but few listened to him, and those who did failed to understand. The seed fell on stony ground and would not grow, but Mendel never doubted that it was good seed.

We can imagine the feelings of the members of the Brünn Natural History Society as they came together one winter night in 1865 to hear one of the world's great scientific papers. No one of the forty members realized the importance of the occasion. To many it was just another talk. Perhaps there was a special reason for attending this particular meeting. Father Gregor Mendel, one of the Augustinian monks from the local monastery, was to read a paper on *Experiments in Plant-Hybridization*, and though the effort might be neither very interesting nor informative, still this sort of thing in a clergyman should be commended.

Intellectually the speaker did not enjoy much of a reputation. He was only a *supplent*, that is an extra teacher, who in spite of all his time in school had failed twice in trying to secure an ordinary teacher's certificate. He was not even licensed to teach in a high school, and here he was, standing up before the local intelligentsia to tell about his experiments with edible peas, conducted in a little corner of the monastery yard.

While the crowd assembled to listen to his essay, Mendel sat waiting with his paper, written in a beautiful hand, before him. If we could talk to his friends in this audience, they would tell us of his background. They would tell a story of his early poverty. He had his roots in Austrian Silesia where the family's condition was so low economically that his father had to work without pay three days of each week on public works, a relic of feudal days. By a series of great sacrifices the boy had been given an education.

First he attended the local school, where the pupils learned something of bees and fruits. The priest in charge of this school was rebuked on this score by the school inspector, and in the report to the archbishop this unusual course of studies was termed a scandal. As a result of this scandal, bees and fruits became a major interest in the boy's life.

Later he was sent to a high school twenty miles from home as a half-ration student. The understanding was that his parents would supplement the bill of fare at the school with occasional boxes of food from the farm. They suffered some reverses, but he was able to eke out the barest existence by tutoring a little. Sickness, brought on no doubt by the combined assault of worry over money and his next meal, overtook him three times during his student days.

He had gone on to the priesthood and was ordained at the age of twenty-five. It immediately became evident that he was unsuited for parish work. His tender nature recoiled at the sight of human pain and misery, encountered at every turn in his parochial duties. Soon he worked himself into a position where he taught Greek and mathematics. Meanwhile he prepared in his leisure to pass the examinations that would give him professional standing as an instructor. At twenty-eight he was examined for certification to teach science. He failed. His superiors felt that he should be given a chance to study with professors, instead of teaching himself, and so he spent about two years at the University of Vienna, where he applied himself to science exclusively. After his return he secured employment at the Brünn Modern School and applied for permission to take the examination that would make him a certificated teacher in a high school. Surely there would be no difficulty now, after all his experience at teaching and his study at the University of Vienna.

Gregor Mendel at about the age of thirty-four was admitted to the examination.

Nobody knows what happened, but when he came back to the monastery, sadness was written on his face. Nobody had the nerve to probe into his wounds. If he ever told his friends, they guarded the reasons very carefully. It is certain that the certificate was not granted. We can only surmise what the causes of his failure were. It may have been that the examining board, with open texts upon their knees, chose to "roll" him for some inscrutable reason.

They may have made the examination so difficult and specific that he could not answer their questions. Or it may be that Mendel ardently defended his personal views in opposition to a canonized opinion of an examiner. Mendel was easily capable of this, having certain stubborn, peasant traits. At any rate the report went the rounds that he had crossed the doctor who had examined him in botany and had maintained his views with too much vigor. He made no further attempt to pass the examinations, but returned home and, fresh from his humiliation at Vienna, significantly began his experiments in botany, which lasted for eight years, when he was interrupted because of the prevalence of the pea weevil. But his experiments had been sufficiently extended, he felt, to offer certain conclusions.

And this material was what he presented to the members of the body of local scientists in Brünn (now Brno). We can imagine the scene. The president announced that they were privileged to hear the results of Father Gregor Mendel's experiments with edible peas. He would not be able to finish the paper at this meeting, but he would conclude his remarks at the following session. Father Mendel looked out over his glasses at the crowd and began to read. There was no preparatory joke to capture the benevolence of his hearers. Everything about his manner indicated an intense seriousness, for now he was to make public the fruit of his long study.

Instead of attempting to study the problems of heredity by crossing different species, Mendel had struck on the idea of simplifying the matter by crossing plants, which showed contrasting characters within the species, with others of the same species. Thus he noted seven pairs of contrasted characters in peas. Some peas had wrinkled surfaces and some smooth, some had green cotyledons and some yellow, some had long stems and some short, and so on. He had crossed these opposite characters, covering the cross-fertilized plants with bags to make certain that no bees or insects would disturb the pollen and thus frustrate his experiments. He had taken infinite patience and kept the most exact records.

Mendel discovered that no matter what resulted in the first generation, even though one of the characters seemed to have disappeared totally, the contrasted characters reverted to type in the second filial generation. For example, when peas having green pods were crossed with those having yellow, both green and yellow podded peas appeared in the second filial generation. This reversion to type worked itself out in definite proportions; dominant tendencies were proportioned to the recessive as three to one. This ratio was predictable. Then he became more obscure when he began to explain what happened when more than one pair of contrasted characters entered the crossing.

Those who knew botany were disturbed by all these mathematical ratios. Some of the members had had difficulty in keeping their attention on what the priest was reading. Others who had dined only a short time before had a hard time fighting off sleep. A few heads had bobbed at the lectures, but everybody managed to join in for the applause. Some added a few extra claps, remembering that after all this was a monk talking about science. He at least had refused to become a medievalist. Such men should be encouraged, even though, of course, the effort might be ill-advised and out of the approved, scientific grooves.

Mendel was pleased with the applause. He mopped his brow while waiting for any question that might be put to him. He had no fear that he could not defend his position. Hadn't he read widely during the years of his experiments? Hadn't he bought Darwin's works as they had appeared? He could show his annotated copies. But nobody asked a question. They weren't interested. Could it be that they were ignoring his work? The order of business was resumed. A prominent professor of botany led a discussion on Darwin's *Origin of Species*, published some six years before. There was something of a rebuke in the professor's choice of a subject, for whereas Darwin had shown the variability of species, Mendel had attempted to show the constancy, if not of species, then at least of certain characters within a species.

Mendel was sad again this evening as he returned to his monastery. "How did the talk go?" we can imagine his fellow monks asking him. "Nobody paid the least attention to it. So many years I have studied about the heredity of peas, and then the learned members of the Society for the Study of Natural Science never even ask a single question. Well my time will come one of these days."

But he was cheered when he remembered that his paper would be published. Certainly the learned authorities in the great centers to which exchange copies of the proceedings were sent would recognize his ability and the truth of his conclusions. One hundred and twenty copies of the transactions were sent to as many intellectual centers, where librarians had them catalogued and put up with the other dusty numbers, in the hope that some day by some chance someone might call for them. But nobody read the work, and Mendel's paper seemed bent for oblivion. Mendel waited. Nobody reviewed his work. But still he said, "My time will come one of these days."

Here was a plain instance of a case in which the parading professional had tripped over his sword. The conclusions of a brilliant amateur passed unnoticed before the eyes of the learned world. If a noted scholar had written the paper, it would have been read, but Mendel was obscure. He was not an authority, and hence the leaves of his contribution remained uncut.

Soon an event occurred in Mendel's life which changed its whole course. Three years after he read his famous paper, he was elected abbot of the monastery of Altbrünn. In the educational world he was only an extra teacher of physics in a high school, but, in the eyes of his fellow monks, he was worthy to be their leader. He accepted the new duties and at first imagined that he would enjoy sufficient leisure to pursue his private studies.

For a time he did, but he was soon deceived. The executive duties of his office robbed him of his leisure. His plants bloomed and died with little more than a fleeting visit from the busy abbot. He had been interested in bees, too, but this interest was also dropped. Probably he gave up his studies because he could not count upon having the time for any experiments that he might have in mind. He took some recreation, however, for he travelled about over Europe a great deal. This proves how incorrect it is to imagine that he led a cloistered life within monastic walls.

Mendel took his duties as a prelate seriously, an instance of which is seen in his contest with the state over a period of ten years. In 1874 a law was passed that ecclesiastical benefices and religious communities should make specified contributions to the fund used for defraying the expenses of religion. The ruling was not anti-religious but aimed at more equally distributing the church's means among its less fortunate ministers. Mendel's stubbornness now came to the fore. With an unbelievable tenacity he fought this exaction to the very end of his life. Finally the government officials were forced to become drastic and collected rents ordinarily received by the monastery. In this way accounts were balanced. Mendel became an embittered man, especially when even the brethren within the monastery opposed his policy in the tax dispute. To their way of thinking he did not manage the affairs very diplomatically. This is proved by the fact that immediately after his death the difficulties with the government were settled.

He now began to suffer from kidney trouble, a condition that was not helped by his devotion to nicotine. He started using tobacco at the suggestion of a physician who told him that smoking would keep him from becoming too fat. But the habit grew on him so that he was known to smoke twenty cigars in a day. But he still remained fat. Friends of his bishop might smile when they remembered that, as a young cleric, Mendel had said that his lordship possessed more fat than understanding, a remark that reached the episcopal ear.

There were few genuine mourners when he passed away, for his stubborn opposition to the taxes had served to lessen his previous popularity. When he was laid to rest, everybody thought that this was the end of Mendel. They knew that he used to say, "My time will come one of these days," but they felt that he had only been bolstering up his courage. When he was in the tomb some sixteen years, he burst his winding sheets and, like Lazarus, came forth from the dead, as he had prophesied he would. About the turn of the century, three scholars working independently on the problem which Mendel had studied in his forgotten paper, came to conclusions that verified what he had done. By the merest chance his study was discovered.

From that time to the present his name has been held in honor in the annals of science. Mendel's experiments have become the corner stone of the science of genetics, and elaborate experiments, inspired by this amateur, have been carried out with plants and animals.

It is unfortunate that Darwin never came upon Mendel's paper. A careful search of the great scientist's library by his son failed to reveal any trace of the work. Darwin might have revised certain of his views when confronted with such telling evidence. But Mendel was born before his time. "Great as was the advance in cytological genetics during the later half of the nineteenth century," wrote Professor E. M. East of Harvard in a paper written in honor of the centennial of Mendel's birth, "one can not imagine an appreciation of the Mendelian type of work by any of the investigators. Their minds were too carefully focussed on the individual fact. Either Darwin or Galton would have seen the truth clearly; but then Darwin and Galton were amateurs who were not trammelled by professional connection with the guild of biologists."

Here then is another instance of an inspired, but in his day unappreciated, amateur pointing out a higher ground to the professionals.

VI

THE STONEMASON OF CROMARTY
HUGH MILLER

"Mr. Miller is one of the few individuals in the history of Scottish science who have raised themselves above the labors of a humble profession, by the force of their genius and the excellence of their character, to a comparatively high place in the social scale." — *Sir David Brewster.*

THE STONEMASON OF CROMARTY

HUGH MILLER

ALONG the eastern coast of Northern Scotland, the little town of Cromarty guards the entrance to the Bay of Cromarty. Nature is strong and unfettered in this region; to the north are the wild highlands, to the east the treacherous North Sea.

Hugh Miller, growing up in Cromarty at the beginning of the nineteenth century, seemed very definitely to belong to this wild region, for he, too, was untamed. He was a problem child. The gossips in the town lamented the fact that the boy's father had been drowned at sea, for he had been a strong man and would have "settled" the boy easily. But his young mother could do nothing with him. She could only wonder why providence had taken her two daughters and left her this son, who was already bringing disgrace upon her by plundering orchards and organizing a gang that was always up to some deviltry. She worried about him constantly.

He was a bright boy but he was not doing well in school. How could he, when he played truant three-quarters of the time? After a year in what was called the Old Dame's School, he passed into the grammar school of the parish where one poor schoolmaster herded one hundred and twenty lads and thirty lassies along the road to learning. Amid the bedlam that prevailed, the teacher seems to have preserved his sanity by taking special interest only in those who showed interest.

Hugh came under his notice as being a capable lad

who read a great deal, and for this reason he was promoted to the "heavy" class where he would take up Latin. But this new study required application of a kind that did not please him. It was much more interesting to read the translations of these Latin books and the biblical stories of the adventure of Joseph, Samson and David.

Some of the parents felt that their children were not getting the best possible training in this overcrowded school, and so a subscription was taken up to open another. To this institution Hugh Miller was sent. The new dominie had fewer students and could therefore keep them busier than they had been in the old school. Moreover, the new teacher knew that his school must surpass the leisurely, undisciplined and antiquated methods of the parish school, or else he would lose his position.

Young Miller, rebel at heart, was not willing to conform to these progressive ideas. In the Old Dame's School he had been taught to pronounce his letters one way, but the new dominie had a new method. He tried to teach the boy the approved pronunciation, but Miller stubbornly refused to change. The teacher determined to chastise such defiance. But his robust student of fifteen was not willing to submit to any punishment, and once the struggle began, there was some danger that the teacher himself might receive the whipping.

The students looked on anxiously. This was a test case and would determine how far the new master's methods and influence would extend. If Miller whipped him, rebellion would be general in the future. The two clinched and tried to throw each other. Miller stumbled over a desk. The schoolmaster pinned him down on the floor and pummelled him unmercifully. The crowd of boys was a little crestfallen when they saw that their leader was getting a terrible drubbing. Finally the dominie let him up. The boy took his tam-o'-shanter and never attended school from that day on.

Now Hugh was something of a poet. He had been writing verses for three years. Immediately after his brawl with the dominie, he hurriedly composed a lampoon entitled *The Pedagogue*. A few lines of this sustained hymn of hate will show the unusual talent of this problem boy.

> With solemn mien and pious air,
> S-k-r attends each call of grace;
> Loud eloquence bedecks his prayer,
> And formal sanctity his face.
>
> All good; but turn the other side,
> And see the smirking beau displayed;
> The pompous strut, exalted air,
> And all that marks the fop, is there.

In spite of his rhymes and his reading, it was the common conviction of the gossips that he would never amount to much. Not only had he defied the school authorities but he had turned atheist as well. Some terrible fate must surely overtake so wicked a youth.

After leaving school, he was faced with the necessity of working to make a livelihood. Choice of employment was limited. After surveying the limited opportunities, he decided to be a stone-mason because its seasonal unemployment would give him some time to read and write. He was apprenticed and set out to his first day's work in a quarry. His heart was heavy. But soon he became interested in the firing of the gunpowder with which rocks were blasted. He forgot his blistered hands in his eagerness to see the nature of the rocks.

There were strange markings on the uncovered ledges of stone. Some looked like the ripples of waves, others were cracked as though they had been the bottom of a dried-up pool. In these deposits stones that were rounded and worn rolled down with the blastings. It appeared to him that these stones had once been tossed about in water, but how would this high point have been the bottom of a body of water? There was nobody whom he could ask such questions; there were not even any books that he might consult. These mysteries became the subject of his thoughts.

The quarrying was too expensive at this point of the Bay of Cromarty, and the men were transferred to a lofty wall of cliffs overhanging the northern shore of the Moray Firth. Here he saw, laid out before his eyes, the crust of the earth where the story of its strata could be read as from an open book. A better place for the study of geology could not be found in any part of Europe. Yet he had nobody to enlighten him and he could only attempt to solve the puzzle unaided.

He picked up a nodule of limestone and cracked it open. Within it there was a delicate piece of nature's sculpturing, resembling one of the volutes of an Ionic capital. He opened a second. There was the imprint of a fish. In another there was a bivalve, in another a piece of wood. Was there anything so wonderful in all the world?

How lucky he was, he told himself, to take up this trade of a stone-mason. The other workmen were not interested in such things, but one, with whom he chatted about rocks, told him about stones called thunderbolts

to be found two miles distant. These possessed remarkable virtues in curing bewitched cattle. When he
had a free afternoon, he visited the spot. He knew at
once that these were not meteors, for a relative who
had sailed to Java had brought home a meteor, and these
stones were entirely different from that. Later he
learned that their real name was belemnite.

By the end of his first year of apprenticeship, his interest in geology was thoroughly awakened. But still he
was working in the dark. What a student with a text
before him can learn in an hour was to cost him years
of speculation. During his fifteen years as a mason,
whether travelling about from one place to another as a
journeyman or working in his own town, geology was
the interest that made a life of toil bearable. His keen
eyes were always on the alert to see what new fossilized
wonder nature had to show him. This study ennobled
his life and kept him from becoming a "Man with the
Hoe," a dull slave at a boresome task.

It soon became clear to the gossips of Cromarty that
Hugh Miller was no ordinary stone-mason. During
periods of unemployment, he applied himself to books.
Writing continued to be the passion of his life. He had
his poems collected and published at his own expense.
His poetry had its limitations, though one of his efforts
has sufficient merit to find place in the Harvard Classics.
Not only did his literary work create a good impression
in his native town, but his character had so developed
that even his former critics were bound to admit that
they were mistaken. He had been thrown with riff-raff
and had not been tainted.

While working at Edinburgh, for example, he was
associated with workmen whose interests were entirely

sensual and whose hero was the man who spent in riotous living the most money in the shortest time. He could not be induced to join their debauches. On one occasion he did drink some spirits. Upon returning to his room, he found that the page of Bacon danced before his eyes. This experiment left a deep impression upon him. Then and there he made a resolution to avoid alcohol, a resolution which he kept. Yes, the village gossips were forced to admit that for once their prophetic gifts had failed them. Certainly he was growing up to be a model man, a poet, a good workman, a friend of the minister and a defender of the kirk.

It is characteristic of the rise of Hugh Miller that he made his advances by sudden leaps. Of these there are three. As a young stone-mason in Cromarty, he lived without any ambition to make a name beyond the confines of the parish. Then a Miss Lydia Fraser, a young lady of culture and intelligence, came to the village. She met him and told him how beautiful his poetry was. Then ambition stirred within him.

This girl was not indifferent to him, in fact it was quite plain that she admired him, but how could he hope to win a wife so far above his station economically and socially? Granting that she would have him, how could he dare marry so lovely a creature until he could supply her with those luxuries which had always meant nothing to him, but which she must have to live in the manner to which she was accustomed?

The girl's mother was profoundly interested in this new acquaintance which her Lydia was encouraging and, fearing that "her daughter might bestow her heart and hand on a mechanic, commanded that the intimacy should be broken off." This was a sorry state of affairs, but the lovers still had their pens. They wrote long, restrained epistles, in which they relieved the anguish of their souls by reciting their woes. Hugh tried to keep from brooding by composing a book on the scenes and legends of Northern Scotland.

The man who had been so happy before with his books, his writing and his fossils was now thoroughly unhappy. He was willing to advance in the world, but he could see no ledge on which to set foot. Then this man, who had displayed no talent for arithmetic in school, was offered the position of accountant in the bank of Cromarty. With some distrust in his ability, he accepted the appointment, for this was the advancement and the security of income he needed before he could at all impress Miss Fraser's mother. After five years, Hugh married Lydia, the first and only woman he ever loved. The spirit of the marriage is shown by the fact that he gave his wife a Bible, inscribed with verses of his own, for a wedding present.

His second leap to higher ground was occasioned by a dispute between the congregations of the Scottish Church and their patrons, who appointed whatever ministers they wished without consulting or considering the wish of the people of the parish. To Miller this was a form of tyranny, a curbing of the free spirit of man. The devout young accountant would fight this throttling of freedom. He addressed to Lord Brougham, who had dismissed the claims of the Scottish Church, a pamphlet in which he defended the cause of the congregations.

The nervous vigor of his style obtained a wide hearing for the cause. Both Gladstone and O'Connell praised the protest. Those who were organizing the "Witness," which was being planned as the organ of the Scottish

Church, were attracted to this young banker in Cromarty and offered him its editorship.   He accepted the position with as much self-distrust as he had that of accountant at the Cromarty bank.   Immediately the paper gained a wide circulation because of his fearless articles.

It was through the columns of his magazine that he attained renown as a geologist, the third leap in his life. He had long been studying fossils, and this was his chance to write up his studies in a popular style.   A month after the articles were begun, he was recognized as a geologist.   Here the amateur's years of study produced fruit.   These papers were later collected into a book *The Old Red Sandstone*.   In this the stone-mason really enlightened the scientific men of his time.   They had long maintained that the Old Red had no fossils or that at best it contained very few.

Miller proved that this formation, far from being barren of fossils, was really very rich in them.   These he described in detail, even doing the illustrations with his own pencil.   He had followed Agassiz, the great authority on fishes, in much that he had written, but he had made his own original contributions, in particular, about certain armored fish.   Among these was the winged fish, having a head lost in its trunk, a humped back covered with bony plates, and two wings extending from its "shoulders."

The members of the British Society for the Advancement of Science met shortly after Miller's articles on the Old Red began to appear, and they were lavish in their praise of his work.   One scientist maintained that he would give his right arm to possess the literary skill shown in Miller's masterly descriptions.   Agassiz proposed that one of these species which the amateur scientist had discovered should be called Miller's winged fish, and today it bears the scientific name *pterichthys milleri*.

Miller now became a recognized popularizer of geology. His next work was the *Footprints of the Creator;* for the American edition of this treatise Agassiz wrote a preface. His last work was *The Testimony of the Rocks.* In these volumes he attempted to reconcile the Biblical with the geological account of creation. A fundamentalist in religion, he labored unceasingly to prove the validity of the account of creation as told in Genesis. He had his difficulties, but at least to his own satisfaction he pointed out that the six days of creation were really six geologic ages. These days were successive revelations made to the mind of Moses.

"Rightly understood," he wrote in reference to the account in the book of Genesis, "I know not a single truth that militates against the minutest or least prominent of its details." He believed that everything was specially created by God. For this reason he opposed the Development Theory, which maintained that more complex beings developed from primitive organisms. In fact, his *Footprints of the Creator* was a reply to *Vestiges*, an unsigned work which had brought this theory to the public attention.

Darwin was to go much farther in his *Origin of Species*, but Miller died three years before it appeared in 1859. Had he lived, we may be sure that he would have gone to the front to fight Darwin and his theory of evolution. Miller, however, never realized that a later generation would be using his fossil discoveries to substantiate a theory which he would have termed both pagan and unscientific.

His sixteen years as an editor was a period of grinding toil, a prodigal outpouring of nervous energy. This began to tell on his health. In the composition of his last work he exerted himself beyond endurance. He complained to his doctor of intolerable pains in his head. He was having trouble putting two sentences together. Was he losing his mind? The modern doctor might suspect a tumor of the brain, but in 1856, the physician suggested that he should have his barber cut off some of his great shock of hair to cool his head.

He began to fear that robbers were interested in breaking into his little museum to steal his fossils. When he went to bed he kept a pistol and sword within reach. In fact he had always carried a brace of pistols with him since the days when he was in the bank at Cromarty, and he had not discontinued the practice after becoming an editor, because he feared that some one of his many antagonists whom he had lashed with his satire might seek revenge.

When he awoke, on the last day of his life, he imagined that he had walked out to his museum during his sleep. This fear and the burning pain in his head drove him to self-destruction. He rose from his bed, crazed with pain. He scribbled a brief note of love and despair to his wife. Then taking one of the pistols, he killed himself. By a curious irony the only one upon whom he ever used his weapon was himself.

His passing was regarded as a public calamity in Scotland. Eulogists proclaimed that his works would always be regarded as classics, ranking with the work of Addison, Hume, and Goldsmith. His books were widely read on both sides of the Atlantic and even translated into many languages. When Walter Scott died,

Hugh Miller was said to be the greatest Scotchman alive. Today his volumes gather dust on neglected shelves. Most of the encyclopedias carry an account of his life and works, but the Encyclopedia Britannica conspires in his oblivion by refusing even a line to his achievements.

VII

A JANITOR RISES TO REMARK
ANTON LEEUWENHOEK

"He was merely an ordinary shopkeeper, holding a few minor municipal appointments, in the little old town of Delft. In the world of science he was no better than an ignorant and bungling amateur — self-taught but otherwise uneducated." —*Clifford Dobell.*

VII

A JANITOR RISES TO REMARK

ANTON LEEUWENHOEK

THE modern man of science often understands very little about the making of those instruments he uses with so much skill and precision, but the early scientists were frequently under the necessity of making the instruments by which they made their discoveries. To Herschel there was something very fascinating about the grinding of lenses for his telescopes. It is still a fascinating interest to amateurs, and thousands of people at this very moment will tell you that lens-grinding is their hobby.

Among Hollanders of the middle seventeenth century there was considerable interest in lens-grinding. Men wanted to explore the sub-visible world, objects so tiny that they could not be observed by the unaided eye. One day, a young Hollander named Anton van Leeuwenhoek — perhaps it was while he was learning the linen merchant's trade in Amsterdam — peered through one of these magnifying glasses. It may have been a flea that he examined, for this seemed to be so popular an indoor sport in those days that men called the instruments flea glasses. Then and there he was enchanted with the detail, and desire was born in him to see more and more of this great, undiscovered, invisible world. All around him were men who were setting sail to explore strange, distant lands. Here immediately under a microscope was the world that he would explore.

The Thirty Years' War was over, and Holland was ex-

periencing a post-war boom.   A little over twenty years
of age, with the trade of the linen merchant learned, Van
Leeuwenhoek returned to Delft, his home, and set up
in business.   There were sources of revenue beyond his
haberdashery.   Before he was thirty he had been appointed Chamberlain of the Council Chamber of the
Worshipful Sheriffs of Delft, a position which carried
with it an annual stipend of about two hundred dollars
for opening and closing the chamber when it was in session, and heating and cleaning the building.   Later he
was licensed as a surveyor and still later was elected
wine-gauger.

But there was sorrow in his life during these years
after his return to Delft.   Of his five children only one
survived infancy.   Little did Anton realize, as he sat
beside the deathbeds of these four infants, that the
hobby in which he was indulging at the time, the making of powerful microscopes and the observing of "little animals," was the first chapter in a series of discoveries that would give children like his own an immunity
against those dreaded diseases of infancy.

Through his forties he kept up his interest in examining everything microscopically.   To do this, he made
better and better lenses and mounted them between
plates of brass, silver or gold.   He was so absorbed in
his interest that he made special lenses to examine a
great variety of objects.   To many who knew him he
seemed to be gratifying a selfish collector's instinct.
Why should a man want to make hundreds of lenses and
refuse to sell them?

But soon citizens began to take notice when distinguished foreigners inquired for the residence of
Leeuwenhoek.   The word had gone abroad that his mar-

velous microscopes should be seen by all travelers who went to Delft, but the warning was added that a letter of introduction, preferably from the Royal Society, was absolutely necessary. The janitor was becoming famous. It was all because another noted citizen of Delft, named De Graaf, had told the secretary of the recently formed Royal Society of Great Britain about this fellow citizen who made microscopes revealing animals smaller than any that had ever been seen before. To prove his boast, he enclosed a letter from Leeuwenhoek.

The secretary was enthusiastic about this new observer and begged him to send on more descriptions of his work. Anton was flattered. He replied, giving three reasons why he had hitherto published nothing: he had no literary style, he did not know the arts or learned languages, and he did not gladly suffer contradiction or censure from others. But he accepted the invitation and began the lengthy correspondence that was to last for over half a century.

Van Leeuwenhoek soon began to feel his importance when the Royal Society elected him a full member. To him that was "the greatest honor in all the world." Verkolye painted his portrait — still extant — in which he is shown with his diploma. In all simplicity he asked a friend if he now should appear self-effacing in the presence of a doctor of medicine?

Picture this large-boned man, just passed fifty, stooping over a little table. All around the wall are cases in which there are the lenses that have made him famous. Then there are rows of microscopes with specimens in position so that he may examine them whenever the fancy strikes him. Imagine him examining an infinitely

small bit of stuff on the end of a needle. His daughter
Maria enters.

"Father, there is a young Irish doctor who would
like to see you."

"What does he want? A doctor! What I think
of some of these doctors! I suppose he wants to see
my marvelous microscopes."

"He is a handsome young man, father."

"What difference does that make, Maria? I can't
have my time taken up showing these things to every
leech who happens to stop in Delft. These microscopes
are mine. Why don't they grind lenses for themselves?
Does he have a letter of introduction?"

"Yes, he says he is representing the Royal Society."

"The Royal Society, eh? That's different. Tell
him to come right in."

The conversation soon turns to be the subject of
microscopes.

"I was wondering if I might have the pleasure of seeing through some of your marvelous lenses."

"Certainly, most certainly. Here you may see the
cells of wood."

"Marvelous," exclaimed the doctor.

"And through this glass, doctor, you may study the
sting of the bee."

The doctor examined it carefully. All the while
Leeuwenhoek kept his hand upon the instrument.

"Remarkable, remarkable!" exclaimed the doctor.

"And here is another through which you may examine
one of my own hairs."

"Very curious, indeed," commented the doctor.
"But you have other lenses more powerful than these.
I should like to see the little animals about which you

have written so that I can convince some of the more skeptical members of the society when I return to England."

"So there are skeptics still in the learned society of scholars?" the janitor said in a melancholy tone. "It would gratify me very much, if I could show you the instruments through which I study the little animals — thousands of them in an inconceivably small bit of water — but I can't do that. If I were to let you look through my best lenses, you would come to know as much as I know. This is the only reward I have for my pains in searching out these mysteries of nature."

The doctor was embarrassed. He listened, however, with great attention, but in his mind he was saying to himself:

"A man, doubtless of great native ability, though he knows no languages. How he trusts his own thoughts! What extravagances he utters because he does not know the progress that scientists in other countries have made."

Later on in the year, a person far more illustrious than the Irish doctor visited Delft. Word was sent to the Leeuwenhoek home that the Landgrave of Hesse would honor him with his presence. Again we can picture Maria, all aflutter, entering the room where her father was writing one of his long communications to the Royal Society.

"The Landgrave of Hesse is coming to see you, father!"

"The Landgrave of Hesse? A German. I hate Germans! I suppose he wants to see through my microscopes. I can't imagine a landgrave interested in the secrets of nature."

"Shall I show him in when he arrives, father?"

"I suppose. The landgrave interested in science. . . bah!"

Again Anton showed a few specimens that he kept in readiness for the inspection of visitors—the cells in wood, the sting of a bee, a hair. As he exhibited his lenses, he held them in his own hand, fearing that the landgrave might pocket one. From the corner of his eye he watched the landgrave's attendant.

"I should like to see," said the landgrave, "through one of those more powerful instruments you have."

"I'm sorry, excellency, but I cannot let you see through those. Nobody uses those except myself. I keep them locked. I don't trust people—Germans in particular."

"Indeed! Then I'll buy several of your best. What price must you have for your microscopia?"

Anton smiled in a superior way. "You must surely know, excellency, that I never sell any of these instruments or give any to anybody. Nor do I intend to do so. If I did, I would be everybody's slave."

"But how would you be a slave," asked the puzzled landgrave, "if I gave you a generous price for your instruments?"

"I'm sorry, but I sell nothing. I need all these instruments. Go to the lens-grinders. I don't trust people—Germans in particular."

When George III expressed his desire to see the planet Uranus, Herschel packed up his seven-foot telescope and waited at court until the king was ready to observe the newly discovered planet, but illustrious rulers who wanted to see through Leeuwenhoek's microscopes came to him. Some little concession was made to Peter the

Great of Russia, when the janitor went to meet him on a barge outside of Delft where they conversed familiarly for two hours. Dukes and princes might come and go, but none ever peered through his very best lenses. Of the hundreds of lenses he had, he gave away only two — and those to Queen Mary of England. He resolutely refused the Royal Society's request for instructions as to how he built his instruments, though by his will the society received twenty-six of the less powerful sort after his death.

Leeuwenhoek felt perfectly justified in not permitting anybody to look through his best microscopes. If men wanted to see what he saw in his microscopes, nothing was to prevent their buying lenses or making them themselves. Leeuwenhoek might well chuckle while suggesting that they make their own instruments. He knew what patience a man had to have in order to grind and polish lenses until they were entirely satisfactory, and then mount them properly. That was not learned in a single day.

There would be a lot of glass spoiled before they would make a satisfactory instrument. And they would lack the patience to study what they might see under the microscope. No, these curiosity seekers must not be allowed to look through his lenses. Probably they would not see what was there anyway. They might even contradict him, and, if there was anything in the world he could not stand, it was contradiction. If they wanted to know what he saw, let them read his many letters to the Royal Society.

But those who had read his letters were still more curious. Men of education noted that the style was naïve, garrulous and unliterary, but these faults were insignificant when they considered the contents of these communications. The following quotation furnishes a splendid instance of his style and substance. It is from his communication on bacteria in the mouth, the first chapter in the history of oral hygiene.

'Tis my wont of a morning to rub my teeth with salt, and then swill my mouth out with water; and often, after eating, to clean my back teeth with a toothpick, as well as rubbing them hard with a cloth: wherefore my teeth, back and front, remain as clean and white as falleth to the lot of few men of my years, and my gums (no matter how hard the salt be that I rub them with) never start bleeding. Yet notwithstanding, my teeth are not so cleaned thereby, but what there sticketh or groweth between some of my front ones and my grinders (whenever I inspected them with a magnifying mirror), a little white matter, which is as thick as if 'twere batter. On examining this, I judged (albeit I could discern nought a-moving in it) that there yet were living animalcules therein. I have therefore mixed it, at divers times with clean rain-water (in which there were no animalcules), and also with spittle, that I took out of my mouth, after ridding it of airbubbles (lest the bubbles should make any motion in the spittle): and I then most always saw, with great wonder, that in the said matter there were many very little living animalcules, very prettily a-moving... These had a very strong and swift motion, and shot through the water (or spittle) like a pike does through water. These were most always few in number.

The second sort ... spun round like a top: and these were far more in number.

To the third sort I could assign no figure: for at times they seemed to be oblong, while anon they looked perfectly round... They went ahead so nimbly, and hovered so together, that you might imagine them to be a big swarm of gnats or flies, flying in and out among one another. These last seemed to me e'en as if there were, in my judgment, several thousand of 'em in an amount of water or spittle (mixed with the matter aforesaid) no bigger than a sand-grain; albeit there were quite nine parts of water, or spittle, to one part of the matter that I took from betwixt my front teeth, or my grinders.

I have had several gentlewomen in my house, who were keen on seeing the little eels in vinegar; but some of 'em were so disgusted at the spectacle, that they vowed they'd ne'er use vinegar again. But what if one should tell such people in future that there are more animals living in the scum on the teeth in a man's mouth, than there are men in a whole kingdom? especially in those who don't ever clean their teeth, whereby such a stench comes from the mouth of many of 'em, that you can scarce bear to talk to them; which is called by many people "having a stinking breath," though in sooth 'tis most always a stinking *mouth*. For my part I judge, from myself (howbeit I clean my mouth like I've already said), that all the people living in our United Netherlands are not as many as the living animals that I carry in my own mouth this very day: for I noticed one of my back teeth, up against the gum, was coated with the said matter for about the width of a horse-hair, where, to all appearances, it had not been scoured by the salt for a few days; and there were such an enormous number of living animalcules here, that I imagined I could see a good 1000 of 'em in a quantity of this material that was no bigger than a hundredth part of a sand-grain.

But perhaps this condition did not exist in the mouths of others, he thought. In truly scientific fashion he made other examinations; in one of these cases he noted the antiseptic qualities of alcohol.

I have also taken the spittle, and the white matter that was lodged upon and betwixt the teeth, from an old man who makes a practice of drinking brandy every morning, and wine and tobacco in the afternoon; wondering whether the animalcules, with such continual boozing, could e'en remain alive. I judged that this man, because his teeth were so uncommon foul, never washed his mouth. So I asked him, and got for an answer; 'Never in my life with water, but it gets a good swill with wine or brandy every day!' Yet I couldn't find anything beyond the ordinary in his spittle. I also mixed his spit with the stuff that coated his front teeth, but could make out nothing in it save very few of the least sort of living animalcules herinbefore described time and again. But in the stuff I have hauled out from between his front teeth (for the old chap hadn't a back tooth in his head), I made out many more little animalcules, comprising two of the littlest sort.

While many professionals in universities were paging the superstitions of Galen and repeating them to students as the inspired medical wisdom of the ages, an amateur had leaped two centuries ahead of his time to the day of Koch and Pasteur.

Four years before the birth of Leeuwenhoek, an English physician had discovered the truth about the circulation of the blood. His idea did not take hold at once. Old Galen's doctrine had been approved teaching in the schools for fourteen centuries, and it was not to be upset in a moment by any young upstart of an English doctor. What was this new babble about the heart's being the center of the blood system? we can imagine the traditional school inquiring. Absurd surely! Who was Harvey to oppose the great Galen? Hadn't Galen clearly stated that the liver was the center of the blood system and that blood oozed from it to every part of the body, that the veins contained blood and the arteries air, that the blood was cooled by the lungs? The world couldn't be wrong for so many centuries.

But Harvey proved that Galen's theory was absurd,

and that the doctrine taught for so long was nonsense. The English physician came to his conclusions without a microscope. It was left for Leeuwenhoek to observe the blood actually in circulation.

Old Anton found some frog eggs and brought them home to be examined under his microscopes. As soon as the eggs were hatched, he began to observe the tadpoles in every imaginable way. When the tadpole was eight or ten days old, he saw something small inside it that moved continuously. The liquid that was driven out of this little throbbing part began to take on a red color. Then putting the tadpole, head first, into a tube, he focused his instrument on its tail. A look of amazement spread over his face.

"This surpasses all the things I have seen in my life," he cried. The blood was being forced from the middle to the surface of the tail through vessels of hair-like fineness, which were bent back in a curve to carry the blood to the interior of the tail and then to the heart. He began to count very slowly. "More than fifty circulations in that tiny tail," he exclaimed.

At last he saw the end of a problem that had vexed him for many years. He did not, however, regard his researches as completed. He must look at this many more times and examine other like animals to be certain of his conclusions. Then he put a very small minnow, head first, into a tube and observed its tail. Again his microscope told the same story. The blood passed from the arteries through the capillaries into the veins. What Harvey had reasoned out, Leeuwenhoek had seen with his eyes. He wrote a long letter to the Royal Society about his studies of the circulation of the blood but told the fellows of the academy that he was not yet content.

He would examine the circulation of the blood in other animals to discover if the process had universal application.

But this doctrine was so amazing. Perhaps even the learned members of the Royal Society might not believe it. Being of a suspicious nature himself, he asked men of unquestioned integrity — an ambassador to England and a noted professor of anatomy — to certify to the truth of his observations. If the world would not believe Anton van Leeuwenhoek, a janitor, it must believe an ambassador and a professor.

Many of the criticisms that professional scientists make of amateurs may be made of Leeuwenhoek. What others were doing in his field of research did not much interest him. First of all, he could know little about their work, since he read nothing but Dutch, then regarded as the language of illiterate fisherfolk. But he did not care what others were doing. He was consulting his own pleasure and not the good of the world when he made his investigations, and he often stumbled into his discoveries by accident. His letters to the Royal Society are filled with ramblings that are often senile, observations that are often childish.

Leeuwenhoek's career is in strong contrast to that of the modern scientist, who, when he discovers something of benefit to humanity, is generally willing to share his secret. Perhaps if he had been more generous in his discoveries, he might have shortened the long fight that man was to wage with his deadliest enemies — germs. Certainly he made very splendid microscopes, but it was probably his technique in using them that made his reports so excellent, possibly a special method of throwing light upon the object he was examining. At any rate the secrets of making and using his excellent microscopes went with him to his grave. He never knew that he was committing a crime against humanity. He never realized the deadly importance of his secrets. Like a small boy he maintained that this was his peep show. He would tell you what he saw, but let you see for yourself — never. No! not for money either.

"No money," wrote this amateur when close to ninety, "could ever have driven me to make discoveries, and I'm only working out as 'twere an impulse that was borne in me, and I imagine I never meet with any other people who would spend so much time and work in searching into the things of Nature."

A friend of mine, whose mother's family has lived for centuries in Delft where the family tomb in the Old Church is beside Leeuwenhock's, tells me that in his youth he and his fellows often passed by the tomb of Leeuwenhoek without a second's thought, and went over to the tomb of a great warrior. In his mind the martial glory of these heroes was then something to wonder at. A lifelong interest in science has taught him to see far more splendor in the achievements of the untutored Dutchman's long fight to wrest from nature her secrets than in the exploits of generals who led armies to great battles.

VIII

A SCIENTIST BATTLES POVERTY
JEAN HENRI FABRE

"Yes, ignorance may have its advantages; the new is found far from the beaten track. One of my most illustrious masters, little suspecting the lesson he was giving me, taught me that some time ago." —*Jean Henri Fabre.*

VIII

A SCIENTIST BATTLES POVERTY

JEAN HENRI FABRE

IF, after considering Leeuwenhoek and his "little beasties," we unroll nature's scroll further, we come upon the insect world of Jean Henri Fabre. One could compare these two men at length. Both finished their schooling at a very early age and, self-tutored, rose to distinction by tireless research, lasting from early life to beyond ninety. Leeuwenhoek wrote the accounts of his discoveries in a simple, garrulous style, often introducing matters entirely irrelevant to material he was describing. Fabre avoided the learned terminology of his insects and often humanized his theme by writing of them as if they were human, introducing all the while those biographical notes that have made his volumes so personal.

To one reading his intimate pictures of their lives it seems that these insects are mighty heroes engaged in enterprises that are being told in epic style. He heroized the insect world, and for this reason Victor Hugo called him "The Insects' Homer." Neither Leeuwenhoek nor Fabre was interested in what the rest of the world was doing in the same field. Fabre admitted that he read the opinions of others very little; his library filled only a few shelves. His great book was nature, whose leaves he turned over for hours without experiencing the least weariness or boredom. He attempted to justify this attitude:

I have made it a rule to adopt the method of ignorance in my investigation of the instincts. I read very little. Instead of turning over the leaves of books, an expensive method which is not within my means, instead of consulting others, I set myself obstinately face to face with my subject until I contrive to make it speak. I know nothing. So much the better; my interrogation will be all the freer, today tending in one direction, tomorrow in another, according to the information acquired. And if by chance I do open a book, I am careful to leave a section of my mind wide open to doubt.

Fabre might have been a professional scientist, teaching in a noted university, if he had not been so poor. But poverty stood by him like an evil angel all through his life. He was born of poor parents in Provence. His father tired of the toil of a peasant's life and decided to seek his fortune by opening a café in the city. But poverty stalked behind them wherever they went.

It was hardly to be expected that Jean's education would make much progress under these circumstances. His elementary training had been received in a wretched shack, used at different periods to shelter men, chickens and pigs. By one way or another, his education progressed to the Latin poet Virgil. Then disaster overtook the family, and he was forced to leave school to earn the bare necessities of life at jobs as varied as selling lemons and laboring on the roads. He despaired.

After a time the clouds lifted. In competition for a scholarship in the normal school at Avignon, his name led all the rest. After a time his teachers at the school thought that he was not making the best of his opportunities, and he did not rouse himself from his lethargy until he was charged with idleness. The truth was that he was not idle. Rather he was preoccupied with the sting of the wasp or the fruit of the oleander.   Although his teachers were quite uncomplimentary about his standing, Jean was not lacking in diligence, even though he had failed to conform to the standard pattern.

With about the equivalent of an American high-school training, young Fabre began to teach at Carpentras at a salary of about one hundred and forty dollars for the entire school year.   He was dissatisfied and hated the place generously.   He told himself that he must get out of this swamp by some means or other.   As he saw it, the only means of ascent was through the study of the physical sciences and mathematics.   If he would learn specified material in these fields, he could present himself for examination and thus receive his degree without attending a university.

He began to instruct himself by instructing others. With the most primitive apparatus he taught himself and his students chemistry.   He collected oxygen for the first time in the presence of his class.   He learned algebra by instructing another.   A trustful student came to him and said that he must know something of that subject to compete in an examination.   Would he teach him enough?   Fabre did not know the first principles of the subject, but he also knew that he must not confess his ignorance too frequently, if he were to succeed in his profession.   If he could only get a text-book on the subject, he was sure he could digest it without a teacher. But the only person who would have such a book was a fellow teacher much older than himself.

Fabre knew that it would be of no use to ask him for the loan of the book.   The only safe way was to remove it from the professor's sanctum.   This could easily be done, for the keys to the rooms were all alike.   With a rapid heart he approached the professor's door, used his own key, lifted the algebra text from the shelf, and returned quickly to his own room. He read through the book as though he were reading a tale of adventure. He gave the boy the requisite lessons and returned it to the shelf from which it had never been missed. It is hardly necessary to note that, if Fabre had been caught at this low business, the world might have been poorer by one scientist.

Another one of his colleagues was an ex-soldier, who had on several occasions failed to pass the examinations for the baccalaureate in mathematics. This man patronizingly undertook to teach Fabre so that he, too, might take these examinations. Before they had worked together long, Fabre was doing the teaching. Both presented themselves for examination. Both passed. Fabre continued on since he was ambitious to receive the licentiate in the same way. Here again he was successful.

Now surely, he thought, he would outdistance poverty. A good appointment must now come as a regard of this industry. But no offer came. Meanwhile his expenses had increased. He had married at the age of twenty-one, and his sorrows in life had begun in real earnest when his first child died. Though his correspondence at this time breathes resignation at the loss, he was bitter because his ability was not recognized by promotion. He had won his licentiate and was entitled to advancement, as even his superior admitted. Instead he and his wife were forced to lead a hand-to-mouth existence.

It was intolerable. Not only did he receive a trifling salary, but he was obliged to wait for his money long after it should have been paid. It was maddening. He had his degrees and was made "to conjugate verbs for a pack of brats!" and then, after earning his pay, he had to wait around for it like a beggar. He often determined to resign when the school term expired, but in spite of his threats, he always returned to his gloomy situation after the vacation.

One day, however, an appointment arrived in the mails. He was to teach physics at Ajaccio on the island of Corsica at about three hundred and fifty dollars a year, over twice what he had been receiving. Poverty was lagging behind a little now, though, to be sure, there would still have to be a great deal of economizing. When the family landed at Ajaccio, they knew that things would be much more pleasant here than at Carpentras. This was a wonderful place to study nature. Almost immediately he began making a collection of rare shells, but he had to forbid himself the study of nature. If he became too interested in that, his work in physics would surely suffer.

It was here that the teacher of physics received his first and his only lesson in biology. A professor from the University of Toulouse visited Ajaccio. When he could not find a room, Fabre offered him hospitality, which the professor appreciated at the time. As the polished professor was leaving some such conversation as this must have taken place:

"I want to thank you, Monsieur Fabre, in the name of my colleagues of the University of Toulouse, for the kindness you have shown me and also for the rare varieties of shells you have collected for us. You have been most hospitable to me; believe me, I shall not forget it. If you are ever at Toulouse, be sure to give me the

pleasure of being your host. You have been most hospitable."

"We have done nothing, monsieur. Our home has
been honored by the presence of a scientist."

"You are interested in science, aren't you?"

"Yes, but I dare not yield to the temptation to study
biology. My work is in physics and mathematics."

"Indeed? Let me give you a first lesson. Let us
examine a snail. But we have no scalpel, no dissecting
needles. Perhaps we can use the madam's scissors and
two ordinary needles, and bring a dish of water."

The young teacher of physics looked on while the
great professor dissected a snail and explained its structure to him. The lesson was brief, but intensely
interesting. Later in life, when Fabre himself was becoming recognized for his studies of insects, he called on
the famous professor. That worthy could recall neither
the famous lesson nor the pupil who had shown him so
much hospitality.

Before Fabre was long on the island of Corsica, he
contracted a fever and was forced to return to France.
When he was well, he was given an appointment at a
smaller salary at the *lycée* in Avignon. Here he gave
twenty years of unstinting service to education, but not
once did he receive a raise in pay or rank. His salary
remained at three hundred and ten dollars a year, though
he later received an additional two hundred and thirty
dollars from the city for taking care of the museum.
His family now numbered five children.

Nobody ever tried more desperately than Fabre to
forge ahead in the teaching profession. He was always
working, if not in school, then at some data for a paper.
If the people of Avignon would not recognize his ability,

he would call attention to himself by his publications.
When he was thirty-two, he contributed an important
article on the habits of the cerceris, a hunting wasp, and
the cause of the long preservation of the beetles with
which it feeds its young. He had dreamed of advancement. And he was recognized. The University of
Poitiers invited him to become a member of its faculty,
but when he reckoned the cost of moving his large family and discovered that the salary remaining would be
less than a dollar a day, he was forced to decline the
offer.

He did not realize how futile his ambitions were until
some days later when the inspector of schools dropped
in to observe his work. After the students had been dismissed, the inspector lingered in the room. Fabre,
anxious to exhibit the fruits of his instruction, showed
some mathematical drawings to the visitor. They were
done exceedingly well. The inspector handled them
mechanically and tossed them aside, saying:

"I understand you have ambitions to teach in a university."

"Yes, I should like that."

"Have you any money?" the inspector next asked.

Fabre stiffened a little. People were always talking
about money. Then he admitted that he was poor.

"Then," said the inspector, "give up these dreams.
The salaries are so small that you would be doomed to
live in poverty. Now if you had a private income ——
I know about your research and your papers, but you
would be poorer at a university than you are here.
Penury in a frock-coat, monsieur, is a tragedy."

Then it was poverty that was blocking his advance
again. If money were necessary for a university post,

he would make it by embarking on a commercial venture. One of the principal industries of the district was the extraction of a dye from the madder root. He would study out a simpler process. Just as he was ready to reap his profits, the slave's hope of freedom vanished. Chemistry produced the dye synthetically.

He had one splendid opportunity within his grasp and he fumbled that. The Minister of Education, Victor Duruy, was aware of the knowledge and teaching ability of this modest, retiring scholar in Avignon. Duruy arranged to have him made a Chevalier of the Legion of Honor. While Fabre would be in Paris, an interview could be arranged with Napoleon III. Perhaps the emperor would engage him as a tutor for his son. When Duruy wrote to Fabre about the proposed honor, the peasant was reluctant to go to the capital, but Duruy, who appreciated the temper of genuine scholars — he himself was the author of a noted history of Rome — ordered him to come.

Fabre was not at all excited by the fact that he was to receive a great honor. He came to Paris, with his old broad-rimmed, black hat and his worn suit. Napoleon chatted with him privately for a while. Fabre had nothing to say, not because he was abashed in the presence of the mighty but because he felt that there was nothing to be said. It was clear to the emperor that such a man as Fabre lacked the social graces, the poise that the instructor of his son must have. Here was the chance that Fabre had wanted for years, but, instead of appearing at his very best, he was dreaming of Avignon. The opportunity had come too late. Already he was definitely set in a way of life and was not to be changed.

Once the interview was over, Fabre was immediately

ready to return home. Duruy was amazed. To come all the distance from Avignon to Paris and then to return without seeing the sights of the capital! Didn't he wish to see the museums for which Paris was noted throughout the world? No, he saw enough of museums in Avignon. He took care of one himself. Besides these things were all dead. He was interested more in things that were alive, even though they were only insects. Moreover this populous center was too confusing for him. He must return to his wife and family.

And so the man who had wanted to go forward in life, with a strange lack of vision, turned his back on the mighty and returned to his tasks in Avignon, where he continued to feel that fate had denied him opportunities. But little did he suspect that trouble was ahead of him even in Avignon.

The political party in power was attempting to secularize education and, as a part of this program, instruction in science was given to girls. Fabre agreed to conduct this work in Avignon. Certain spinsters in the town were sure that there was something scandalous in this new learning. There was grave danger to maidenly morals in this liberation of the female mind. Fabre tells us the story:

You can see how heinous my crime was: I taught those young persons what air and water are; whence the lightning comes and the thunder; by what device our thoughts are transmitted across the seas and continents by means of a metal wire; why fire burns and why we breathe; how a seed puts forth shoots and how a flower blossoms: all eminently hateful things in the eyes of some people, whose feeble eyes are dazzled by the light of day.

The little lamp must be put out as quickly as possible and measures taken to get rid of the officious person who strove to keep it alight. The scheme was darkly plotted with the old maids who owned my house and who saw the abomination of desolation in these new educational methods.

Fabre had taught science to girls as a part of the anti-clerical program, and, with the return of the clerical faction, his resignation was being sought. He was disgusted, but he did not attempt to fight back. If they wanted his resignation, they might have it. Besides he was weary of teaching for a pittance, weary of this constant wrestling with poverty. If he could only have the leisure to write some elementary manuals in science, he knew that he would earn at least as much as he made at teaching.

After so many years of explaining nature's mysteries to young minds, he had acquired a skill in making them clear and interesting to children. He could never understand why writers of manuals made their books so unnecessarily uninteresting. But he would have to have quite a sum to live before receiving any royalties, and where could he go for a loan? He could not ask Duruy, for he had fallen before the political assaults of the clericals. Fabre turned to John Stuart Mill, with whom he had become acquainted when the latter had taken up residence at Avignon in sight of the grave of his wife. The philosopher gave the teacher a generous loan, and the Fabres with their household effects took the road to Orange.

Eight years passed. His text-books were enjoying considerable success. His debt to Mill was paid, and there was something laid aside. Then all of a sudden the family was moving again. Once more the landlord had his finger in the matter. In front of the Fabre home

were two rows of plane trees. These his thrifty landlord cut down. Fabre, who loved these trees, was ex-
asperated and decided that in the future he would live
upon his own acres.

Thanks to the vogue of his manuals, he was able to
buy a piece of property near the village of Sérignan.
He sang a psalm of delight as he took possession of the
place. His struggle with poverty was over; he was
independent; his dreams were realized. His desires had
been very modest indeed, for the place he had acquired
was a wretched piece of land from an agricultural point
of view. For his purpose, however, this dried up, un-
fertile, stony tract was ideal, since it was the rendezvous
of many insects he had long desired to study. He was
fifty-seven now, an age when most men begin to think
of death or retirement. But Fabre's life had only begun. His wife, who had struggled with him all through
the years, died shortly after their coming to Sérignan.
After mourning for a decent interval, at the age of three
score, he married a young woman, who in a short time
brought three more Fabres into the world.

Here at Sérignan he set about making those experiments which were to find place in the ten volumes called
the *Souvenirs Entomologiques*, written during the next
twenty-eight years. Other scientists had typed and
filed the classification and description of the insects, but
this did not interest him as much as observing them in
their natural surroundings and writing the diaries of
their private lives. He had the leisure now to lie for
hours, sometimes under a blazing sun, observing the
habits of ants or wasps, of spiders or beetles or bees,
prying into their homes, spoiling their work or teasing
them, to note their reactions. To him this prying into

nature's secrets was the most interesting thing in the world.

It was often urged upon Fabre that he write out a theory of the origin of instincts, thus synthesizing much of the analysis that he made through the many years of his life. But he resolutely declined so bold an undertaking, saying that man knows nothing about anything, that he would not presume to sound the depths of the ocean because he had stirred a few grains of sand on the shore. Fabre had seen many theories come and go in his long life, and he did not covet the mantle of the prophet.

"Theoretical rubbish heaps up," he wrote, "and the truth ever escapes us." Yet in the matter of instincts, he lent all the weight of his authority to support the view that there is a distinct line of cleavage between instinct in animals and intelligence in man, thus opposing the view that instinct is simply a lower level of intelligence. In the long range of his experiments, he seems to have found nothing that disturbed him in this conclusion.

He was one of the really great scientists who opposed the evolutionary theory advanced by Darwin. Although Darwin referred to him in the *Origin of Species* as "the inimitable observer," and in personal correspondence suggested certain experiments with mason bees, which Fabre painstakingly carried out, Fabre never gave Darwin's book a hearing. He began it, but did not long continue, claiming that it bored him.

At the age of eighty-four, he ceased publishing. Again the spectre of poverty appeared. The income from his texts had fallen off, and the popular studies he had written at Sérignan had not yielded much in the way of royalty. In desperation the poet of science

wrote to his friend, the famous Provençal poet, Mistral,
that he would appreciate finding a buyer for certain
paintings of mushrooms that he had made long ago.

The poet was touched by the destitution of his friend.
A great scientist in want! He would tell the world
about this neglect. The response to Mistral's plea was
immediate and generous. The government gave him
a pension, defending its neglect by stating that his condition had been known, but that Fabre's sensitiveness was
so great that the matter required extreme delicacy.
From neglect he now passed into the glare of publicity.
He complained of the excessive attention he was receiving. By a curious irony, the General Council of
Vaucluse voted him scientific instruments, when his
work was over.

Fabre was capable and he knew it. It was the lack of
early recognition, coupled with the constant struggle
against poverty, that saddened a great part of his life.
He was constantly letting remarks about his disappoint-
ment escape him. "I have known some," he wrote,
"who, having achieved skill in turning somersaults, have
prospered better than the thinker." Certainly he was
not given the recognition that he deserved at a time
when he could make use of it, a recognition that was
frequently conceded to less capable men, who studied
the methods of getting on.

Men with half his intelligence realized that advancement comes not solely on the basis of ability, but through
the quality of one's personality, through valuable contacts, carefully fostered. Fabre paid no attention to
"selling himself." He never seemed to relax, had no
time for frivolity. Not only this, but he seemed to pay
little attention to the social graces which no one who

would rise can afford to neglect. He had no time for social calls, and absolutely refused to change his wide-rimmed black hat for the more formal dress required on occasions. People came to regard him as queer.

But if earlier in his life Fabre had received an appointment in a university as a professional entomologist, with no worry about securing a means of livelihood, his name probably would never have crossed the borders of France.

IX

FROM INDIGO TO EXCAVATION
HEINRICH SCHLIEMANN

"Schliemann is an outstanding example of my repeated contention that the enlightened amateur beats the solid expert every time." — *Emil Ludwig*.

IX

FROM INDIGO TO EXCAVATION

HEINRICH SCHLIEMANN

No MAN ever set the compass of his life and proceeded with more directness to the goal of his ambition than Heinrich Schliemann. Though he journeyed much over land and sea he always approached nearer to the vision he had in his mind from youth.

What was this vision? It was the ancient city of Troy. He had his father to thank for the inspiration, for when Heinrich was a little fellow, his father took him upon his knee and told him the age-old story of Homer. How Paris had stolen Helen, and Menelaus and Agamemnon had set sail from Greece to bring her home again. How the war lasted for ten years, how Achilles sulked in his tent, and Ulysses outwitted the Trojans by means of the wooden horse.

"But where is Troy now, father?" he would ask. "Nobody is sure, my boy. Some of the teachers say one thing and some another. This happened a long, long time ago. The city was burned, the sand storms covered it over, and men have forgotten where it was."

The tale laid hold of the imagination of the boy. The father was pleased at this early interest in things classic and gave him for Christmas a book in which the events of the great epic of Homer were illustrated. Whatever unfavorable criticism may be written of his father — and considerable has been written, for he was sensual, financially irresponsible and irascible — he must be given

credit for lighting a fire in the boy's mind which was
never extinguished. At eleven he was packed off to an
uncle's home where he studied some Latin. As a Christmas gift, the son sent the father a brief Latin essay on
the fall of Troy.

But this relationship between father and son did not
move on as pleasantly as these early incidents seem to
indicate. At fourteen the boy had left home to work
for a grocer. The vision of the Troy that he had
promised himself he would discover must have been
somewhat dimmed while he worked from dawn to dusk
at tasks that were hard and boring. His ambitions were
somewhat revived when he heard a drunken scholar re-
cite a hundred lines of Homer. "What a beautiful language!" Heinrich exclaimed. He seems to have had
no scruple in bribing the minstrel with drink to repeat
the performance several times.

One day Schliemann was missed at the grocer's
counter. His days of selling a pound of this or a pint of
that were over. Later his memory failed him when he
tried to remember why it was he left his sixteen-hour-a-
day job. Perhaps there were several reasons. He had
spat blood while lifting a heavy cask. Then, too, he
was not getting on well with his father — a circumstance
hardly to be wondered at since the latter was making a
fool of himself to the disgust of his son. Perhaps it was
his determination to show his father that he could make
his own mark in the world. But there was also a love
affair that had been broken off by the girl's parents, who
disapproved of Minna's betrothal to a poor son of a
reprobate minister. All these factors may have contributed to young Schliemann's resolution. He might
not be strong physically, but his day would come, and

when it did he would make so much money that they would all be glad to say, "I knew him when——"

If it had not been for these adversities, he might have turned into a vagabond, but opposition only made him more determined. He would show the world.

Being out of a job, he went to school and studied book-keeping for nearly a year. Then he was off to Hamburg to find work. But his lack of experience and ill health hindered him at every turn. In desperation he signed up as a cabin boy on a brig bound for South America. When the ship was off the coast of Holland, it capsized. For four hours he held on to a cask in the raging sea until he was tossed up onto the Dutch shore. This experience over, he decided to live the prosaic life of a landlubber.

His good fortune now begins, never to desert him. At Amsterdam where the inspired amateurs, Leeuwenhoek and Spinoza, learned their trades, he eventually found work. He was only an office boy, but what an office boy! When he was sent out on messages he spent his time declining nouns and conjugating verbs in foreign languages, stealthily reading some passage in a foreign tongue or translating sentences he would need when he, too, would be a merchant. Languages would multiply his personality, increase his opportunities. He knew that he must first improve his knowledge of his mother tongue, and he took lessons in German. His interest in English led him to attend services in an English church where he slowly repeated to himself the words spoken by the preacher. His memory grew sharper every day. In his first year in Amsterdam he studied French as well as English, in his second year, Spanish, Italian, and Portuguese.

A young man of such talents and ambition could not long remain unnoticed. At twenty-two he was employed by an importing firm and straightway proceeded to climb to the top over his seniors in service. When he was two years with his company, he was made its representative in St. Petersburg.

This new appointment involved the necessity of learning Russian. It wouldn't be hard to learn the language, but where in Amsterdam could he find an instructor? He unearthed a Russian book and began. Even if he had no tutor, he must enjoy the flattery of a listener. A Jew, who knew nothing about the language, was glad to lend a patient ear for two hours each evening at four francs a week. Perhaps Schliemann didn't have the correct accent, but what of it? He kept on shouting in the hope that this might atone for faults of grammar.

If he had only known it, he might have saved the francs he paid his ignorant listener, for the circle of his audience was wider than he imagined. People in the same house rebelled at this ranting in Russian. The landlord asked him to continue his studies elsewhere. He did so, but again he was ejected. There was nothing thin-skinned about Schliemann. This was his method, and he would stay with it. When merchants from Russia appeared some weeks later, he was able to converse with them.

When Maria in *Twelfth Night* berates Aguecheek as a fool, Sir Toby springs to his friend's defense. "Fie, that you'll say so! he . . . speaks three or four languages word for word without book . . ." If so much learning excited Sir Toby's admiration, his superlatives would die of exhaustion should he try to recommend Schliemann's ability at languages. By the time he was twenty-five, he could speak twenty languages "word for word without book." Later he added others until the number reached thirty-five.

How did he do it? First of all he was no pail to be filled by the teacher's toil. Instead of letting the instructor conduct the lesson in the usual method, he began by asking questions. Soon he had the several hundred words necessary for connected narrative. Then he wrote little compositions which his teacher corrected. This material he memorized, shouting it aloud because he intended to speak it. In fact it was the utility of language study that spurred him on. On every page he memorized he saw future customers rising before him. Their orders might repay him many times over for his trouble. Later, when learning languages became a passion with him — and the more of them he learned the easier was the next one — he would study some he would never use, but that was after he was financially independent.

Once in Russia, the agent found that he could make much more money if he went into business for himself. He prospered at selling indigo, and the vision of his ancient Troy seemed to grow brighter. But he must not dwell on it. A fortune must be made before undertaking so expensive a project. Gold must be piled up before the gold of a buried city could be reached. With intense application he set to work. That did not mean, of course, that he must chain himself to one place. St. Petersburg was his address for the next twenty years, during which time his *wanderlust* drove him to many parts of the world, once even around it.

He was doing well in Russia when word reached him that his brother Louis, two years his junior, had died of typhus in the gold fields of California. Heinrich had tried to do something for his brother by teaching him several languages and later offering him several hundred dollars to set up in business. But Louis had scornfully refused so slight a sum. He wanted to be taken into business with Heinrich and, to force his hand, wrote a letter in which he dramatically threatened to take his own life, signing the statement with his blood. Promptly Heinrich sent his brother in Holland enough money to return to Germany. With some cash in hand the brother decided to postpone his suicide and sailed for America just when the gold rush to California was in progress. He had Heinrich's gift for making money and in two years was worth thirty thousand dollars.

When Heinrich heard of his brother's wealth, his respect for him increased immeasurably. Then word came of the brother's death. Schliemann was interested in the wealth that Louis had left. He had helped his brother and he felt that no one could challenge his right to inherit the fortune. He decided to go to California. When Heinrich made his first voyage to sea, eight years prior to his brother's death, he was penniless. This time he went not as a cabin boy but as a prosperous merchant, though not yet thirty. But he must have felt himself a re-incarnated Jonah when eighteen hundred miles out of Liverpool the engine of the ship broke down. A sail was fitted up. It was over two weeks before the ship put in at an Irish port.

Schliemann was vexed but not vanquished. Again he booked passage, and this time the god of the sea relented. When he presented himself as claimant of his brother's fortune, he discovered that Louis' partner had absconded with the money. He could sue, but he was too nervous a man to become involved in the law's delay and too prudent to risk a fruitless session in the courts. Instead of bemoaning his loss, he opened a bank in California where he bought gold in eight languages. He stayed in America a year and a half during which he contracted fever twice and doubled the thirty-five thousand dollars he had at the outset. The vision of his buried Troy now seemed brighter.

Returning to Russia he found, like Midas, that everything he touched turned to gold. Every year showed a great increase in his income. In one year he doubled his fortune. But in spite of increasing wealth, he claimed to be unhappy. The truth was that he had been luckless in love. Once he had acquired means, he had decided to renew his suit for Minna, a girl he had known at home. To his sorrow he learned that she had married several days before hearing from him. This wound healed quickly. In a year he was raving of the divinity of one Sophie, but his pride was hurt when a soldier of fine physique was preferred to him. Then he was distracted by Katharina. He married her to his sorrow. In ten years there were three children, and Schliemann took it amiss when informed by his wife that she would have no more.

His wife didn't seem to understand him, a difficult task to be sure. They did not waste much sympathy on each other. With him the making of money had become an obsession; he was constantly preoccupied with business matters. If the interest of the moment was not business, then it was a new language, which he was learning by his noisy method. Heinrich was internationally minded; Katharina was quite satisfied with Russia and rebelled when he wanted her to follow him to foreign cities. To her nothing was so dull, stupid and wasteful as going to Asia Minor to excavate a buried city. Most certainly she wasn't going. She was a Russian; in Russia she would live and die.

Though he was unfortunate in love, his business contacts continued to be more and more successful. Luck was always on his side. On one occasion, during the Crimean War, the docks at Memel were totally destroyed by fire. Crushed, he told himself that he would have to start again at the very bottom to rebuild his fortune, for practically all his wealth was tied up in materials that had just arrived. Later, word came that his merchandise alone had escaped. His goods had arrived when the warehouses were overstocked and had to be stored elsewhere. Because the Crimean War was in progress, prices of war materials soared at the time. He disposed of his goods at a great profit and later piously wrote in his memoirs, "Divine providence often protected me in the most marvelous manner, and more than once."

Heinrich had postponed the study of Greek to his middle thirties because he knew that Greek literature would interest him so much that his work would be neglected. Now that his capital insured a large income, he began to talk of retiring to take up his life ambition, the location of buried cities. He began Greek as he began everything. Soon he was forming his theories about the location of ancient sites. Business began to interfere with his study. He attempted to retire when he was thirty-six, but a law suit brought him back, and he was not able to free himself from the shackles of business until six years later.

He ended his old life and began the new by making

a journey around the world. With the instincts of a business man, he immediately filed his report to the world in a book on China and Japan. Arriving in the United States, he felt perfectly at home. California was admitted to the Union in 1850. Since Schliemann had been in the state at the time, he became a citizen of the United States by simply declaring his presence. He was not a man to slip through the country in disguise. On his former visit, he had called on President Fillmore, chatted with him for an hour and a half and met his family. Now he called to see President Johnson. He bought stock in various railroads in America and rode over the lines with the feeling of a director. He was taking no broker's word for anything; most men in his opinion were rogues anyway.

Paris now became his address. To his Russian wife he sent all kinds of bribes. He wrote of his palatial quarters — the theatre, luxuries, the education of their children — but she was cold to all these promises. When pleading was of no avail, he stormed. He would cut her off penniless, leave the children barely enough for their education and divorce her.

Meanwhile he kept up his intensive studies. Greece and Troy were visited. Promptly he issued his report in a work outlining his theories. Professionals, of course, quarrelled with the conclusions of this amateur. His positive spirit always made enemies, though his ability was recognized by the University of Rostock, which conferred on him the Doctorate of Philosophy.

Schliemann believed so whole-heartedly in his theories that he determined to spend money to prove them. But first he must remarry, and before that there must be a divorce from his chilly spouse in cold Russia. For this divorce he would go to the United States. About this time the divorce laws of the State of Indiana were undergoing revision. He had enough money, it appears, to retard the revision. Perhaps it was to avoid the impression that he was in Indianapolis only to divorce his wife that he bought a house and an interest in a starch business there. Once divorced, he wrote to a friend in Greece that he was again free. Would he pick a Greek wife for him? The reply was immediate. Nothing could be easier. In fact his friend would not be obliged to go outside of his own relationship to find a suitable girl.

When this strange wooer appeared in Athens the word spread on all sides that the wealthy German had come! Too bad he was so old — surely thirty years older than Sophia — but he had money and that was something a good Greek girl should consider. Quickly she was dressed in the finest clothes to be found. She must look her best for this was the chance of a lifetime.

Schliemann's swift glance saw that the girl of sixteen had undeniable charm. The parents noting this were highly pleased. It was a cautious business. Schliemann, the merchant, liked the bargain, but he thought that perhaps after all there should be a little romance in these new espousals. He inadvertently asked the girl why she was marrying him. With a childlike simplicity she told him the truth; he was wealthy, and, besides, her parents had told her this was the right thing to do.

This unexpected frankness chilled his ardor. He was a merchant, but he drew the lines at buying a wife. Did her parents think a wife was a slave? He would look around for himself. One hundred and fifty candidates quickly presented their credentials, but the business of selecting a wife from such a multitude was too nerve-racking a task for his impetuous nature. Meanwhile Sophia's relatives were active; the misunderstanding was cleared up.

Despite this unromantic method of wooing a wife, the marriage turned out happily, doubtless because of the humble nature of the bride. She did her best to meet Heinrich's ideal of what a wife should be. She adored her husband as a god and yielded to him in everything, even to the style of furniture in her own room.

Now he was ready to excavate the Troy he had dreamed of discovering since his father held him on his knee and told him its story. He appeared in the Troad with his Homer in hand. The epic would help him identify the spot of the city of Priam. Some scholars were amused to think that anyone should believe Troy ever existed, to say nothing of consulting the poems in order to settle the location of the city. Most of the scholars who believed that there was a Troy held that it was near the modern Bunarbashi.

When the German merchant appeared on the scene, he was sceptical. He paged his Homer and, trusting entirely in the text, said that this was not the spot. The Troy of Homer was near the sea, but this location, though ideal for a citadel, was too far inland, a journey of several hours. The warriors couldn't have crossed many times from the ships to the walls within the course of a single day, if this was the site of the citadel. This place was too far from the coast. Moreover it was too steep toward the river to permit Achilles to pursue Hector around the walls three times.

Calvert, the American consul at the Dardanelles, is entitled to the credit of showing Schliemann the site near the modern Hissarlik, only three miles from the sea, where Troy was eventually excavated.

For a score of years he worked at Troy intermittently. The first two campaigns were not very encouraging. Scholars paid little attention to his project. But during his campaign in the third year, on one never to be forgotten day in the annals of archaeology, the Schliemanns noted that a pick had pierced the top of a chest. The men were dismissed. Doctor Schliemann had suddenly remembered that this was his birthday.

When the rejoicing workmen had gone, the Schliemanns quickly got to the contents of the chest. "Ah!" said Schliemann, "this was Priam's treasure. Look at these necklaces, jewels, ornaments of all kinds. That golden goblet must weigh over a pound. Hold your shawl, Sophia, and we will fill it before anyone discovers us. The Turks will never see these things. What appreciation have they of such rare ornaments? The idea of dividing this treasure!"

"Isn't it wonderful?" Sophia exclaimed.

"You will wear the beautiful ornaments worn by Helen of Troy, my dear. These treasures are priceless."

The hoard of about eight thousand seven hundred gold objects was smuggled to Greece. Their joy was too great to be concealed. Upon hearing that Schliemann had failed to surrender half of what he had found, the Turks ruled that he must pay ten thousand francs. Always theatrical, he paid five times the amount and promptly wrote a book on these Trojan antiquities.

For his dishonesty with the Turks, he paid dearly. When he later sought permission to continue his excavations, there were all kinds of obstacles put in his way.

After a great deal of red tape, the privilege of digging was granted. When he came to Dardanelles, the Governor of the Troad kept him cooling his heels for two months on the pretext that the permit must be confirmed. Schliemann raged. When he was allowed to proceed with his work, an official was sent along to take care of Turkish interests. This man harried Schliemann so much that he decided in his anger to give up the work — at least for a time. But first he would tell the world in a letter to the *London Times* what he thought of the Governor of the Troad. The Governor was transferred.

He now crossed over to Greece and began excavating at Mycenae. But his deception of the Turks did not enhance his reputation among the Greeks. Here too he was hedged in with the restrictions of officials. He was allowed to dig under certain conditions, but he could retain nothing of what he discovered. He was forced to content himself with the exclusive privilege of publishing for a period of three years whatever he might discover. Again the professionals said that he would find nothing, for he was excavating in the wrong place.

This was hardly a bargain from a business man's point of view, considering the expense to which he went in bringing these records of antiquity to light. He employed one hundred and twenty-five laborers at a wage of about forty-two cents a day. Not only did he expend money, but he and his wife wore themselves out superintending the work from early morning to dusk, in scorching sun or in a wind constantly blowing dust into their inflamed eyes. But they were amateurs in love with their work and they did not mind the expenses or the weather. In spite of all these annoyances, he could imagine nothing more interesting than the excavation of such a glorious city where every object revealed a new page of history.

He was, of course, successful, as he knew he would be. Immediately he sent a telegram to George, King of the Greeks:

With extreme joy I announce to Your Majesty that I have discovered the tombs which tradition, finding echo in Pausanias, has designated as the sepulchres of Agamemnon, Cassandra, and Eurymedon, and their comrades, slain during a banquet by Clytemnestra and her lover Aegisthus. . . I have found in the sepulchres immense treasures of archaic objects in pure gold. These treasures are sufficient in themselves to fill a large museum, which will be the most wonderful in the world, and which during the centuries to come, will draw to Greece thousands of strangers from every country. As I work for the pure love of science, I naturally make no pretensions to these treasures, which I give intact to Greece with keen enthusiasm. May God grant that these treasures may become the corner stone of an immense national wealth!

Schliemann was not a man to hide his light under a bushel. His telegram to the king certainly showed little restraint, but he had reason to glory, for his treasure was the greatest that any excavator had ever found. In the five tombs there were many funeral offerings of priceless value — diadems and pendants, bracelets and rings, crosses and vessels, breastplates and masks — all of gold.

Schliemann had difficulty in deciding to what nation he would leave his Trojan treasures. To the Greeks? No! They had heckled him too much while he was slaving to promote the wealth and glory of Greece. To the English? Perhaps. The treasures were in London for a time. Finally he was prevailed upon to give

them to the Berlin Museum. The city in gratitude made
him a citizen of Berlin, a rare honor.

From his youth to that day in 1890 when he fell exhausted in the streets of Naples and died among strangers
without uttering a word, his life was a constant fever
of activity. One might expect that at his age he would
be more inclined to stay at home with his wife and their
two children, Andromache and Agamemnon. But his
restless energy gave him no peace. He wanted to see
everything, to know everything. With this temperament went certain faults. He was irascible, blunt, preju-
diced. His impetuous nature hurried him to the end of
an enterprise.

Since he was primarily interested in Homer, he ruth-
lessly tossed out everything until he reached the lowest
of the nine cities. In his haste he had passed the Troy
of Homer, now known as the sixth city, and had gone to
the bottom — to the early Aegean civilization, hitherto
unknown. Archaeologists have often criticized this
haste, but he was a pioneer in archaeology, and the technique of excavation was not worked out at that time.
Today the University of Cincinnati is busy sifting the
material tossed aside by Schliemann, as he hurried to get
to the very bottom of the pile.

But after all his limitations and eccentricities are recited, there still remains a character of generous impulses,
a mind of insight and originality.

X

BANKER HISTORIAN

GEORGE GROTE

"It is a coincidence so striking as almost to put the English university system itself on the defensive, that neither Grote nor Gibbon owed anything to Academic training. Gibbon indeed spent fourteen months at Oxford: — 'the most idle and unprofitable of my whole life.' George Grote, the son of a London banker, ended his school days at sixteen, when he left Charterhouse. He had been grounded in Latin by a devoted mother at five years, however, and he took with him to the bank little or no mathematics, and an enthusiastic love for metaphysics, classical literature, and history, which proved to be lifelong." — *The Warner Library.*

X

BANKER HISTORIAN

GEORGE GROTE

DURING the year when Schliemann began his digging at Troy, another business man, turned scholar, was ending a long career in England. This was George Grote, who, though trained in banking, had written a history of Greece in a dozen volumes.

Looking at Schliemann's background, one would hardly prophesy that this merchant would ever startle the learned world. It was equally improbable that Grote would ever distinguish himself in the field of scholarship, for his career had been decided by his father at birth. The Grotes were bankers, and this boy would be a banker, too, just as his father and grandfather had been. Who could believe that the oldest son would ever desire to be anything else? So it was that at the age of sixteen young Grote found himself at a desk in his father's bank.

Grote had sent his son George to be educated at Charterhouse because the headmaster agreed with the Egyptian proverb that a boy's ears are on his back, and he hears when he is flogged. As he sat at his desk in the bank, the recent graduate of Charterhouse could attest to the severity of the discipline maintained there. He could still hear the headmaster saying:

"Master George, I assure you that this matter pains me far more than it does you, but my duty is clear; so is your infraction of the rules of Charterhouse. You admit, then, that you were out of bounds?"

"Yes, sir."

"Where were you?"

"At the tavern, sir. Since tomorrow is our leaving day, I thought you would not take it amiss ——"

"Take it amiss! Do you not perceive that your infraction of the discipline is more to be censured since tomorrow is your leaving day? This is an outrageous breach of conduct and, if left unpunished, may become a low precedent in this school. You did well to tell me the truth, for my senses are not so dull as to fail in detecting the odor of spirits on your person. You are more guilty than the others because you organized this brawl."

"But really, sir, we drank but little and sang ——"

"And therein your conduct emulated that of the low spirits who frequent such resorts. You will bend, please."

The father had wanted discipline for his boy and in that respect he had made no mistake in choosing Charterhouse. But since the elder Grote had nothing but contempt for the impractical life of the scholar he made a mistake in sending his boy there, for Charterhouse had an entirely classical course of study. The boy was already almost spoiled for business. As he worked with his accounts in the bank, he envied those classmates of his whose parents had permitted them to continue studying, and often dreamed of how much more interesting it would be to turn the pages of Greek authors than those of dull ledgers. His sojourn at Charterhouse awakened in him a fondness for classical learning that was never to pass away. There was, however, a thick vein of common sense in his nature. He kept on at his accounts and spent his leisure with books.

Circumstances in the Grote home seemed to lend themselves to study. The mother, who had been something of a gay belle in her day, had lost much of her interest in hospitality after her marriage. Her sparkle was further dulled by her acceptance of Calvinism. To escape the severity of home life, her husband occasionally went out to drink some ale with friends who were not welcomed by Mrs. Grote. George accompanied his father in this relaxation, but he did not enjoy these drinking bouts. They were a dismal murder of time. He was making friends of a sort different from the cronies to whom his father had introduced him. These were philosophers — important men in their day and still remembered — Ricardo, the elder Mill, and Bentham.

His interest in books was deepened by the unhappy turn of a love affair. He was twenty-one at the time. Harriet Lewin, two years his senior, seemed to him the fairest creature that ever breathed, but he lacked the courage to tell her. Young Grote had to confide in someone. He knew that either his father or mother would frown on such frivolity. Recently he had become very intimate with a reverend gentleman of the district who, being a splendid classical scholar, had helped him in his studies. Grote had the profoundest respect for him and told the divine his feelings toward Miss Lewin. But the reverend gentleman now assumed the role of the villain in the melodrama.

"Miss Lewin's heart and hand are engaged to another," he said.

George was crushed. He could never be happy again, he told himself. Life had suddenly lost all its importance. His father saw that his son was going through a crisis and a few questions brought on the confession that he had fallen in love. The elder Grote's ideas on the subject of love had undergone considerable revision since his marriage. Catching his son in a moment of despair, he compelled him to promise never to marry until he would receive parental approval. To George it made no difference what promise he made, since he had lost Harriet.

But Harriet, off on a yachting vacation, heard of the episode, and when she returned, the reverend gentleman was unmasked. The heart and hand of Miss Lewin were not engaged, though the reverend gentleman himself had vainly endeavored for months to compel her to receive his addresses. George was a happy man again. Immediately he appealed to his father to release him from his promise.

"Indeed not," said the father. "You are too young. It would be too expensive. Have nothing further to do with the Lewins."

If he studied before, his interest in books was now redoubled. Three years passed, and during that time he applied himself to a vast quantity of heavy reading in the classics, history, philosophy, political science, German, French, Italian. Then there were long discussions with his philosopher friends. He was developing rapidly into a thinker, the wound in his soul was healing. Then one day by chance he came upon Harriet, as she was waiting in her carriage. He talked to her for ten minutes, but the young philosopher was so confused and uneasy that he uttered scarcely one rational sentence.

"She looked lovely beyond expression," he wrote. "Her features still retained the same life and soul which once did so magnetize me; I never have seen it, and never shall see it, on any other face."

The vision of Harriet in the carriage would not leave his memory. He must bring the matter up to his father again. Wasn't he too old to be submitting to this tyranny? The father relented. The son might marry in two years, but there must be no visiting in the meantime. The lovers found some satisfaction in writing each other the minutest details of their unhappy lives, but they could not bear the agony of separation for the two years the elder Grote had stipulated. They eloped.

When the ceremony was over, they returned to their separate homes. After several weeks the groom summoned up enough courage to tell his father. The elder Grote forgave his twenty-six-year-old son and settled him in a house next to the bank so that the thought of it might never leave his mind. It was not a healthy place, and this may have been the reason why the first and only child lived but a week. The mother contracted childbed fever, which left permanent traces in her health.

About this time the idea of writing a history of Greece occupied his attention. His wife claimed credit for suggesting it to him. She said to him:

"You are always studying the ancient authors whenever you have a moment's leisure; now here would be a fine subject for you to treat. Suppose you try your hand."

Grote had a great sympathy for the Greek city states where democracy flourished, and he early defended it very capably against Mitford, a historian who had assailed Greek rule by the people with the evident purpose of furnishing a horrible example to those who were at the time agitating for the reform of the ballot, a question that was just coming to a head in England. Grote was for representative government in England, where members were still elected to the House of Commons by an ancient system which granted representation to a cemetery, and denied it to large industrial cities. Grote, who had for years been discussing theories of government with his radical friends, and who felt that the democracy of Athens was an ideal, could not quietly observe this fight for more equal representation.

During the long period of his wife's convalescence after the birth of their son, he worked by her bedside, composing his first published work on Parliamentary Reform, in which he assailed the theory of class representation current in England. His sympathy with popular issues was more and more bringing him to the fore as a candidate for parliament. His wife was not adverse to this, but she felt that the *History of Greece* should first be completed. In her diary she wrote: "The History of Greece *must* be given to the public before he can embark in any active scheme of a political kind." Despite her italicized *must*, he stood for parliament, and was successful.

Immediately he distinguished himself by his speech on the ballot. Liberals hailed him as a new champion; his speech was given wide circulation. Twenty years after its delivery, Lord Brougham told Mrs. Grote that he had heard the great orators of the century, and he had made up his mind that the two best speeches he had ever heard in parliament were Macaulay's first speech on the copyright question and Grote's first speech on the ballot.

Grote was not a practical politician. He was too much of a philosopher, too much of an individualist. When he was returned to parliament for the last time, he won by so narrow a margin that he decided not to run again. Besides it distressed him to think that his history had been neglected during those eight years. His scholarly studies had to be dropped for affairs at the bank or the business of parliament. The years he had spent in the House of Commons had ripened his genius. The political questions debated in the ancient assemblies had more meaning to him now. What he had written years before was put aside, and he began his history anew. His fresh plan was so elaborate and the project so absorbing that he decided to sever his connection with the bank to which he had given thirty years of his life.

Grote came to his new work with the enthusiasm of an amateur. Now he was free to devote himself to a task he had wanted to perform for the past score of years. To his new labor he brought the training of the successful man of business. An instance of this transfer of training was the regularity of his industry. As though he were a clerk in his bank, he sat down at his desk regularly each day and spent a definite number of hours at his work. There was no temperamental complaint from him that inspiration was lacking. He was at his desk to receive it if it came. His wife felt he was at his desk too much, and, in order to keep him from turning into a recluse, she constantly planned recreations for him.

Such industry quickly bore fruit. Three years after his retirement the first two volumes of his history appeared. In these the instincts of the banker were evident. He examined the credit basis of the great legends of Greece. Some scholars were of the opinion that the great Greek myths were a veil concealing events that really occurred once upon a time. To Grote myth was a past that never was present. He tells the legends, but makes it clear that there is nothing worthy of credence before the date of the first Olympiad, 776 B.C. Later scholars have proved that this traditional date is unfounded in fact. Grote's acceptance of it is an instance of how a sceptic may in a careless moment lapse into belief.

With steady industry and a godlike calm he completed his elaborate plan. In the next ten years he produced ten volumes, bringing his series to a close with the generation taking its name from Alexander the Great — 300 B.C.

Nothing that had ever been done could at all approach the extent of this digest of Greek history. Professional scholars might well look with envy on this row of volumes and note that its author had never attended a university. But if they were jealous, they were likewise generous in giving him the recognition that was his due. When the work was nearly finished, Oxford made him a Doctor of Civil Law. Mrs. Grote described his feelings in these academic surroundings:

Grote, personally, was a *little* nervous on finding himself in the thick of the academic throng for the first time in his life; all the circumstances of his own literary career having run in a channel so distinct from that in which college men travel, he felt like a stranger introduced into the privileged fraternity. But I am bound to add that he returned from Oxford full of grateful and complacent feelings; the cordial welcome given to the non-academic scholar seemed to tell upon his mind, whilst his classic taste was moved to lively relish by the few sentences of elegant Latin addressed to him on his reception by Lord Derby, of which he expressed much admiration.

Surely any scholar would feel that his dreams were amply realized in such honors, and that he might sit back and gaze with satisfaction at what he had done. It was not so with Grote. After the history was finished and subsequent editions revised, he began his *Plato and Other Companions of Socrates,* which appeared in three volumes after nine years' work.

Honors now came thick upon him. Cambridge made him a Doctor of Laws and Letters. Although he had never been a student in college, he was elected to the presidency of University College. At seventy-five, two years before his death, Gladstone, himself an inspired amateur in the classics, offered him the title of peer, an honor he felt forced to decline. At his death he was buried in Westminster Abbey, beside that great historian of Rome's decline and fall, Edward Gibbon.

Mrs. Grote published an interesting biography of her husband, though she gave too much space to the chronicle of her illness, the trips she took in the interest of her health, the foul weather, and their perpetual moving from one house to another. As a personality, she has more color than her husband. He was the quiet thoughtful scholar, she his business manager. A sarcastic critic might refer to George Grote of the House of Commons as "the member for Mrs. Grote," and Sydney Smith, on seeing her with a rose turban on her head, might remark that he now understood the meaning of the word "grotesque," yet there is no doubt she was an ideal partner for "her historian," as she called her husband.

She felt it her duty to see that he did not overwork, and to this end she insisted on his taking recreation. With some difficulty she trained him to be a gracious host ; he even grew to enjoy whist.   But she did more than keep him from nervous breakdowns.   She discussed his books with him, found a publisher, read practically all the proofs of his history.   Like most men who become great, George Grote had a helper who labored with him not for fame but for love.

XI

ENLIGHTENING THE DOCTOR
STEPHEN HALES

While we congratulate ourselves on having attained to an understanding of the principles of ventilation, on having abolished typhus fever from our hospitals, prisons and ships, on having devised apparatus for sustaining life in irrespirable and deadly atmospheres, let us never forget that the initial stages in the comprehension of these things were worked out not by any high-placed, well-paid, public official, but by a modest amateur, the scientifically minded, country clergyman, Stephen Hales.— *D. Fraser Harris.*

XI

ENLIGHTENING THE DOCTOR

STEPHEN HALES

IF we search for a layman with the proper credentials to make him an inspired doctor, we encounter ·difficulties. The reason for this is obvious. The ideal doctor knows a considerable number of fields; he is a composite of many professions. Moreover, at least in modern times, a man must be properly licensed before he is permitted to practice, for the sick show a strange prejudice in expecting a physician to do his preliminary cutting on cadavers before assailing the quick flesh. Although among medical doctors there are no inspired amateurs of sufficient stature to consort with these amateurs of other fields, still in the history of medicine there are men from other walks of life who have made contributions to the knowledge of the human body and the means of curing its ills. There is a well-known statement supporting this view in Oliver Wendell Holmes' essay *Scholastic and Bedside Teaching:*

Medicine . . . learned from a monk how to use antimony, from a Jesuit how to cure agues, from a friar how to cut for a stone, from a soldier how to treat gout, from a sailor how to keep off scurvy, from a postmaster how to sound the Eustachian tube, from a dairy-maid how to prevent small-pox, and from an old market-woman how to catch the itch-insect. It borrowed acupuncture and the moxa from the Japanese heather, and was taught the use of lobelia by the American savage.

Priestley created wonder in the minds of his parishioners

by visiting a brewery to determine the nature of the gas in the vats of fermenting beer, but this was in no way comparable to the various non-clerical interests in which the Reverend Stephen Hales indulged. These ranged all the way from hints to housewives on cooking to plans for ventilators of ships and prisons. As a youth his recreation had been the study of anatomy, chemistry and botany. After he left Cambridge and was made a perpetual curate of Teddington in 1708, at the age of thirty-one, he had that security of income and leisure for reflection which made it possible for him to continue his scientific hobbies.

There is no evidence to prove that Parson Hales was any more neglectful in ministering to his flock than other clergymen of that day. In fact, it would seem that he performed his duties very exactly. Certainly he was a little stricter with his parishioners than was customary in his church in those days, for he made women do public penance.

The poet Pope, who lived near him and who knew him personally, wrote of "plain parson Hale" in one of his Epistles, paying tribute to "his exemplary life and pastoral charity as a parish priest." And Alexander Pope was the last man in the world to praise any man who was undeserving, least of all a minister. As it was, the poet found reason to censure him for his experiments on living animals. "How do we know," the poet asked sarcastically, "that we have a right to kill creatures that we are so little above as dogs, for our curiosity, or even for some use to us?" Apparently the march of progress in this instance was being led by a churchman.

Hales is remembered for his observations on blood pressure, the first study that was ever made on this popular subject of conversation. His rather crude experiment was performed on a mare. The animal was tied down, the artery in its left thigh opened and tied off. Into this artery he inserted a brass pipe to which a second brass pipe was fastened, which in turn was joined to a glass tube nearly nine feet high. When the binding of the artery was loosened, he observed that the blood rose eight feet and three inches above the left ventricle of the heart of the animal. Here is the fountain head of that bit of science which has disturbed you — or will disturb you — when your physician tells you that your blood pressure is either too high or too low.

While he did not hesitate to practise vivisection on animals, he was profoundly interested in saving man the pain of the surgeon's knife. Those who have read the secret diary of Samuel Pepys will remember something of the operation which men suffered when surgeons of his day cut for the stone. The coming of the doctor with his retinue of stalwart helpers, whose duty it was to hold the patient still while the cutting was being done, was like the descent of an armed band upon the home of a defenseless peasant. There were no anesthetics then and the pain suffered was intense. In those days of imperfect diagnosis, it sometimes happened that the cutting failed to reveal a stone. In such cases the physician might hand the patient one from the supply in his pocket, kept for just such emergencies.

The Reverend Hales applied himself to the study of solvents for bladder and kidney stones. The Royal Society thought so well of the paper which he presented on the subject that its members awarded him the Copley Medal, the most noted distinction which it was within its power to confer. Some of the learned gentlemen of the society knew from experience the suffering connected with cutting for the stone; those who had not suffered the operation probably feared it as much as Pepys did. To a man they were anxious to reward any scientist who made any progress in lessening the necessity of the knife.

No surer evidence of the integrity of the medical fraternity can be given than its interest in preventive medicine, whereby doctors deliberately strive to keep people from incurring infection and illness. It is in this phase of medicine that Reverend Hales was particularly interested; for his work on ventilation, in which he proved the value and necessity of fresh air, he takes a place as one of the great sanitarians of all time.

People of Hales' day had little knowledge of the value of fresh air. Many houses had been constructed with as few windows as possible. One reason for this was that a man's tax depended on the number of windows in the home. The ever unpopular tax collector had fallen into special odium in England because of the hearth or chimney tax, whereby property value was judged by the number of grates in the house. During the reign of William III, this tax was supplanted by one which could be computed without the appraiser's invading private dwellings. The bigger a house, the more windows it had. Therefore the rental value of a home was determined by the number of its windows and openings. People are as clever in dodging taxes as authorities are in inventing them, but in this case the means they took of avoiding the tax, that of having few or no windows, was a most unhealthy artifice. Men began to live in dark, damp, foul-smelling chambers. Particularly foul was the air in prisons where there were other reasons for not having many windows.

To be sentenced to a jail in those days was not an opportunity for a man to get caught up in his reading but frequently a sentence to a death, almost certainly resulting from jail fever. When several notables died at the trials held under these conditions, the matter of remedying this situation was taken up by a committee of the Royal Society, which handed the problem over to Hales, the logical man to consider it, for he had for some time studied the importance of fresh air and the harmful effects of breathing foul air over and over again.

His theories were tested at Newgate Prison where his invention, a windmill, operating bellows by which foul air was drawn from the cells, was mounted on top of the roof. The beneficial effects were immediate, the death rate dropping over fifty per cent. After his apparatus was installed in Savoy prison, where the average death rate had been about seventy-five a year, only four prisoners died of jail fever in the ensuing three years.

Hales was also interested in combating that scourge of life at sea, the scurvy. This began with bleeding gums, after which the teeth fell out, the skin became blotched, the ankles and wrists swelled. The sufferer really rotted to death. In spite of his reputation, certain naval officers treated him with scant courtesy when, at the request of enlightened authorities, he presented himself to help them solve their problems. But Hales convinced seamen that they could not sleep in crowded, ill-ventilated quarters and remain in good health. One captain of the period publicly expressed his enthusiasm for the ventilators in this way:

"Two hundred men aboard for a year, pressed from

gaols, with distemper all landed well in Georgia. This is what I believe but few transports or any other ships can brag of nor did I ever meet the like good luck before which, next to Providence, I impute to the benefit received by the ventilators."

Of course the credit for curing the scurvy does not go to Hales, though his emphasis on fresh air as essential to the health of seamen was a contributing factor. As far back as 1617, a naval physician had pointed out the value of lemon juice in preventing this disease, but it was really left for Captain Cook to demonstrate to physicians the value of these forgotten suggestions.

Ministers have often been criticized for obstructing the path of science, but this charge cannot be levelled at Stephen Hales, for he was far ahead of his day in matters scientific. Anything touching life was of absorbing interest to him. The process of growth in plants fascinated him, and his studies in this field were so penetrating that he has been called the founder of experimental, botanical physiology. Indeed, some few years ago, the American Society of Plant Physiologists honored his name by creating the Stephen Hales Prize in Plant Physiology. So great was his interest in animal life that he practised vivisection in spite of criticism. In the case of human life, his profession demanded that he interest himself in the life of the spirit, but he seems to have saved his genuine enthusiasm not for matters touching the supernatural life but rather the natural life of man.

XII

THE LENS-GRINDING PHILOSOPHER
BENEDICT DE SPINOZA

"He developed heterodox religious opinions,
which led to his excommunication by the Amsterdam rabbinate in 1656. Therefore he settled down
to lead the picturesque but difficult life of a
philosophic saint, grinding lenses for a living and
devoting the leisure of his short life to the composition of an *Ethics* 'demonstrated in the manner
of geometry.'" — *Benjamin Ginzburg.*

XII

THE LENS-GRINDING PHILOSOPHER

BENEDICT DE SPINOZA

IN A very broad sense every sane man may be said to be a philosopher. He has some principles by which he guides his course through life's arguments and perplexities. Generally his ideas are not original. Often they spring from his allegiance to some organization sponsoring mass thinking. When such a man discusses the universe, we say that he is philosophizing. He is speaking in the manner of a lover of wisdom, though in reality his statements may be far from true.

But in a technical sense a philosopher is a prober of causes who attempts to solve the riddle of this painful world, the power or law that sustains it, and the purpose of it all. He is interested in man's nature, his place in the universe, his duties and obligations. These questions offer difficulties to the philosopher. The theologian will not confess himself at sea in these issues, for he maintains that these courses have long ago been charted by revelation.

Benedict de Spinoza was an amateur philosopher. He had no academic background; indeed, it would have been quite impossible for him to gain a university degree in the middle of the seventeenth century because universities were closed to Jews. He never held a chair of philosophy, though he was offered the opportunity to teach that subject at the University of Heidelberg. He never gave any lectures, yet his ideas have been a potent force in shaping the thought of many lecturers since his time.

Though Spinoza could furnish no university credentials, he was not on that account untutored. His father had sent him to the synagogue school when he was seven, and this instruction, consuming a generous portion of the day, continued until he reached the age of twelve. In this period he completed the reading of the Old Testament in Hebrew and was introduced to Hebrew grammar and the Talmud.

Spinoza's father, though constantly plagued with ill fortune, was able to keep his bright son in school. At thirteen he was sent to the Tree of Life Academy. Here Baruch—later he used the Latin equivalent, Benedictus—studied the sacred text and then the commentary, and was a joy to his father and the elders, who took it for granted that he would grow up to be an illustrious rabbi in Israel. But there were difficulties in the sacred writings which, he felt, could not be solved. Other scholars before him had seen many intellectual objections. He read their guides for the perplexed, but the perplexities still remained. He reverently pointed out his difficulties to the rabbis; but to the young thinker the replies were not answers.

It is often difficult to trace the seeds that later develop into apostasy. Sometimes it is difficult for the one who has had the experience of a change of faith to trace its origin and growth for his own satisfaction. When one considers the sheltered life led by young Baruch, his aloofness from the gentiles in Amsterdam, and the restricted range of subjects in the curriculum of the academy, his development is as difficult to explain as that of a botanical sport which suddenly appears among a hundred thousand flowers, all of the same variety with the exception of one which possesses an absolutely different characteristic.

There were many things to keep Baruch from deserting the ranks of Israel. He knew that he would never be welcomed wholeheartedly by gentiles. Then, too, he would always be regarded as vile by those whom he had deserted. He could hardly forget the penance — he was eight years old at the time — that had been meted out to Uriel Acosta when the latter sought re-admission to the synagogue after his desertion.

That unfortunate man had bared his back for the lash; afterward, as the righteous left the temple, he lay prostrate at the portal to be tramped under foot by his more orthodox brethren. Wild with pain, he armed himself to kill those who had humiliated him. But he was unskillful in the use of weapons, and when his aim missed, he turned his gun on himself. All these considerations must have flooded Baruch's mind, as he contemplated surrendering the faith for which his fathers had suffered for centuries. He shrank from being a stumbling-block to the piety of others about him, but everything within him rebelled at living this life of allegiance to ideas in which he did not believe.

Baruch's interest in the ancients had led him to take Latin lessons from a director of a private school who had once been a Jesuit. There was some adverse criticism from pious Jews in Amsterdam when this became known. The misgivings of the children of Israel were not unfounded, for Baruch's new professor had been through a religious crisis in his own life and was interested in disseminating the ideas derived from his meditations. It is not impossible that it was he who opened up the sealed compartments of Baruch's mind by telling him, between declensions and conjugations, of the "new learning."

The Jews of Amsterdam were shocked when they learned that this promising youth, who had practically lived in the synagogue, had taken up his residence at the home of his new teacher. The rabbis had disapproved in the first place when he had enrolled to study Latin. Gentile learning was vain. Hadn't one rabbi done penance forty days and forty nights to purge his mind after learning this language? Indeed there had been rabbis who had studied Latin, but to live under the same roof with the gentile teacher. . . Yet the leaders of the synagogue treated their erring brother with great consideration. They were aware of the capability of this young man of twenty-four. They knew that many seemingly conscientious objectors can often be made to see, by the light of the glint of money, a point of view hitherto unacceptable.

Spinoza was told that if he returned to the performance of his religious duties, he would be granted a stipend of about four hundred dollars a year. He would eventually be admitted to the rabbinate and become a leader in Israel. But Spinoza was not to be won so easily from his conclusions. The rabbis shook their heads gravely, remembering certain temptations that had been in their own minds, and mourned for youth's impetuosity. Spinoza made it clear that he had no price and thereupon returned to live under the roof of the gentile. The rabbis did not act hastily, but it was clear to them that they had no choice but to excommunicate this rash youth, if only to discourage others who might be contemplating a similar career of sin.

About this time an unsuccessful attempt was made on his life, and he left the city for a village just outside of Amsterdam. Then his excommunication was made public. The rabbis declared that they had for a long time been aware of the frightful heresies which he not only professed but taught others, that he had been accused and convicted in their presence. "Therefore," they wrote, "we excommunicate, expel, curse, and damn Baruch de Espinoza." The decree angered Spinoza, and he futilely answered the condemnation.

The young heretic felt his isolation very keenly when he found himself cut off from association with his kinsmen. He was not yet so detached as to be indifferent to the scorn in which he was held by the Jews about him. His former friends were now forbidden to communicate in any way with him, to show him any kindness, to stay under the same roof with him or approach him within a specified distance. Those who would keep their souls clean must avoid him as if he were a leper.

Before his break with the synagogue, Baruch had not been obliged to worry about his means of subsistence, but now he must earn his bread. The student looked out upon an unfriendly world and wondered how he could wrest from it the bare essentials which even the philosophers must have. After a few unhappy weeks at the village outside of Amsterdam, he returned to the city. The blood of merchants was in him, and he considered for a time the idea of devoting himself to a business career. In the preface to the *Improvement of the Understanding* he relates his temptation to "take the cash and let the credit go," but after a sharp struggle he reasoned that if he were to obtain happiness, it would be more certainly reached through indifference to the accumulation of external goods.

Once back in the city, he began to earn his living by grinding lenses. This was a rather unfortunate choice of occupation, for he was tubercular, as his mother had been, and this work kept him in his room, away from the fresh air and sunlight, breathing glass-dust into his lungs. He kept up the trade, however, for a score of years and died with his polishing tools in hand.

It was quite natural that he should become the high priest of a group of liberal-minded merchants in Amsterdam. These men were amateur theologians and philosophers who loved to discuss high themes. Baruch was welcome in their circle. He had studied the Scriptures in a most thorough fashion and had read the commentaries. He could shed light when light was needed. Moreover the young Jew inspired their respect, for he had had the courage to suffer for his convictions. They had the pleasure of his company for four years, and then he decided to move to Rynsburg, forty miles away.

The motive of his leaving is uncertain. It may be that the philosopher could not find the seclusion necessary for the work he wished to do. Then, too, he may have been taunted by his former co-religionists, and this explanation gains some value when we consider that the town to which he went was the center of the Collegiants, a sect of few dogmas and abundant tolerance, welcoming members of any creed. Their ministers were in a sense amateurs, being endowed, in the opinion of the faithful, with no greater power than any one of the brethren. This breadth of tolerance must have pleased a man whose sensitive soul had suffered so many sharp thrusts from the Jews of Amsterdam.

It may be that he found the years of his life, which he knew would be brief, slipping away from him without that work done which his nature urged him to perform. When he attained the seclusion necessary for sustained thinking on profound subjects, he immediately began writing *A Short Treatise on God, Man, and His Well-being*, which was followed by his unfinished essay *On the Improvement of the Understanding*. These writings were not intended for publication but for the private inspiration of his Amsterdam disciples who circulated them in manuscript.

Students at the University of Leyden, not far from Spinoza's home, soon discovered him. In their enthusiasm for speculation they made their way to Rynsburg to discuss philosophy with him. They, too, were interested in the newer thinking typified by Descartes, and Spinoza was not unwilling to spread the new gospel. His fame went abroad. The solitude he had hoped for in Rynsburg was vanishing. His leisure was further limited by the fact that he had undertaken the instruction of a not too intelligent student, who was to live with him.

Spinoza had begun the composition of *The Ethics*, but he could not work with this pupil in the house. To improve the student's mind he dictated to him a section of Descartes' *Principles of Philosophy* in the form of geometrical propositions. Later, while on a visit to Amsterdam, his friends urged him to sit down and finish the work for publication. Since he was not in entire agreement with Descartes, he had some scruples about it at first but in the end consented. The book brought him immediate recognition.

In the hope of gaining protection against attacks from

the religious, he moved closed to The Hague. Here he took up his tools and began to grind his lenses by day; at night, from ten o'clock far into the morning, he labored over his *Ethics*.

About this time Holland chose to forget the service of its Grand Pensionary, Jan de Witt. At the first sign of military reverses, a fickle populace began to cry out for the return of the House of Orange. Calvinist clergymen were at pains to point out the godless men with whom De Witt associated, and, of course, among this number Spinoza was included. The latter saw that much of the trouble then disturbing society was due to a religious intolerance that refused dissenting minds the right to express their views freely.

Feeling that he might be able to effect something in the cause of freedom by publishing some rational ideas on the Scriptures, government, and liberty of thought, he interrupted his *Ethics* to write the *Short Treatise on Politics and Religion*. The work was published anonymously and has often been printed with a false title to escape discovery. There is a copy extant with the title, *The Art of Sailing Against the Wind*. When this tract, regarded as diabolical in its day, was finished, he again turned to the labor of writing his *Ethics*.

And so he continued to toil unceasingly at polishing his lenses and his ethical propositions. So intensely did he apply himself that often he did not leave his room for days at a time. Finally, his masterpiece, *The Ethics*, a closely connected structure of cold geometrical propositions was finished, and so was his life. With his manuscript he set out for his friends in Amsterdam. But enemies heard that a new book of his was forthcoming, and they raised such a storm of protest that he thought it unwise to have it printed then and returned with it to The Hague. His life work was over. He could drive his frail body no farther, but he worked to the very end.

In 1677, in his forty-fifth year, after giving instructions about his manuscripts, he died resignedly and peacefully, as he had lived. Many a prayer of thanksgiving was uttered by the devout at his passing, and the opinion of the century that succeeded his death is pretty well summed up in the words of a preacher who passed his grave and said to his companion, "There is Spinoza's grave; spit on it."

It is not difficult to understand why a minister would suggest dishonoring the grave of Spinoza, for his explanations of the Bible had opposed the necessity of revelation, miracles and prophecies. In his mind much of the miraculous in the Scriptures had resulted from a literal interpretation of its poetry. Moreover he did not accept the Christian dualism of spirit and matter; there was no spirit but only matter.

On these grounds many proceed to atheism, but Spinoza refused to be classed as an atheist. To him everything was God. Man not only lived and moved and had his being in God, but he was a part of God or Nature — terms which were identical to him. Man, therefore, had within him no spiritual principle independently surviving in a future life. This was not a roseate prospect for those who believed that the virtuous would be decorated in the next world and the wicked burned. He scorned the idea of doing good for a prize and avoiding evil to escape punishment.

Moreover man could not merit reward or censure because he was not free. His actions are predetermined by causes over which he has no control. If one knew all the causes, remote and proximate, of an action, it would be apparent that he was determined to this action. So the delusion of freedom rises out of man's desires and volitions. If a stone cast into the air were suddenly given consciousness and found itself moving, it would conclude that its motion was the result of its own power. Man, too, is impelled by forces of whose nature he is ignorant and, therefore, concludes that he is directing his own course.

Hearing this, the orthodox Christian would assert that there would be small reason for living if this were true. Spinoza replied that, because one was not destined to live forever, he saw no reason why he should not enjoy as much of life as lay before him. The sun does not shine always; yet we enjoy it when it does. He held that there was no definite aim or purpose in man's existence. Man would naturally pursue happiness, which consists in the intellectual, not the sentimental love of God. This was equivalent to the understanding of nature and really furnished man with science as a pursuit that would bring happiness. Man's greatest good, then, lay in the realization of the relation of his mind to God or Nature. If one is in tune with the universe and views all things from the aspect of eternity, he will enjoy the happiness that is proper to his nature.

The philosophy of materialism may produce the selfish, anti-social criminal, but there was nothing base in Spinoza. Few lives have been holier than his. Indeed many a saint has ranked below him in self-restraint. He chose a life of self-denial deliberately, not as a means of expiating the waywardness of his youth, as did Augustine and Ignatius. As a young man, Baruch was not guilty of those follies which drive men in their old age

to sackcloth and ashes.   His self-control has awakened
the admiration of many who will not accept a single point
of his philosophy.   There are traces of impatience in
his letters, but the provocation was ample.

Once he became excessively angry.   Jan de Witt had
gone to see his brother in prison, and both were brutally
murdered by the mob.   When Spinoza heard of this, he
was determined to face the rabble and speak his indignation.   His landlord asked him what he would say.
He would paint a placard on which he would write the
words, "Base Barbarians," and wave this before them.
The landlord simply turned the key in the door of his
tenant's room.   The philosopher quickly regained his
composure and uttered words of resignation that remind
one of Christ's prayer on the cross for the forgiveness
of those who "know not what they do."

Spinoza was an ascetic in his own life, but he had not
the fanaticism of those who would maintain that simple
pleasures, indulged in solely for enjoyment, are unlawful
for the man who would be virtuous.   He believed that a
reasonable man should enjoy pleasure within bounds,
that no indulgence should be carried to the point of
excess, since this would be unreasonable and ultimately
lead to unhappiness.   He wrote in *The Ethics*:

I say it is the part of a wise man to refresh and recreate
himself with moderate and pleasant food and drink, and
also with perfumes, with the soft beauty of growing plants,
with dress, with music, with many sports, with theatres,
and the like, such as every man may make use of without
injury to his neighbor.

Spinoza did not have the means to enjoy all these
things, but he generously conceded their use to those

who could afford them. He believed that the best things in life were free. One of his early biographers estimated that during one month he had allowed himself only a pint of wine. Sometimes, when tired, he would smoke a pipeful of tobacco with his landlord.

Considering the intolerance of his age and the groups of mass thinkers he offended by his teachings, he fared very fortunately. Many a man has lost his life for espousing doctrines such as those Spinoza advanced, but by some miracle he escaped physical punishment. He did not die by the violence of a mob, nor were fagots put under him that his life might be taken without the shedding of blood, nor was he ever sent to prison. It is a marvel that this outspoken champion of free thought died naturally. Perhaps we may attribute his escape to the quiet virtue of his life, which must have impressed even zealots who would have gladly crucified an infidel in the thought that they were offering God a pleasing sacrifice.

XIII

TODAY'S AMATEURS

XIII

TODAY'S AMATEURS

THE interests of these inspired amateurs have ranged from gases to philosophy, but not every study between these two terminals is represented in these pages. Still there can be little doubt that every field of study would reveal its inspired amateur upon investigation.

No mention has been made of men who pursued one of the fine arts with success, though they were trained in other fields. Examples of these are plentiful. Consider, for example, how many physicians have devoted their talents to literature: Chekhov, Rabelais, Schiller, Oliver Wendell Holmes, Sir Arthur Conan Doyle, Sir Robert Bridges, and Sir Thomas Browne. Nor has mention been made of inventors, men of great resolution and ability, who have perfected some device or machine in a field entirely foreign to their daily work. Here, too, the doctors have their representatives in a most unexpected field. Gatling, who invented the gun named after him, and Guillotin, famed for reviving the guillotine, were both physicians. Other professions could offer their candidates, too. But the number of amateur inventors is so great that a list of these would hardly create wonder.

The selections of amateurs have been made from scientists and philosophers who dealt with studies rather than devices, with the theoretical rather than the practical. Thus in the field of botany Mendel finds a place instead of Burbank. The latter was practical and literally donated a great number of new varieties of fruits, berries, flowers and trees to man. Yet he had not the scientific temper, being interested in practical matters rather than in theory.

Though our selections have been made from the dead, there are many inspired amateurs abroad today. This is especially true in the arts. The radio has devoted much attention to the work of amateur musicians, and this has brought to the public attention a great number of finished performers. The depression has promoted this, for it gave people the leisure to pursue some such avocation. Yet distinction here is much easier of attainment than it is in the realm of science or philosophy.

The question may be raised whether the professionally untrained man has a chance in our time of accomplishing anything noteworthy in scientific studies. People are always ready to admit that in former generations the opportunities of making an original contribution were more numerous than they are in the present. To a great extent this is true, for the development of necessary equipment in certain fields of science makes it rather improbable that the "private gentleman" will engage in any work so costly, and it is still less probable that he will light upon anything that has escaped the professional eye, if he applies himself to these problems.

It must be admitted that it is much more difficult to be an inspired amateur astronomer in our day than it was in the days of Herschel. The heavens have been swept too frequently to admit of the probability of an amateur's discovering what professional astronomers have missed; yet only recently two comets have been discovered by amateurs. In the field of chemistry, so thoroughly combed each year for dissertations by hundreds of students and by the host pursuing research for private ends or corporate interests, there is little chance that an amateur will ever advance the frontiers of knowledge. The same condition obtains in physics.

Yet there is danger in such an attitude. If one argues by analogy, he may maintain that the professionals are too many laps ahead of the amateur in the race of discovery. Such comparisons are more clever that cogent. The same statements were made by professionals of a former age when they addressed the amateur. The feeling of the guild toward the intruder has never been cordial. Relatively considered, the amateurs whom we have discussed were impeded by difficulties just as serious as those that face the modern amateur. In spite of all the equipment and preliminary knowledge necessary, tomorrow's possibilities of success may equal yesterday's.

We are inclined to look upon the discoveries of a former age as primitive; we forget that what every schoolboy now knows was once a puzzle to profound thinkers. If a route has been discovered, it is easy to point it out. Perhaps those principles that have been laid bare in our own time have required no more native genius or intense concentration than the earlier elementary conclusions. It is characteristic of each generation to place itself on an intellectual pinnacle and maintain that succeeding ages will never mount higher.

We are inclined to smile at the theories advanced in science a century ago, forgetting all the while that the generations to come may smile, as they read some of our accepted scientific theories. We are greatly amused as we turn the pages of magazines showing the fashions of only a generation ago; in later ages some historian of the curious and the naïve may include our theories in his narrative.

Even in those fields, then, which have been so thoroughly investigated, it is not safe to admit that the full limit of development has been reached. The great scientific advances made thus far in the twentieth century should teach us caution in this matter. It may well be that science is still in the larva stage and has not yet taken to wing. We may be at the threshold of unimagined discoveries. This is at least a more enlightened policy than that short-sighted attitude of one legislator, living in the middle of the last century, who maintained that, since all the fundamental inventions were discovered, there was no longer any need of keeping the patent office open. Amateurs of brilliant intelligence may yet make valuable contributions to the history of man's struggle up from superstition, ignorance, and barbarism.

While it is true that certain fields of science have been carefully typed and filed, there are other sections of knowledge which offer unbounded possibilities. All the fossils in the earth are certainly not studied and catalogued. There are problems in geology the solution of which may be found in some amateur's garden. The microscope, which Leeuwenhoek loved so much, will still continue its book of revelation. Zoologists know that there are many thousands of animals, from the lowest to the highest orders, which await study and classification.

There are buried civilizations awaiting the shovel of the archaeologist, who may produce evidence completely altering our positive interpretations of ancient civilizations. There are still many mysterious ills which afflict the human body, many of its functions are imperfectly understood, many remedies yet to be discovered. Some clear-eyed amateur may look into the face of one of these enigmas and see what others have not seen, even though they have gazed a lifetime.